WITHDRAWN

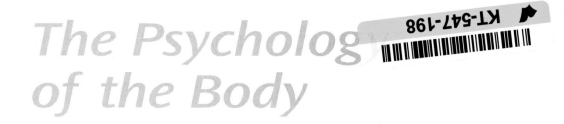

The Psychology of the Body

Our Commitment to You

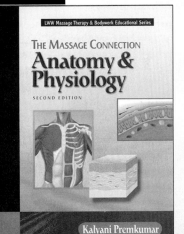

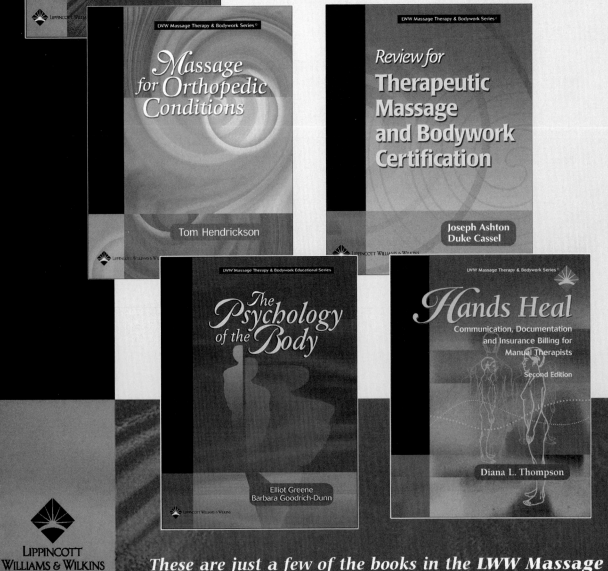

LIPPINCOTT WILLIAMS & WILKINS IS DEDICATED to enhancing massage therapy and bodywork education by providing you the best resources with the **LWW Massage Therapy & Bodywork Educational Series**.

LWW strives to find the leading experts in the field of massage therapy to write extraordinary books covering topics crucial for massage therapy students and practitioners. We then combine the text with outstanding visual presentations to create superior resources for you! It is our goal to help you become more knowledgeable and better prepared for your future in massage therapy and bodywork.

The Psychology of the Body

Elliot Greene, MA, NCTMB

Co-Director of the Washington Institute for Body Psychotherapy
Private Practice
Silver Spring, Maryland

Barbara Goodrich-Dunn, BFS

Co-Director of the Washington Institute for Body Psychotherapy
Private Practice
Silver Spring, Maryland

 LIPPINCOTT WILLIAMS & WILKINS
A **Wolters Kluwer** Company

Philadelphia • Baltimore • New York • London
Buenos Aires • Hong Kong • Sydney • Tokyo

Senior Acquisitions Editor: Peter J. Darcy
Managing Editor: Linda S. Napora
Marketing Manager: Christen DeMarco
Project Editor: Paula C. Williams
Designer: Armen Kojoyian
Compositor: LWW In-house Composition
Printer: Data Reproductions Corp.
Photographer: Molly Roberts

351 West Camden Street
Baltimore, Maryland 21201-2436 USA

530 Walnut Street
Philadelphia, Pennsylvania 19106-3621 USA

Printed in the United States of America

Library of Congress Cataloging-in-Publication Data
LOC data is available: 0-7817-3782-6

To purchase additional copies of this book call our customer service department at **(800) 638-3030** or fax orders to **(301) 824-7390**. International customers should call **(301) 714-2324.**

Visit Lippincott Williams & Wilkins on the Internet: http://www.lww.com. Lippincott Williams & Wilkins customer service representatives are available from 8:30 am to 6:00 pm, EST, Monday through Friday, for telephone access.

03 04 05
1 2 3 4 5 6 7 8 9 10

Why do clients have emotional releases and what causes them? What should I do if a client has an emotional release during a session? Why did my client react this way to the massage? How can I support my clients emotionally in an appropriate and ethical manner? Why am I having an emotional response to my client and what should I do about it?

Nearly every massage therapist, bodyworker, or somatic educator eventually encounters a client who has an emotional release during a session. Sometimes practitioners are overwhelmed, frightened, confused, or unsure how to respond. Others intervene without necessary caution, use incorrect interventions, or act outside their scope of practice. *The Psychology of the Body* explains what an emotional release is, what causes emotional release, and how to respond to emotional release in a responsible and effective way.

We wrote this book for practitioners whose professional methods involve working with the body, but who are not psychotherapists. Our purpose is to provide practitioners with more knowledge and a greater understanding of the psychological issues that can arise from using touch in therapeutic practice. *The Psychology of the Body* covers such topics as:

► Why and how massage and other related forms of practice are a psychological intervention
► The role of touch in survival, growth and development, and emotional healing
► The interconnection of the mind and body and how this explains the relationship between tension and psychological defenses
► How the relationship between therapist and client impacts the healing process, how underlying psychological factors influence the practitioner-client relationship, and how touch affects this connection
► A body-centered explanation of psychological defenses, boundaries and limits, such as scope of practice issues and boundaries concerning behavior on the part of both the client and therapist
► How to identify the boundary line between performing massage therapy and other touch-based methods and psychotherapy and how to avoid violating that boundary
► Exploring the body–mind connection
► How and why emotional release takes place during massage therapy and other touch-based methods
► How to deal with emotional release
► A study of the psychophysical patterns created by emotional defenses and how to tailor your work with a client based on these patterns while staying within your scope of practice
► A review of the major mental health conditions designed for massage therapists and practitioners of other forms of touch-based methods
► Working with mental health professionals, understanding who they are, what they do, and how to collaborate, network, and refer to them

We also have devised exercises that will enable readers to discover how their personal beliefs and psychological makeup influence how they practice.

We perceive there is a strong need for such information in the massage therapy, bodywork, and somatic education communities. Although nearly every practitioner eventually encounters emotional release and complex psychological issues in their practice, this subject is rarely covered thoroughly enough, if at all, in training programs. Our experience is that many practitioners feel unprepared to deal with these issues when they arise in their practices, yet have a strong wish to know more and be better prepared. When we have taught workshops on this subject, students have shown intense interest. School directors have also expressed an awareness of this problem and want to provide better information to students.

The subject matter is approached conceptually and practically. Conceptual issues are discussed expansively, but not to the point of being overwhelming. Practical issues are addressed in the form of suggestions for how to apply the concepts in actual practice and through self-directed exercises. Our approach appeals to understanding, rather than memorization. Jargon and technical terminology are avoided, but definitions are provided to enhance understanding. Previous study of psychology is not required. Ideas are introduced in a common sense manner, yet are advanced in that the concepts are expanded to include complex ideas.

We hope that *The Psychology of the Body* will give you a greater understanding of the psychology of touch and will help you add another dimension to your practice.

Acknowledgments

We are grateful to those who have helped us on the path for knowledge about the mind and body, which we hope we have shared in this book. We thank our clients, students, and classmates from whom we have learned so much, and our many teachers, in particular Dr. Jim Cox, Dr. Malcolm Brown, Katherine Ennis-Brown, and Kevin Andreae.

We have heartfelt thanks and tremendous respect for everyone who made this book possible: Dr. Michael Diamond for reviewing several chapters from his perspective as a psychiatrist and keeping us "medically correct" via a gentle bedside manner; our peer reviewers for their astute comments and suggestions that were incredibly helpful; content editor Laura Bonazzoli whose "tough love" editing helped us produce a better book; artist Armen Kojoyian for managing to take our rather primitive scratchings and complex ideas and turn them into impactful images; photographer Molly Roberts for producing sterling photos and being a breeze to work with; all the people who bravely and generously volunteered to be models for the photos and must remain anonymous to maintain confidentiality of their identities; and the staff at LWW: especially Pete Darcy and Linda Napora who capably guided us through the publishing process from beginning to end, Kathleen Scogna who worked on the development aspects of the book, our production editor Paula Williams who oversaw the transformation of the manuscript into a published book, and marketing manager Christen DeMarco and marketing coordinator Meghan Eng for helping to spread the word.

We also thank all our friends and colleagues who offered support and encouragement on many occasions—especially when it was most needed.

This book is dedicated to our families:

Elliot's—Sara, Bea, Seymour, Lloyd, Alcmene, Carolyn, Ariel, and Lauren; and Barbara's—Danny, Heddi, Abram, and Martina.

Reviewers

W e wish to express our gratitude to the reviewers who read the proposal and drafts of all of the chapters. They provided helpful feedback that has resulted in a stronger book. We thank them all. Some of the reviewers wish to remain anonymous. We acknowledge:

Nancy W. Dail, BA, LMT, NCTMB
Director
Downeast School of Massage
Waldoboro, Maine

Mark W. Dixon, NCTMB, HHP
Huntington Beach, California

Raymond T. Moriyasu, MA, AB
Salve Regina University
Newport, Rhode Island
and
Downeast School of Massage
Waldoboro, Maine

Donald Webb, CMT, NCTMB
Webb Massage Therapy
Towson, Maryland

How to Use This Book

Background

We started teaching massage therapists about the psychological dimensions of touch and massage therapy twenty years ago. The massage school we graduated from asked us to develop a series of classes on this subject because we were trained as body psychotherapists, as well as massage therapists. Students who were practicing massage work were encountering interesting, unexpected results that left them with many questions. The person on the table being massaged sometimes did not report feeling good as the massage therapist might expect; sometimes he or she experienced troubling feelings or even released strong emotions while on the table. Other times after such a massage, the person receiving the massage would experience new insights about him- or herself or wonder what had just happened.

Students often went into massage school expecting massage to stimulate good feelings and reduce tension and stress, yet people being massaged were at times crying, getting scared, trembling, feeling rage, bursting out into laughter, or having memories. Sometimes the person seemed upset or spaced out after such a massage; other times the person seemed to have reached a new level of awareness. Those students who believed that negative emotions were bad or dangerous were particularly disturbed. They often wondered what was going wrong. Shaken by what was happening to the client, their first impulse was to stop what was going on and try to put a halt to any emotional responses. We observed that the students clearly needed a better understanding of what caused emotional release, what was going on during a release, what their own attitudes were about it, and how to work with someone who has an emotional response during massage therapy.

Body Psychotherapy

Several years before we created these classes, while we were training in body psychotherapy, we also took massage training as a better way of understanding the body and the effects of touch. By studying both body psychotherapy and massage therapy, a cross-fertilization occurred in both our thinking and our practice. Due to our training and practice in body psychotherapy, emotional release was not threatening to us, but was seen as an important part of the process of personal change. Our body psychotherapy training gave us the opportunity to observe many group and individual sessions that involved a variety of emotional releases by people with a wide range of characteristics. We saw that although such emotional releases could be intense and sometimes explosive, people came through their emotional releases and benefited from them when they were given correct grounding and support. We experienced emotional release opening a space for new ways of feeling and thinking. It was as if the unlocked, intense emotion also unlocked the mind and heart of the client. We came to understand that emotional release, if properly worked with, could be a positive event that could lead to growth and understanding.

We also understood that not all emotional releases were beneficial. Some emotional release is repetitive or cyclical and does not actually lead the person into deeper awareness, but keeps the person fixed in an unproductive—or even destructive—pattern of thinking and feeling. Some emotional release can be an unconscious performance to gain sympathy or attention. Sometimes emotional release is created by the expectation of the therapist and is not a genuine, spontaneous opening for the client. Only by being present and open to all kinds of emotional expression did we begin to distinguish what promotes healthy change from emotional expression that is harmful or ineffective. It is also important to note that we do not advocate intense emotional expression as a way of life or the solution to all problems. The dramatic emotional expression seen in one phase of therapy will often integrate itself into quiet reflection in another phase.

Emotional release is not an intended goal of massage therapy; however, it can sometimes be a spontaneous byproduct. Since it is something that happens in practice, massage therapists need to be able to deal with emotional release and other forms of verbal and nonverbal emotional expression. While it is true that the massage therapist can set a tone in his or her work that may facilitate this kind of response, the massage therapist can rarely set a tone so that emotional release will never happen.

In teaching massage students about the psychological aspects of working with the body, we wanted to equip them not only to deal with emotional release, but also to improve *both* their analytic and intuitive capacities in choosing the types of methods both physically and psychologically appropriate for each client. In addition, we used body psychology related ideas to train students in forming and maintaining appropriate relationships with their clients. Because so many people come to massage in some sort of psychological need without knowing it, we felt that massage students should understand this and have a bundle of skills to deal with the presence of unconscious needs and expressions.

Scope of Practice

We also felt that understanding the concept of scope of practice was important for massage therapists so that they know what they can and cannot handle. They needed to: (1) know how the body expresses psychological patterns; (2) be able to recognize the types of individuals for whom massage is psychologically contraindicated; (3) be aware of the major mental health conditions and disorders; (4) know when to refer to a counselor, psychologist, or psychiatrist; and (5) know how to create a referral network of these types of professionals.

Being able to effectively handle a client's intense emotional release can be an exhilarating, even intoxicating experience. Teaching massage students to be aware of the potential of psychological inflation on their part—caused by doing such dramatic, powerful work—became important. We needed to teach the difference between being present to psychological release and purposely eliciting it.

This book therefore is an outgrowth of our teaching experiences. We want readers to learn about the phenomenon of emotional release and how to work with it, but at the same time understand and appreciate the limitations massage therapists must respect in using this information. Our goal is to guide readers so that they will neither be afraid of nor indifferent to dealing with psychological issues, nor stray out of the scope of practice of massage therapy. Discussing and understanding what can sometimes be a very thin line between the practice of massage therapy and psychotherapy is a major part of gaining such a balanced perspective.

We will be giving readers a great deal of psychological information; yet we want to be clear that we also respect the boundaries between massage therapy and psychotherapy. We feel that respect for the boundaries does not require keeping this information from massage therapists, but that this knowledge when used appropriately will enhance skills and enable people to be better massage therapists.

Using the information properly is the key. Because of this, we implore each reader to carefully read Chapter 4 in which we discuss the topic of the boundary lines between massage therapy and psychotherapy. The information in this book will not make readers psychotherapists or counselors. Our intention is to expand the capabilities of massage therapists and others who work with people on a bodily level.

We have often been asked how the therapist can know whether he or she is staying appropriately within the scope of practice of massage therapy. One way of knowing that you are staying within these boundaries is that the body remains your primary focus in your sessions and the psyche remains secondary and in the background, even if you subscribe to a holistic approach to your work. Emotional release is a way the psyche comes out of the background and into the foreground, i.e., moving "front and center into your attention." If you allow the psyche to emerge and then sink back into the background over time on its own, your focus is likely remaining appropriate. However, if you find yourself caught up, session after session, in your client's psychological and emotional state, or find yourself introducing psychological questions or interpretations, you may be crossing the boundary into a psychotherapy situation.

The information in this book is intended to help you understand what is taking place during massage therapy sessions, not to give you tools to conduct counseling. Because we will be giving great emphasis to psychological information, this point may not always seem apparent as you read this book, so we ask you to do your best to keep this in mind.

Reading Guide

Contents. Like most books, *The Psychology of the Body* should be read in the sequence of the Table of Contents. Our intention is to give clear and full information for the massage therapist to use responsibly. For this reason, reading this book in the sequence in which it is written is important. Spot reading may cause the reader to misunderstand or even distort the bigger picture.

Terms. Our intended audience for this book is massage therapists, bodyworkers, somatic practitioners and educators, physical therapists, occupational therapists, or other professionals whose work includes the somatic experience. However, in order to be concise, we use only the terms "massage therapy" and "massage therapists" rather than continually repeating "massage therapists, bodyworkers, somatic practitioners and educators, physical therapists, occupational therapists, or other professionals whose work includes the somatic experience and touching the body" when we intend to refer to the profession and the professional. As you can imagine, if we were "politically correct" and included every title, such sentences would become tedious to read! We hope no reader is offended by this practice, as we want to address our entire intended audience.

For similar reasons, when we intend to refer to mental health professionals or their work, such as psychiatrists, psychologists, marriage and family therapists, clinical social workers, psychotherapists, and counselors, we use the terms "psychotherapists" and "psychotherapy."

Photographs. We have obscured the faces of the individuals in the photographs to protect their identity and privacy. We did not ask any counseling clients to be photographed in order to maintain appropriate ethical boundaries. Please note that in some instances, when we are demonstrating techniques, standard draping procedures were not used so that the placement of the therapist's hands would be visible.

Contents

The Psychological Life of the Body

Chapter 1

We often think of our psychological lives as something taking place only in our minds. Until recently, seeing the mind and body as separate entities has been the predominant viewpoint of psychology from the time of its emergence as a separate field of study. This mainstream view, of course, has had a great influence on how people within our society think about and experience themselves and other people. However, others outside the traditional view of psychology have believed during this same time that the mind and body are unified, not separate, entities. They came to their beliefs through experiential and empirical discovery. Now, science is increasingly also supporting their view. More recently, research has produced evidence that the mind and body are literally indivisible.

Much of the scientific understanding of the connection between body and mind has come through the study of psychological and physical trauma and dysfunction. Kurt Goldstein, a German neurologist and psychologist who fled to the United States in 1935, began to articulate this through studying how severely wounded war veterans coped with disabling injuries. Goldstein brought a Gestalt viewpoint (the whole is greater than the sum of its parts) to the study of trauma in place of a solely analytical stance that has traditionally been the method of studying the human organism. He challenged mainstream reductionistic approaches that held that dysfunction results from a breakdown of parts of the nervous system and that treatment involves repairing these affected parts. Goldstein's studies led him to believe that not just the brain, but the *entire* organism works as a whole to cope with disabling injuries. He saw that the nervous system functions as a unitary whole, rather than as a brain commanding the lower nervous system.

More recently, the study of emotional trauma and post-traumatic stress disorder has led medical science to a deeper understanding of the connection between body and mind. People with emotional trauma due to war, disasters, and physical and sexual abuse were often unresponsive to verbal psychotherapy. Studies of how the brain, the sympathetic and parasympathetic divisions of the autonomic nervous system, and a variety of biochemicals found throughout the body act in concert to respond to trauma have led to new thinking about treatment. Researchers and practitioners, such as psychiatrist and trauma specialist Bessel van der Kolk, have advanced not only the scientific groundwork, but have introduced somatic methods to the treatment of trauma. Van der Kolk, for example, has embraced body-based psychotherapies, such as Hakomi Integrative Somatics, Pesso Boyden Psychomotor, and Somatic Experiencing. The idea that "it's all in your head" is no longer viable.

An interest in addiction led neuroscientist and researcher Candace Pert to pursue her investigation of the bodymind connection. She discovered the opiate receptor within the body, a major breakthrough in comprehending how addiction works and why addiction is so tenacious. Pert went further, however. In her book, *Molecules of Emotions*, she describes a biochemical system of emotional communication within the entire body that is parallel with and interacts with the nervous system. She concludes that our emotions and their biological components form a dynamic network linking mind and body.

Studying dysfunction has also contributed to the study of consciousness. Neurologist Antonio Damasio has examined what happens to the experience of feeling, self, and identity of people with anomalous brain injuries. His conclusions in his books, *Descartes' Error: Emotion, Reason, and the Human* and *The Feeling of What Happens: Body and Emotion in the Making of Consciousness*, describe the location of consciousness as being within the entire body, not just the head. Damasio states that emotions and a "felt sense" of the body play key roles in the formation and awareness of personal identity. *We know who we are not only through our minds, but with our bodies as well.*

Best-selling books such as those of Damasio and Pert, as well as similar books, articles, and media interviews, have promoted greater public awareness of the relation between body and mind. The growing recognition of the unity of body and mind has in turn increasingly influenced popular thinking about the psychological life of the body. In recognition of the unity of the body and mind, the term **bodymind** will be used in this book.

Massage therapy often focuses on anatomy, physiology, kinesiology, and massage theory and technique. However, the psychological life of the body affects your relationship with your massage clients and the progress of their therapy. Each client's body needs to be touched according to that client's psychological needs, as their needs are experienced consciously and unconsciously through their body structure. Knowing how clients' different holding patterns and tissue types need different kinds of touch can be invaluable to the massage therapist. In short, listening to what your clients' bodies are telling you emotionally will expand and enrich your practice, elevating it from technique-bound mechanics to artistry.

An understanding of how the psychological life of the body affects massage therapy begins with an appreciation of the nature of massage as an intervention and the psychological aspects of touch. We explore these topics next and then discuss a common emotion-based reaction to massage therapy that we call the paradox of healing. This chapter closes with an overview of the role of the therapeutic alliance in helping your clients overcome resistance and let go.

MASSAGE AS INTERVENTION

Intervention is a word one often hears in relation to psychotherapy. It is also a term associated with confronting a person with an addiction or another problem. However, in this book, we use the term **intervention** to mean any action, verbal or nonverbal, on the part of the massage therapist, which changes the course of a session. A useful way to conceptualize massage is as an intervention in the flow of the bodymind. Without this intervention, the patterns in both the body and psyche are likely to continue along the same course with little change.

Massage intervenes on more than the level of the skin and muscles of the body. It also intervenes in how we organize our past, experience our present, and anticipate our future. It does so because massage affects the entire nervous system, including the brain, spinal cord, and visceral and peripheral nerves, all of which help us to organize our interpretation of ourselves and our world. To illustrate how the body is involved in the organization of experience, let's look at an example from our work with one of our clients.

Leo

Leo had had a hard day at work and was feeling frustrated. He sensed himself breathing shallowly and vaguely felt the bodily location of his frustration as being somewhere in his back. As he experienced this frustration with the present situation, he would find his mind traveling back to other frustrating situations. He also had that "on edge" feeling. He anticipated that things would go wrong, which added to his frustration. In addition, his tense body diminished his coordination, motor control, and concentration, causing him to make mistakes and become even more frustrated. Leo was so caught up in the racing back and forth of his thinking that he could not seem to get out of it.

In a session of massage therapy, Leo's back and shoulders softened. His breathing deepened. But more than that happened: Leo's on-edge feeling diminished. As his back and shoulder muscles loosened, his mind traveled to events that were not frustrating, and after a while, his mind simply became less active. Leo was even able to forget about his problems for a while; when they did return, he saw them in a different light. He felt relaxed, open, and optimistic.

We are sure that every massage therapist reading the above case example would say that they, too, have seen similar responses in their clients. Although you might not have thought about it, what occurred in Leo's session was an intervention: the massage therapy *intervened* in Leo's thinking and feeling through touch. What Leo was thinking and feeling after the session was different from what he was thinking and feeling before the session. The massage intervened in how Leo organized his experience. Although his day had been frustrating, Leo's memory of the day was not filled with frustration. In the present, he felt relaxed and able to deal with whatever came. His attitude toward the future was open and mildly optimistic. The intervention not only changed how he organized his experience, but also, for the time being, it changed a set of habitual patterns. This may sound mysterious at this point. However, it will become clearer as we explore the psychology of touch.

THE PSYCHOLOGY OF TOUCH

Touch is the first sense that makes sense. The fetus is touched constantly in the womb by the amniotic fluid and later, if delivered vaginally, by the walls of the mother's birth canal. As the newborn emerges, he or she is picked up and held and-if fortunate—immediately placed on mother's body in order to feel the security of his or her being through touch. Whereas the infant's sense of vision is not yet organized enough to assist in interpreting reality, touch immediately and directly lets the newborn know that his or her world is secure (Figure 1.1).

The Role of Touch in Survival

The sense of touch is also pivotal to life itself. In the animal kingdom, infant mammals need to be touched to initiate various physiological functions after birth. For example, newborn kittens have to be touched, usually in the form of licking, for their elimination systems to begin functioning. In humans, infants are known to perish from lack of touch.

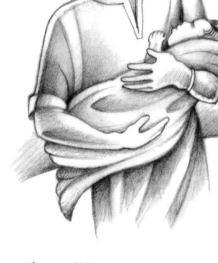

Figure 1.1
The mother transmits the security of her being through touch.

At the turn of the twentieth century, American child care was under the influence of Dr. Luther Emmett Holt, professor of pediatrics at the New York Polyclinic and Columbia University. His booklet, *The Care and Feeding of Children*, was first published in 1894; by 1935, it was in its 15th edition. Holt's influence on parents, doctors, and institutional administrators was extensive and long lasting, similar to that of Dr. Benjamin Spock in the 1950s and 1960s. Holt recommended feeding a baby according to a rigid schedule and warned against spoiling a baby with too much handling. He specifically advised against kissing a baby and warned parents not to reinforce crying behavior by picking up a baby when he or she cries. Sanitary procedures were emphasized over nurturing, to the point of almost eliminating mothering and caring behaviors.

The adoption of Holtian philosophies harmed generations of children, but none more so than those placed in American orphanages. A 1915 study by Dr. Dwight Chapin revealed that mortality rates in American orphanages were at levels of 100% for children under the age of 2 years. In other words, no infant admitted to an orphanage survived. Deaths were officially attributed to "marasmus," which was described as "wasting away"; that is, the babies had no diagnosable illness, but simply failed to thrive.

Around the same time, Dr. Fritz Talbot of Boston visited Germany to examine foundling homes and institutions, searching for ideas to improve survival rates of infants institutionalized in America. While visiting the Children's Clinic in Düsseldorf, Talbot noticed a cleaning woman carrying a baby on her hip while she performed her duties. Talbot was told that the nurses gave to "Old Anna" the babies that seemed most at risk. In essence, Old Anna was the cure of last resort. When Talbot learned that the babies given to Old Anna's care invariably survived, he determined that the cure must be simply the touch and nurturance that Old Anna gave the babies. He returned to America determined to reinstate touch as a therapeutic intervention in U.S. institutions.

By the late 1920s, the importance of touch was becoming more widely recognized, and several hospital pediatricians introduced a regular regimen of nurturing in their wards. For example, Dr. John Brennemann, who had worked at a foundling home that used the Holtian methods and had observed the horrifying mortality rates there, ordered that all babies be touched and nurtured several times a day at the hospital he directed. At Bellevue Hospital in New York City, mortality rates for infants fell to less than 10% after they instituted measures mandating nurturing touch. Gradually, nurturing methods began to be used at hospitals across the United States, and the connection between touch and survival became indisputable (Montagu, 1986).

For infants, the feeling of love is connected to the feeling of safety, of being secure in a strange new world. Touch is the way in which infants directly and non-symbolically experience love; therefore, a continued experience of touch is essential for their survival.

The Role of Touch in Growth and Development

Human growth and development also depend on touch. To the infant and young child, touch is like a powerful form of magic, providing comfort and soothing pain. The child's innocent request that the caregiver kiss a "boo-boo" to make the pain go away exemplifies the magical power that children attribute to touch. If we think of how powerful the touch of the caregiver actually is to a small child, we can better understand that the touch of a massage therapist and the ability to soothe pain can make the therapist seem powerful to a client. Touch also stabilizes the body and guides it in learning new tasks, such as walking, using tools and utensils, picking up objects, running, throwing, and so on.

Several progressive methods of education emphasize the role of touch in helping children assimilate abstract concepts such as mathematics. For example, children learn addition by manipulating buttons or an abacus, or by clapping their hands and stomping their feet in rhythmic counting songs. In fact, the word manipulation originates from the word *manus,* the Latin word for hand, which reflects its association with touch and the ability to contact and control elements in the environment. Someone who is adept at this is often considered able to "handle" things.

Touch can also affect our development in negative ways. Pinching, slapping, punching, restraining, and pushing all are forms of touch that can be used to inhibit certain forms of expression or behavior by the child, to send messages of power and domination to the child, or to express the caregiver's anger and rage at the child. Neglect—the absence of nurturing touch—may be used for the same reasons, and though it leaves no visible scars, can be felt as deeply. Both abusive touch and neglect can arrest a child's emotional development, resulting in an adult who is wary of any form of touch, even nurturing touch. If it is the only form of touch a child receives, abusive touch may even cause a person to actively seek (and sometimes give) negative forms of touch, since he or she feels familiar and, in an odd way, *safer than gentler forms of touch.*

The Role of Touch in Emotional Healing

In addition to its central role in human survival and development, touch can also change a person's emotional responses and help promote emotional healing. In other words, just as it can provoke the development of unhealthful patterns, touch can also be the tool that releases those patterns.

How this occurs is, in a sense, the subject of this book. But simply stated, feelings take place in the body as well as the mind. Indeed, as we have noted, there is no actual separation of the bodymind. The body is the vehicle for expression, which primarily occurs through movement. Expression can take form in movements as small as raising the eyebrows in surprise or fear, or as large as flinging the arms wide apart in uninhibited joy. Movement is the province of the muscular system: a child who needs to inhibit his or her natural feelings, whether for healthy or unhealthy reasons, also unconsciously either inhibits muscles that would express those feelings or activates muscles opposing those muscles of expression. In either case, the effect is the same: using the muscular body to keep the unacceptable emotions "under wrap." Touch can disrupt the patterns of muscular tension intended to inhibit emotions; thus, touch can have the effect of changing a person's emotional responses and promoting emotional healing.

This sounds wonderful—and it is, as long as the client is really ready to have his or her emotional responses change. As is seen in the next section, this often is not the case.

THE PARADOX OF HEALING

Sometimes massage sessions do not go as smoothly as we expect. In general, massage is a requested intervention. How is it then that the same client who requests this intervention also resists it in a variety of ways? The answer relates to the phenomenon that there is a conscious part of the mind that desires change through the vehicle of therapy and an unconscious part of the mind that finds this change to be threatening. This is one of the greatest paradoxes of any therapeutic process: although the client consciously desires change, he or she *may* also unconsciously dread it and thus resist the process. We refer to this as the **paradox of healing.**

The threat to the client's unconscious bodymind can take many forms. Ironically, the biggest threat often is a feeling of a strong sense of aliveness and living fully in the body. Although the person may consciously or unconsciously fear expressing "negative" emotions, a deeper fear exists that the core of the self—what we like to call the *true self*—may be wounded if expressed or exposed to the world. This true self contains joy, excitement, love, vulnerability, and tenderness, as well as anger, sadness, and fear. It is as if these expressions of the true self will get the client into trouble somehow and therefore must be controlled. The more controlled they are, however, the more deadened the client becomes. Feeling a loss of that control can be threatening—even terrifying. Sometimes the harder the client's rational mind works to bring about change, the harder the unconscious works to defend against the change.

Doris

The paradox of healing was dramatically in play behind the scenes during a massage therapy session with Doris, a colleague. Her client was deeply relaxed, and Doris was confident that the session was going well until she began to work on her client's upper back. Suddenly, the energy in her client changed from deeply relaxed to angry. She jumped off the table, got in front of Doris, and accused her of making her feel bad. Doris, not surprisingly, was shocked and scared. She tried to leave the room, but her client barred the door. Fortunately, Doris was an adept talker and was able to calm her client down and get her back on the table. Later, Doris came to us in a state of shock and asked for advice, having no idea why this incident had happened.

We began by discussing with Doris her client's physical tension patterns, the interventions Doris had made, and her relationship with the client. In the course of our discussion, Doris came to understand that her client was not "crazy" and that she herself had done nothing wrong. The tension in her client's

Doris

upper back muscles was apparently invested in inhibiting the expression of certain feelings that were unacceptable to her. As we will discuss later, this was a classic case of what we term "holding back." Her back literally was holding back feelings. When the tension was released, the feeling that was being held back came out. But the client was unwilling to experience the feelings as her own and therefore had accused Doris of "making her feel bad." A deeper understanding gave Doris the ability to return to her client and discuss the experience with her and to continue the therapy.

Doris's example is more dramatic than most. Still, it highlights how the requested intervention of massage therapy can have an opposite effect—in this case, an adverse reaction—from what was intended. More commonly, massage therapists encounter less dramatic responses.

A client who is unconsciously feeling threatened by the therapy, despite how effective the therapist may feel the work is, may derail it by suddenly beginning to cancel appointments, forget appointments, or fail to pay for appointments. In some cases, the client suddenly disappears altogether. Or, a long-term client who has always been satisfied with the work may suddenly begin to complain about it, although the massage therapist is using the same methods. Or, the client and therapist may repeatedly spend an entire session working together to open a part of the body that by the next appointment has tightened up again. Such derailing confronts the therapist with a conundrum: the client is coming to undergo some sort of change for the better, but does not seem to be cooperating in the process. In these situations, the client's lack of cooperation is not overt, but subtle and elusive. In most cases, it is not intentional and the client has no conscious awareness of it.

When they first encounter the paradox of healing, many massage therapists think that they are doing something wrong. They may even take classes or workshops intending to learn more powerful and newer techniques ... but the results remain the same. This is a clue that something beyond the massage therapy is going on. Although the client consciously wants a positive outcome, such as relaxation, stress reduction, or increased ease of movement, unconsciously he or she feels threatened by it and does not want it. For some reason, resistance is working to foil the therapeutic intervention so that everything remains the same, *even if it is uncomfortably the same.*

Tension As Defense

Tension is a fact of modern life, and dealing with tension is in many ways at the core of the work of a massage therapist. Releasing tension often brings relief, a feeling of well-being, and a heightened sense of somatic awareness. However, when tension is associated with protecting oneself from emotional pain, the story can be quite different. When protection manifests as tension, it is critical for massage therapists to understand the role of tension in psychological defense.

Tension Patterns

In your anatomy and physiology courses, you learned about the neuromuscular aspects of tension and that tension—by contraction of the muscles—is essential to movement and maintaining posture. In this book, when we discuss **tension patterns,** we specifically mean neuromuscular contraction that has settled into a habitual pattern that inhibits the client's emotional expression and full range of motion. For clarity, we are not referring to biomechanical patterns when using the term tension pattern.

A tension pattern may have been established in the past as a way of coping with emotionally threatening events by holding or blocking the expression of feelings. Sometimes, such a pattern persists for many years, even though the causative event is long over and may even be forgotten.

One of the easiest ways to see the relationship between tension patterns and emotion is by holding your breath. Next time you bump your elbow, stub your toe, or experience some sort of sudden pain, notice what sound you make and how you are breathing. Most likely, your throat closes around the full scream that a child would make, and you emit a strangled sound. Or, you may make no sound at all—only hold your breath and hop around. Holding the breath is one of the first ways children learn to control the sensation of pain or the expression of emotion. Try holding your breath for a moment now: notice the bodily tension required to do it, the enormous effort and the number of muscles involved in this simple act. Now try breathing while still maintaining this tension pattern. This is essentially what happens in chronic tension patterns in the body: the person learns to block emotions or pain and simultaneously function in a way that is adapted to the block. The adaptation may be so well accomplished that it eventually becomes "invisible," requiring no conscious awareness. It may become apparent only when the person's life is destabilized by some positive or negative event. For example, a man may wonder at his child's birth why he has difficulty expressing his joy, or a woman may wonder as her spouse leaves her why she feels nothing. Such powerful events trigger changes, which, in turn, may lead a person to investigate the causes. What often happens is that *an emotional block in the body eventually fades into the background of awareness and only comes into the foreground when something radical highlights it for us.* Massage therapy can be one of these triggering events that intervene in our habitual patterns.

Hank

One of our clients, Hank, was brought up in a family that did not express anger. Whenever Hank started to become angry, his mother would respond by saying sweetly, "You're not really angry, are you?" This would stop Hank's expression of his feelings, make him question the validity of his feelings, and prevent him from fully experiencing his feelings. To stop himself from expressing anger, Hank tightened his muscles in his arms, shoulders, and back. This tension made angry expressions difficult or even impossible. For example, making a punching motion is difficult if there is tension in the rhomboids. Hank grew into an extremely mild-mannered adult, whose arms, shoulders and back were chronically locked into a painful tension pattern that enabled him to deny his anger.

Recontraction and Armoring

Tension patterns that have a mechanical origin tend to stay changed after they have been worked on and cleared. In contrast, psychologically based tension patterns, even if cleared several times, tend to recur. This happens because, no matter how good relaxation of the pattern feels, it also presents a threat to the unconscious bodymind. As we have seen, unconsciously, the client believes that the pattern protects him or her from intolerable emotions; thus, the client will unconsciously work to reestablish it session after session. When we see such a pattern reform itself, what we are calling **recontraction,** we recognize at once that something frightening or discomforting may be happening for our client. However, because it is outside the client's conscious awareness, we often have no idea precisely what we are encountering.

Recontraction indicates that the particular tension pattern has become what is termed **armoring.** Like a medieval suit of armor, psycho-physical armoring not only prevents "arrows" from injuring the person, but also makes it difficult to move freely and express emotion (Figure 1.2). Unlike the medieval armor, psycho-physical armoring is not passive. Rather, it is highly responsive to events taking place within the person's psyche and in the person's environment, reasserting itself whenever it senses release. Armoring, then, attempts to undo the effects of massage. The person's armor is able to "sense" because it is embedded within the nervous system and is functioning on the level of the unconscious. Since the purpose of armor is to defend against threatening sensations or feelings, it will attempt to reconfigure the tension patterns that the client may be consciously trying to break.

One of the more interesting manifestations of armoring is in defense against feelings of pleasure. Although Western culture outwardly seems to be pleasure seeking, there is among many Westerners a fear—usually unconscious—of authentic pleasure, relaxation, and well-being. Massage requires a form of surrender, a yielding of focused control that opens the person to a greater depth of feeling and, in turn, a more profound sense of satisfaction in the present moment. Some clients who are highly functional in the world depend on their ability to focus mentally and avoid distraction. The intervention of massage diffuses this focus, threatening the configuration of tension that the client believes he or she needs to remain superfunctional. The decision to leave massage therapy is often fueled by the fear of collapsing too much into relaxation and pleasure and becoming less productive—or more vulnerable— as a result.

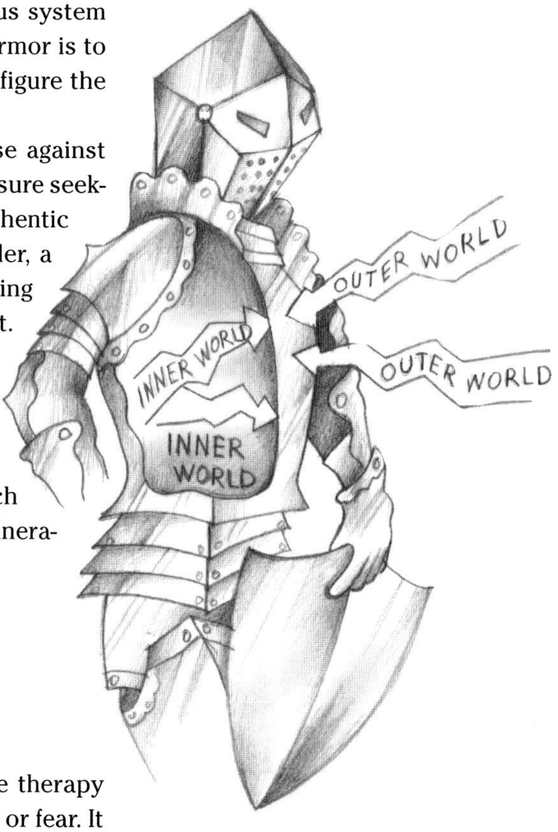

Emotional Release During Massage and Bodywork

Emotional release is a phenomenon in which a client, during a massage therapy session, begins to spontaneously express emotions, such as crying, anger, or fear. It can manifest in deep sobs, yelling, fist pounding, foot stomping, tremors, and large-scale contractions; however, it can also be subtle, manifesting only as a single tear, a shift in breathing, or a change of color in the face. Emotional release occurs when a pattern of tension in the bodymind has been disrupted. Releasing the defensive tension pattern also releases the emotions "held" by the tension pattern, and a spontaneous outburst of emotion can result.

Earlier we discussed the case of Hank, the client who learned to inhibit his anger by tensing his arms, shoulders, and back. We often have feelings that we do not express overtly, but still feel. When Hank's rhomboids were released in massage therapy, they simultaneously released the "brakes" on his feelings of anger. He began to talk about how angry he was that his mother would not let him be angry, and his hands balled up into fists. His voice took on a growling tone. The energy

Armoring
Armoring is defined as any chronic pattern of involuntary tension in the body that dampens or blocks emotional expression, alters perception of the outer world or inner psychological world, diminishes or eliminates kinesthetic awareness, and restricts range of motion. Chapter 7 provides a complete discussion of armoring.

Figure 1.2
Armoring unselectively blocks external and internal stimuli. Armoring is a defensive protection against perceived dangers from both the external and internal worlds. Like an actual suit of medieval armor, psychophysical armoring not only prevents arrows from injuring the person, but also makes it difficult or impossible to express and move freely. Only defensive responses are possible. Also, it is equally difficult to get out of a suit of armor as to get into it!

released from his arms, shoulders, and back rushed through him, empowering him to challenge the inhibiting messages about anger that he had absorbed from his mother.

In Hank's case, as in most we encounter, the inhibition of emotions began in the client's past. However, as the next case example shows, the emotions themselves are not always related to the past.

Joan

Our client Joan was taught by her family that crying was an expression of weakness and something to be avoided. Joan learned as a child to tighten her jaw and push out her chin to stop her tears. In massage, when tension in her jaw and chin was released, she cried. However, her tears were not about her childhood, but about her relationship with her husband. Although the pattern was established in childhood, the content was related to current experiences.

The experience of emotional release may make the client and the massage therapist uncomfortable, but the fear of the release is often worse than the reality. The client typically fears that emotional release will cause him or her to become inappropriately expressive, to embarrass him- or herself, or to lose control in life in general. The therapist may fear that the client will have a nervous breakdown on the massage table, scream at or hit the therapist, or storm out. Our own experience is that in almost all cases the client is able to distinguish appropriate from inappropriate reactions. Emotional release enables *appropriate* expression of emotions that have previously been or would have been suppressed or repressed. If the client does demonstrate difficulty with appropriate expression, a referral for psychotherapy is appropriate.

OVERCOMING RESISTANCE AND LETTING GO

Bruce

Bruce had been suffering from chronic lower back pain that was so severe he could not work more than a few hours a day. Thorough medical exams could not reveal any outstanding organic problems, nor did various medical treatments help. Palpation showed that Bruce's back had extensive chronic knots. Deep-tissue work started melting some of these knots, bringing Bruce great rushes of relief. Waves of sobs began to come out as he talked about how much suffering his back had caused him and how little support and understanding he had received. As the session ended, Bruce spoke with great satisfaction of how powerfully moving the session had been. Elated and hopeful, he asked how often he could come. Yet he proceeded to cancel the next two appointments he had made and failed to reschedule any further appointments.

Six months later, Bruce resurfaced. Through discussions with him about what had happened, the complex causes of his behavior were gradually revealed. As much as Bruce wanted to get better, he had been overwhelmed. As

Bruce

can happen with chronic pain, Bruce had adjusted by numbing himself. Unfortunately, he had found that drugs and alcohol helped with this, which complicated his clinical picture. The release he had experienced during massage therapy had upset the status quo that he maintained through his tension patterns, and thereby had upset the stability he had acquired, admittedly at a very high cost. Bruce was not ready to change, to give up his numbness, so he unconsciously avoided the massage therapy that had offered him his first sense of hope in years. Six months more of suffering were required before he could risk change and return to therapy. This time he was ready.

The tenacity of certain tension patterns can be surprising and frustrating to the novice massage therapist. With experience, however, you will come to realize that the simple application of techniques is not enough to permanently disrupt these patterns. Something more is required; namely, the active participation of the client.

With much work and training in self-awareness, the client can maintain change in the body. Massage is a powerful vehicle for helping the conscious and unconscious minds to communicate. When a protective pattern is opened repeatedly and the client finds that the emotions that the pattern was defending against are actually tolerable and finite, the unconscious mind can begin to accept that the tension pattern is no longer necessary. It can then let go of the pattern and become congruent with the conscious mind, thereby allowing the whole, true self to emerge.

As emotionally based patterns in the body spontaneously emerge to the awareness of the therapist and client, working with these patterns together creates a *therapeutic alliance* between them. This differs radically from "just getting a massage." In forming a therapeutic alliance, the client pledges in some form to contribute his or her active involvement, acknowledging that the massage therapist cannot undo tension patterns without his or her participation. The client must contribute awareness and commitment. Only in this way can the client overcome resistance and let go. In later chapters of this book, we say more about forming and maintaining a therapeutic alliance.

REFERENCES

Damasio, A. (1995). *Descartes' error: emotion, reason, and the human brain.* New York: Avon.

Damasio, A. (2000). *The feeling of what happens: body and emotion in the making of consciousness.* New York: Harvest.

Gerson, M. (1996). *The second brain: A groundbreaking new understanding of nervous disorders of the stomach and the intestines.* New York: Harper Perennial.

Goldstein, K. (1995). *The organism.* New York: Zone Books.

Keleman, S. (1986). *Emotional anatomy: The structure of experience.* Berkeley: Center Press.

LeDoux, J. (1998). *The emotional brain: The mysterious underpinnings of emotional life.* New York: Touchstone.

Montagu, A. (1986). *Touching.* New York: Harper & Row.

Pert, C. (1987). *Molecules of emotion.* New York: Scribner.

Reich, W. (1980). *Character analysis.* New York: Noonday Press.

Van der Kolk, B., McFarlane, A.C. & Weisaeth, L. (1996). *Traumatic stress: The effects of overwhelming experience on mind, body, and society.* New York: Guilford Press.

2

Psychological Factors Affecting Massage Therapy

Touch is psychologically meaningful. We almost always interpret and assign meaning to touch on a conscious or unconscious level. Our meanings are affected by the part of the body touched, the duration of the touch, the amount of pressure applied, the rate of movement of the touch, and the situation in which the touch occurs. Other factors that influence the meaning of touch include previous personal experiences of touch, cultural norms and values, social status, gender, and relationship. Although the way in which each of these factors is influential is fascinating, we will focus on relationship in particular.

When one person touches another, it takes place within the context of relationship. Within that relationship, each person is cast into a role. Some familiar relationship roles are parent-child, teacher-student, friend-friend, boss-employee, lover-lover, physician-patient, stranger-stranger, attorney-client, spiritual leader-follower, and therapist-client. The nature of these roles, in turn, bestows certain meaning to touch within the context of each relationship. Depending on the type of relationship and its component roles, the same touch can take on vastly different import. For example, we may interpret a pat on the head (in most Western cultures) as affectionate when given by a parent to a child, demeaning when given by a boss to an employee, and violating when given by a stranger.

RELATIONSHIPS AND ROLE ASSUMPTIONS

Think about your feelings toward, and relationship to, the following people in your life: your physician, nurse, religious leader, counselor or psychotherapist, personal trainer, acupuncturist or other complementary health care provider, and teachers. You might notice that with many of these figures, you may carry a certain amount of respect, trust, and admiration whether or not you know them well or their professional background. We tend to believe that such people in our lives are wise, superior, and trustworthy and have our welfare in the forefront of their concern. *The role itself constellates these feelings and assumptions.* In contrast, when we enter roles that are reciprocally paired with the ones above, such as patient, client, worshipper, or student, other feelings and assumptions are constellated. You might think, for example, of individuals in these roles as somehow being younger, less knowledgeable, or less powerful, needing help and care, being more dependent, in an inferior position, or needing guidance or leadership, or wanting to grow. Why do we make such assumptions based solely on an individual's role in a particular relational context? And what roles are most influential in the massage therapy setting?

Archetype of the Healer

Most massage therapists do not actively or consciously seek power, and many may not even see themselves as particularly powerful. Indeed, many massage therapists work within models that seek to diminish or de-emphasize their power, viewing the massage therapist as a facilitator of the client's own inner healing forces or conduit for healing energy. Within such models, the word *power* can even take on negative connotations. Despite this, massage therapists *are* powerful figures for clients, who tend to attribute power to them solely because of their role as therapist. Even if the massage therapist does not want or seek out power, clients still ascribe power to the therapist because *power is an intrinsic element in the therapist-client relationship.* To understand why, we need to examine the archetype of the healer and how this archetype contributes power to the role of healer.

Roles such as physician, nurse, religious leader, counselor, or psychotherapist share what Carl Jung, the father of analytical psychology, called the archetype of the healer. Jung found that across many cultures certain roles, such as the magician or shaman; symbols, such as the circle or mandala; and myths carried important psychological powers. He called these universal roles and symbols **archetypes**. Myths and fairy tales are stories in which these archetypes appear in our cultural life. They also appear in popular culture. Fictional characters such as Star Wars' Yoda and real people whose image appears in the media such as Mother Teresa, manifest the archetype of the healer.

The most elemental archetypes are those of the mother and father. Jung identified many other important archetypal figures, such as

---

Box 2.1

THE ARCHETYPAL HEALER

How does the archetype of the healer work in your personal psyche? To find out, begin by listing the healing professionals with whom you personally interact, such as (but not limited to):

▶ Physician
▶ Nurse
▶ Massage therapist, acupuncturist, etc.
▶ Yoga, Tai Chi instructor, etc.
▶ Minister, priest, religious teacher
▶ Fitness instructor or physical trainer

Then ask yourself these questions:

1. Do I always take what this person says as wise or right?
2. Do I allow myself to question internally what this person says?
3. Do I allow myself to question this person to his or her face if I think there is a problem?
4. Do I always do what this person says without question?
5. Do I want this person to like me more than I usually want to be liked by people?
6. Do I want to be this person's favorite or to feel "special" to him or her in some way?
7. Do I think this person is "better" than I am on the whole?
8. Do I think he or she has some "special" knowledge that, if I could learn it, my life would improve?

hero, villain, martyr, trickster, child, wise person, and lover. He pointed out that archetypes exert their influence in the deep background: "Archetypes, so far as we can observe and experience them at all, manifest themselves only through their ability to organize images and ideas, and this will always be an unconscious process, which cannot be detected until afterward" (Jung, 1954–1979, p. 231).

The archetype concept gives an interesting insight into the role of the massage therapist and why it holds such power. The archetype that your physician, nurse, dentist, minister, psychotherapist—even your personal trainer perhaps—carries is that of the healer. It is the archetype of the healer that elicits the respect and awe that you likely feel toward a person in one of these roles. The archetype is also the source of the power you attribute to such people. Box 2.1 provides an exploration of the influence of the archetype of the healer.

The healer archetype, as with all archetypes, is impersonal. This means that the power attributed to the person does not necessarily match the actual person's skills, wisdom, or capacity to heal. In fact, in reality, no mortal human being can be as wise, good, or skillful as the healer archetype. Nevertheless, the archetype serves an important and useful purpose. *It allows the client to believe that healing is possible and that it is possible with the client's particular therapist.* Although archetypal power seems magical, it is a sound psychological concept that a client's belief in the therapist's ability to help the client is critical to therapeutic success. Only through this belief will a client trust, open up, devote energy to working on him- or herself, and go through the difficult times that sometime arise during therapy.

Stefan

Stefan had gotten a lot from his work with his massage therapist, Jill. He had unexpectedly found that massage therapy had made him much more aware of his feelings. He had tremendous respect for Jill and listened carefully to everything she said. Her work with Stefan had been profound.

One day, as they were ending a session, out of the blue Stefan mentioned he had felt a slight pain in his calf while he was just sitting in his easy chair reading a book the other night. Without thinking, Jill said lightly in passing, "Oh, something must have been going on that you couldn't stand." Because the session was ending, they did not pursue it.

The next session, Stefan came in very excited. Before they even started the massage, Stefan told Jill that he had made a great breakthrough. He understood what it was he could not stand. Jill's off-hand remark had led Stefan to think about what he could not stand up to or tolerate in his life. He realized that he was in the wrong profession and decided to investigate changing the course of his career. Stefan was effusive in his thanks to Jill for her remark at the end of the session.

Jill was completely confused. She had to strain to recall what it was she said to Stefan during the previous session. Jill was usually thoughtful about what she said to clients, and she would consider carefully whether what she was about to say would be helpful. This time, however, the remark seemed so innocuous that it escaped her recollection of the session. Jill realized how productive this off-hand remark actually was and, for the first time, how powerful *she* was in relationship to her clients.

This case study is an example of the archetype of the healer. Stefan's belief in Jill stemmed from his unconscious, which viewed Jill as an archetypal healer. To Stefan, everything that came from Jill seemed to be invested with great

Stefan

thought concerning his internal process and well-being. Jill was a benevolent and powerful authority for him. While Jill was an excellent massage therapist, sophisticated regarding matters of healing, and truly caring, she was not endowed with the all-knowing power Stefan saw in her. It was the archetype of the healer *within Stefan* that took Jill's off-hand remark and used it to bring about Stefan's breakthrough. Stefan attributed the process to Jill because he did not yet fully understand that he had the capacity *within him* for his own healing.

However, the healer archetype potentially has a dark and shadowy side that can be harmful. It becomes especially dangerous when the therapist believes that he or she actually *is* the archetypal healer—that he or she *is* all-knowing, all-giving, all-good, and all-powerful—rather than just embodying these qualities. Such identification with the archetype is a *very seductive* form of ego inflation, which causes the therapist to feel that he or she can do no wrong. Personal uncertainties, insecurities, even cautions are erased. Thus, it can be very intoxicating—and very dangerous.

Ego inflation caused by archetypal identification leads the therapist to stop reflecting on his or her own actions, values, and motives in the conviction that everything he or she does is perfect and right. In other words, the ego-inflated therapist does not ground intuitions or impressions in reality. Thus, the therapist's vulnerability to making mistakes increases dramatically. Even worse, archetypal overidentification can lead the therapist to abuse the power the client assigns to him or her. For example, the therapist might direct the client to actions that benefit or aggrandize the therapist, rather than the client, such as selling the client expensive products of dubious value, recommending that the client increase the frequency of sessions, or persuading the client to join a spiritual or social group.

Archetypal identification can be just as possible for a therapist who has no overt spiritual beliefs or framework or for a therapist who incorporates the inflation into a spiritual system or approach. It sometimes announces itself by thoughts such as, "I *am* a shamanic healer-massage therapist," or "I *am* guided by a higher spirit when I touch someone." While it is a fine thing to have one's work inspired by traditional or exotic healing, a red flag is waving when these images give a feeling of power that has an intoxicating quality. However, sometimes archetypal identification can be disguised. No thoughts or images arising from spiritual systems appear in the therapist's psyche. It can be more a feeling of being "golden" (i.e., everything I touch turns into gold), highly talented, and special, but without self-examination or questioning one's actions. Inflation by the healer archetype also causes one to be unaware of the inflation itself. Such archetypal inflation is distinct from simply having healthy self-esteem and confidence.

Polly and Bob

Polly was a massage student. Bob was her instructor and her massage therapist. He was very popular at the school. He seemed to know a lot and was always exploring new and interesting ideas. Whatever Bob said, people around the school seemed to take to heart. Polly felt very lucky to have him also as her therapist.

Polly and Bob

One day after class, Polly saw a group of students clustered around Bob. He seemed to be glowing with excitement. Bob was talking about an investment plan that was bringing him enormous returns very quickly. He told them that with only a modest amount of money paid to him, he could get them involved on the ground floor, when the greatest profits could be made. One person in the group mentioned that he had read an article in the business section of the newspaper that this particular business was highly speculative. "Oh," Bob said, "That's putting negative energy into this and you'll pull this thing down." A hush fell over the group. They had listened in class to Bob talk about the relationship among energy, intention, and outcome. Polly felt excited. She wanted to show Bob that she believed in him. "I think I might want to try this," she said. Polly wrote a sizeable check on the spot.

Any number of investment advisors would say that this is a terrible way to make an investment decision. However, Polly felt that Bob was a very wise and special person who would never involve her in anything that would harm her. For Polly, if Bob said it, then it had to be reliable.

Bob believed that this investment scheme was a "can't miss-sure thing." Things had gone exactly according to the formula given to him by the man who had brought him into the plan. He was already getting dividends after only a few weeks. Besides this, Bob felt really good about himself. His professional and business endeavors were going so well, he felt as if he could do nothing wrong. Everything he had put into taking myriad trainings, reading so many books, following every trend in healing, receiving so much massage, becoming a renowned therapist, and building his school was paying off. Bob believed he had figured out how life worked. He thought he could hardly fail.

Besides Polly, Bob convinced several other students and clients to invest with him. He felt very good about it, because he was helping people he cared about become more prosperous. It seemed like a win-win situation to him. He was going to make money from the investments his students and clients made, while they would make some money, too. Even more important to Bob, he was teaching them how to live better, more positive, lives.

Bob kept receiving dividends. Polly received a couple of dividend checks, but then they stopped coming. Polly told Bob about this during a session. "You're thinking negatively about this," he said, as he worked on her back, "You know how we create our own realities." Polly felt terrible about herself. She had doubted Bob, who had only her welfare in mind. She had failed to follow his wise guidance. She decided to be patient and follow Bob's advice to think positively. Despite this, no more dividend checks arrived.

As we saw in Stefan's case, Polly also unconsciously saw the archetype of the healer within Bob and gave great credence to everything Bob said. However, in this case, it was *Bob* who was caught up in the shadow side of the archetype of the healer. The unquestioned belief that everything he did was positive for his students and clients, along with his belief that he had found the secrets of how life worked, was evidence of the ego inflation caused by overidentification with the archetype. In turn, this caused Bob—despite his best intentions—to mishandle his relationship with his student-client.

As stated in the beginning of this section, clients assign power to the therapist whether the therapist wants it or not. Denying that clients imbue the therapist with such power will not make it go away. The therapist needs to become attuned to the client's attributions of power and use it on the client's behalf, that is, to advance the client's therapeutic process. The power of the healer archetype, as with all archetypes, exists for a purpose. By imbuing people in our lives with such archetypal power, we assign them vital roles in our development. *We need to believe that those to whom we go for healing can heal* (caring, helping, guiding, etc., can be substituted for the word healing here). When we invest archetypal power in someone, it is the person seeking to be healed who "gives" the power to heal to the healer. In this sense, this power does not "belong" to the therapist, since the healing force comes primarily from within the client.

Jung liked to say that when an archetype, in a sense, takes hold of us and inspires us, that it is especially powerful. If we accept and build on Jung's idea, we can say that the nature of the massage therapist-massage client relationship gives it special power. But it is not only the special nature of the therapist-client relationship that makes it powerful, it is also the fact that it *is* a relationship.

Relationship As the Heart of Therapy

The *relationship* between the therapist and the client, besides the work itself, is also part of the therapeutic process. To go one step further, *the therapeutic relationship is a key to healing and the effectiveness of the therapeutic process*. The importance of this observation cannot be overemphasized. Many studies and texts by members of a variety of the helping professions on the subject of what makes therapy effective have found that the relationship between therapist and client is a critical factor—in many cases surpassing the effect of the type of techniques used. For example, Whiston and Sexton (1993) found that the literature on the therapeutic relationship suggests that it is the single most powerful predictor of therapeutic outcome, whereas a study of body psychotherapy clients by West (1994) found that clients reported that the quality of their relationship with their therapist was more important in their work than the techniques that were used.

In *How Clients Make Therapy Work*, psychotherapist Arthur Bohart states:

The most important thing the therapist generally has to offer the client is a relationship. However, this is not because the relationship is curative (although it can be). Instead, the relationship is helpful for two reasons. First, a good relationship involves the client in the process, and client involvement is what energizes whatever goes on in therapy. Second, the relationship provides a context or workspace where clients can generatively work . . .(pp. 19–20)

Bohart's statement can certainly be applied to massage therapy. The most healing aspect of a series or course of massage therapy sessions, especially in the longer term, can be the relationship between client and therapist. The massage therapist can facilitate this through building a trusting relationship by being non-judgmental, reliable, and supportive.

Here are some ideas of how to enhance the therapist-client relationship and play the role of massage therapist better. Make eye contact when talking to clients. This gives a nonverbal cue to the client that you are centered and focused on them and their issues. It also gives the client a message that you are confident in your abilities and knowledge. In contrast, averting eye contact is a sign of submissiveness or avoid-

Box 2.2

SOURCES FOR LEARNING MORE ABOUT COMMUNICATIONS AND INTERVIEWING SKILLS

Please note that several of the books listed below have been written for mental health professionals. Although these books contain much information about communications and interviewing skills that can be used effectively and correctly by massage therapists, some of the information and methods may not be appropriate for massage therapists to use because doing so may violate scope of practice rules. Keeping in mind the dividing line between massage therapy and psychology/psychotherapy is imperative when deciding which information you can use. Chapter 4 has an extensive discussion of this dividing line.

We have included short annotations to give you an idea about what each source offers, as well as the skill level of its content.

Bolton, Robert. People Skills. New York: Simon & Schuster, 1979. *This is more of a "how to" book than an academic textbook. The author emphasizes how to use these skills for interpersonal communication and collaborative problem solving in personal life, more than professional work. Intermediate level.*

DeJong, Peter, and Berg, Insoo Kim. Interviewing for Solutions. Pacific Grove, CA: Brooks/Cole, 1998. *Much of this book may not be appropriate for massage therapists, but Chapter 3, Skills for Not Knowing/Basic Interviewing Skills, should be. Besides covering fundamental skills, the authors' philosophy of "not knowing," that is, learning how to "let the client take the lead" is interesting and useful. Intermediate to advanced level.*

Egan, Gerard. You and Me: The Skills of Communications and Relating. Pacific Grove, CA: Brooks/Cole, 1977. *Much of this book may not be appropriate for massage therapists, but Section II, The Skills of Listening and Responding, should be. Listening skills are a critical part of communications. Intermediate to advanced level.*

Fanning, Patrick, McKay, Matthew, and Davis, Martha. Messages: The Communications Skills Book. Oakland, CA: New Harbinger Publications, 1995. *This nontechnical book thoroughly presents all the building blocks of communications skills and is worth using for the exercises alone. Basic to intermediate level.*

Martin, David G. Counseling and Therapy Skills. Prospect Heights, IL: Waveland Press, 1999. *Much of this book may not be appropriate for massage therapists, except for Chapter 2, Learning to Hear; and Chapter 3, Finding the Words. These chapters have good information on listening skills and forming properly worded statements. Advanced level.*

Murphy, Bianca; Dillon, C. Interviewing in Action. Pacific Grove, CA: Brooks/Cole, 1998. *This excellent textbook is used in a number of graduate study courses, however discerning massage therapists can use much of the information. Advanced level.*

(Continues)

ance, which detracts from the role of therapist. To facilitate eye contact, sit on the same level as the client. This also nonverbally cultivates and reinforces a sense that you want to relate to the client as an equal, rather than a superior. When greeting and talking to the client, observe a "personal space" around the client. The size of the personal space varies depending on the individual and his or her culture. In American culture, it is usually about three feet. Some therapists have a tendency to invade the client's space, which can cause discomfort for the client. Although we know that our clients are coming for massage, and therefore being touched, ask permission in some manner before approaching or touching. For some clients, this may be the first sense of empowerment that they experience. Furthermore, because of the intimate nature of massage, the client's sense of safety and control are paramount. For example, for clients who have been abuse victims, violating their personal space may make them feel intimidated or threatened.

Keep conversation professional and refrain from divulging personal information, especially discussing your own personal problems and issues. Inappropriate conversation can undermine your role as therapist and can be a boundary violation (we discuss boundaries in Chapter 4). On the other hand, encouraging the client to communicate with you, especially to tell you how he or she feels about your touch (e.g., too light, too heavy, just right, please repeat that), can be very important. Some clients need to be "given permission" to disclose how they feel. While the client is speaking, especially while sharing personal information, make gestures, such as nodding your head, to provide nonverbal cues to the client that you are engaged in listening and responding. By the way, such gestures need to be honest reflections of your inner state, not merely mechanical, glib, or *pro forma*. Professional dress also affects a client's impression of you in your role of therapist, although what amounts to proper dress depends somewhat on the client's image of a therapist. For example, wearing a white coat or smock may fit the role for one client, but may put off another client, who associates it with and dislikes the medical establishment.

In contrast, wearing a neat polo shirt and athletic pants may fit the image of a sports massage therapist, but discomfort someone who associates massage with energy balancing. As trust is established, these parameters can be appropriately relaxed.

To the casual observer, the relationship between a massage therapist and client may seem minimal and not so significant because it is primarily nonverbal, physical work. Also, very little analysis or talk about the relationship usually happens during massage sessions. However, all interactions, both verbal and nonverbal, converge to form the relationship between therapist and client. Therefore, *the massage therapist's ability to appropriately form and guide the relationship can have profound effects on the course of the work.*

Good communications and interviewing skills will clearly strengthen your ability to guide the therapeutic relationship with your massage client. We encourage you to do so. Because several good sources for learning communications and interviewing skills are available, and this is not the main focus of this book, rather than say more here we will offer a list of sources in Box 2.2 that will help you in this area.

Box 2.2 (Continued)

SOURCES FOR LEARNING MORE ABOUT COMMUNICATIONS AND INTERVIEWING SKILLS

Rivers, Dennis. The SEVEN CHALLENGES: A Workbook & Reader About Communicating More Cooperatively. *If you feel you are a beginner, this is a good place to start because it presents basic concepts in everyday terms. Also, it is free of charge! Available at:* http://www.coopcomm.org/workbook.htm. Basic level.

Thompson, Diana. Hands Heal: Communication, Documentation, and Insurance Billing for Manual Therapists. Baltimore: Lippincott Williams & Wilkins, 2001. *The first chapter, Communication and the Therapeutic Relationship, gives a good overview of the subject from a massage therapy perspective. You may want to read this chapter before reading more specific or advanced books as it digests ideas from some of the books on this list. Basic level.*

The Three Worlds of Relationship

The client and the massage therapist bring their personal histories, hopes, dreams, expectations, fantasies, beliefs, and values into the massage room. These may not be consciously acknowledged or verbally stated, yet they can influence the progress of therapy as much as—or more than—the pain, injury, tension patterns, or other physical factors on which the client and therapist usually focus. Dealing with unspoken psychological factors is a tall order for any massage therapist, especially for the novice practitioner. The following discussions should help increase your awareness of these factors and of your ability to integrate them into your work.

To use a concept from existential psychology, for each person a relationship involves the simultaneous coexistence of three realities: my world, the other person's world, and the world we create through our interaction. In the therapeutic relationship, this becomes the therapist's world/reality, the client's world/reality, and the world/reality that is created through the interaction of therapist and client.

We often use this framework when massage therapists see us for supervision, that is, guidance about their work (we discuss supervision at length in Chapter 3). First, we ask the massage therapist being supervised to describe what took place during a session from the perspective of the client. Second, we ask him or her to describe what took place from the perspective of the therapist. Third, we ask the massage therapist to describe what took place within the interaction between client and therapist. The challenge for the therapist is to understand, be aware of, and track these three spheres. This supervision exercise helps develop this ability. The sections that follow deal with each of these "worlds."

Box 2.3

INFLUENCES FROM TEACHERS

To help you reflect on what biases may have influenced you, try asking yourself the following questions. Observe whether your teachers underemphasized or overemphasized these issues or omitted these issues altogether. You may need to repeat these questions for each teacher if you have been influenced by more than one teacher.

▶ What reading assignments were you given related to psychological issues?

▶ What did your teachers teach or tell you about emotional release on the table?

▶ If people had emotional releases during your training, how did your instructors handle them?

▶ What did your teachers teach or tell you about modalities that emphasize emotional release?

▶ What were your teachers' attitudes when they talked about those modalities?

▶ What did your teachers teach or tell you about the relationship between client and therapist?

▶ What values about massage did your teachers impart indirectly, i.e., without necessarily stating them explicitly?

THE THERAPIST'S WORLD

Both therapists *and* clients have unspoken factors that influence the progress of massage therapy. We are purposely starting with the therapist's world, rather than the client's world. This is because it is our observation that massage therapists and students frequently place much more attention on what is going on with the client, rather than on themselves. As we will see, the therapist's beliefs and personal psychology are influential and deserve equal attention in understanding the dynamics of therapeutic interactions.

Beliefs and Values

What the massage therapist comes to believe about what is an effective massage comes from many sources. A major source is massage education. This education may be broad, taking in many modalities; or it may be narrow, focusing primarily on the benefits of one or two modalities and perhaps also rejecting others. Clearly, teachers have an enormous influence on the didactic knowledge that students learn. However, teachers also have great psychological influence on what students believe and value.

As discussed earlier in this chapter, a teacher plays a role that has a powerful impact on the student. Whatever biases arise out of a teacher's personal psychology can be consciously or unconsciously passed to the students. This is more obvious on the conscious level, because the teacher usually overtly states his or her ideas about psychological issues. On the unconscious level, however, how the teacher approaches psychological issues and how he or she communicates this to students reflect the teacher's attitudes and feelings. For example, if a teacher has a psychological trait of neediness, the teacher may place an emphasis on massage being soothing and catering to the needs of the client, or the teacher may imply that ending a massage with the client not completely satisfied is bad. Other teachers may resist dealing with or talking about *any* psychological phenomena and emphasize technique alone. Since most students usually model their teacher to some extent, they "absorb" this as a tenet for massage. Box 2.3 helps you to assess any biases you may have picked up from your teachers.

Your religious and spiritual beliefs may also shape your beliefs about massage. For example, if your spiritual values emphasize transcending personal emotional pain, you may also believe that expression of feeling contradicts transcendence and should be avoided. As another example, if your spiritual values hold that negative emotions are personal weaknesses, you may also believe that your clients should not express such emotions. Another example is that you may be part of a spiritual system that believes in self-sacrifice and altruism, which might lead you to be always loving and supportive at any cost or in any circumstance.

Another influential belief can be simply stated as, "What is good for me is good for you." This may be conscious or unconscious on the part of the massage therapist, and it is a dangerous belief to hold unchallenged. For example, while deep tissue work may be highly beneficial for the therapist, it may be completely inappropriate for certain clients. Similarly, while the therapist may prefer subtle, light energy work, some clients may need deeper, very physical work. In the realm of psychotherapy, a common observation is made that therapists need to be aware of the tendency to have clients work out the *therapist's* problems. For example, if the therapist is having a personal problem with anger, he or she may believe many of the clients have problems with anger and have them work on anger issues. This is not automatically a bad thing. Sometimes it can allow the therapist to gain insight into the needs of clients who may indeed be similar to the therapist. However, in many cases, what works for the therapist is not what will work for the client.

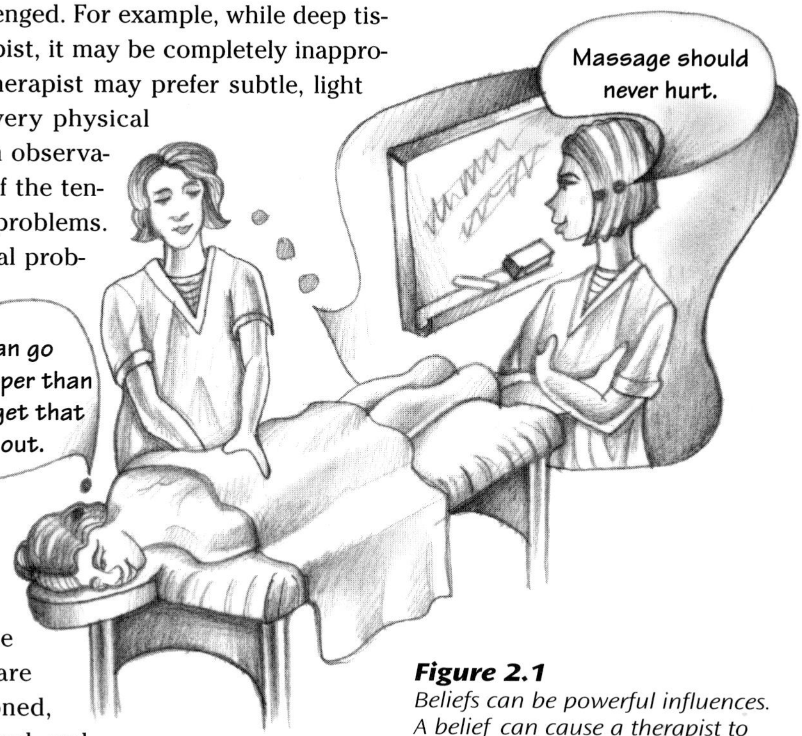

Another area of influential beliefs could be termed **rigid beliefs;** these are beliefs that are strongly held, rarely examined or questioned, accepted as universally true, almost never changed, and applied in all cases. Rigid beliefs often have a "should" embedded within them or implied by them and can have any origin. Some examples of a rigid belief are: "Massage should never hurt," "People should not have emotional release during a session because it is harmful," or "Everybody needs touch all the time." Rigid beliefs often are invisible to the believer and are consequently rarely examined because they are so strongly accepted to be absolute truth (Figure 2.1).

One's personal, psychologically based beliefs clearly also have a major influence. What one's family has both said and conveyed about the expression of feeling creates the foundation of these beliefs. In addition, how we have responded to situations and events in our childhood creates beliefs about feeling and expression. Let us take, for example, the belief that the expression of anger should be avoided at any cost. This could have any number of origins in the family. Parents might have overtly stated that expression of anger is wrong or may have nonverbally conveyed that message by never showing anger or irritation. On the other hand, one might have experienced a family in which there were few limits on the expression of anger. This may have led to a conclusion that anger is always destructive or that anger is the primary way to express oneself. The same could be said about any variety of feelings and expressions. Box 2.4 helps you to assess the influence of family members and significant others on your personal beliefs about feelings.

There is no single right way to feel about feelings. However, the massage therapist must know his or her own beliefs and understand them, know where they are coming from, and not attempt to impose these beliefs on the

Figure 2.1
Beliefs can be powerful influences. A belief can cause a therapist to miss a cue.

Box 2.4

INFLUENCES ABOUT FEELINGS

What did your family or adults who influenced you communicate about these feelings?

▶ Sadness	▶ Fear	▶ Shyness
▶ Anger	▶ Doubt	▶ Sorrow
▶ Joy	▶ Confidence	▶ Grief
▶ Excitement	▶ Depression	▶ Rage
▶ Shame	▶ Playfulness	▶ Terror
▶ Pride	▶ Fun	

Now go back to these feelings and think about how *you* feel about feeling or expressing them.

Box 2.5

PERSONAL BELIEFS AS INFLUENCES

These are examples of personal psychological beliefs that could influence the therapist's view of the client. How do you imagine each of these could influence your view of your client and how you might respond to your client as a therapist?

- ▶ **I can't deal with anger**
- ▶ **I can't deal with neediness**
- ▶ **I can't deal with sadness**
- ▶ **I like feeling spacey**
- ▶ **I need to control everything**
- ▶ **Feelings are too messy**
- ▶ **I am right . . . always**
- ▶ **Feelings are a sign of weakness**
- ▶ **It is good to always be feeling and to express feelings in any way**
- ▶ **Too much excitement makes me nervous**
- ▶ **I can't stand to see people hurting**
- ▶ **The answer to everything is love**
- ▶ **Saying no is mean**
- ▶ **To be a feeling person is to be a more spiritual person**
- ▶ **Transcending your feelings is being more spiritual**
- ▶ **When someone expresses feelings, I have to take care of him or her.**

Now go back through these beliefs and see if any sound familiar. If so, then see if you can get a sense of how your belief(s) influences how you work as a therapist.

client nor permit these beliefs to distort the therapist's perception of what is taking place within the client. This can be difficult and tricky. *Self-knowledge* is the key: the more a therapist learns about his or her personal psychology, the less likely the therapist is to impose his or her beliefs on clients or allow them to distort an understanding of the client. Box 2.5 helps you to assess any personal beliefs that may influence your work with your clients.

Finally, another substantial set of beliefs that can have a significant influence on how we work as therapists involves how we envision healing and change.

How Do You Envision Health?

We all have some sort of internalized model of health. Parts of it may be formed through deliberate, careful thought, whereas other parts may be formed from casual or subconscious assumptions and impressions. As a massage therapist, you need to be aware of what your model is and how it influences your internal and external responses, thoughts, and feelings. This is because both your model and your way of applying it will greatly affect your work and your capacity to develop therapeutic relationships with your clients.

For example, although it is helpful to have an internalized model from which to draw, if our model of health is rigid or if we try to superimpose it on our clients, we may become blind to our clients' unique interpretations and manifestations of health. Imposing a model can be like making the foot fit the shoe, rather than the other way around. Even worse, what is healthful or therapeutic in our model or our opinion may be ineffective or even harmful for another person. Being aware of and open to this possibility is critically important for the therapist.

Noticing the positive projections (see definition in Chapter 3) we make on those we think are living a healthful lifestyle can be useful. Along the same vein, observing what your internal and external responses are to people who do not fit into, attain, nor seek out this model can also be important. How would you respond, for example, to a client who admitted to shoplifting, or to driving while intoxicated? Even relatively minor situations, such as a client who uses profanity, smokes, or eats junk food, can be opportunities for introspection and self-discovery.

Understanding your responses when people do not meet your model of *emotional* health is just as vital. For example, if forgiveness is a value within your model and your belief is that everyone must reach a state of forgiveness no matter what injustice has happened, you might experience some difficulty when working with clients who are angry and do not want to forgive the people with whom they are angry. Your response to this situation could be to try to get them to change their mind, tell them that this is just a stage and they will eventually come around, or tell them they will not be able to progress until they forgive. Or, you might generate a subtle air of disapproval in the room. All such responses potentially invalidate their feelings, which could cause a number of problems, such as damaging trust within the therapeutic relationship. A subtle, but essential, difference exists between imposing how someone "should" feel based on a model and understanding and offering alternative ways of feeling and dealing with a situation.

One way to make your own model of health more concrete and conscious is to examine your thoughts regarding body and mind that contain the word "should." Deliberately thinking through your own "shoulds" will help you see whether you really believe that your shoulds form a healthy picture. You may discover that many of your shoulds related to physical and emotional health are formed from introjections (see definition in Chapter 3). You may also find that your shoulds do not present a coherent, consistent, integrated model at all.

When examining your shoulds, you need to be very honest with yourself. What you *really* believe is what will come through in your practice. After you have made an honest list of your shoulds, you can decide whether these beliefs do authentically form your model of health or whether they are a hodgepodge coming from various sources. Box 2.6 helps to identify your "shoulds."

Perhaps in your training, your instructors gave you a model about how change happens in the body. It is less likely that they spoke directly about a model of how change happens in the bodymind. Because many massage therapists are not taught integrative models of therapeutic change, they tend to construct their models of health from personal observation and study, self-help books, novels, movies, self-help groups, religion, spiritual and secular gurus, and even from relatively brief statements made at workshops. Such models are not formed systematically, but patched together, often in a subconscious, unexamined way.

How Do You Envision Therapeutic and Personal Change?

A therapist's model of therapeutic change can be as influential as his or her model of health.

Box 2.6

IDENTIFYING YOUR "SHOULDS"

Which of these statements do you believe? Place a checkmark next to all that feel true to you. Please note that sometimes "shoulds" are hidden within statements as absolutes. For example, "A healthy person should always be happy" may appear in your thoughts as "A healthy person *is* always happy," but it is still a "should."
A healthy person should:

- ☐ always be happy.
- ☐ express his or her anger.
- ☐ have a spiritual discipline.
- ☐ always forgive.
- ☐ not think too much, but come from his or her heart.
- ☐ be intuitive.
- ☐ have work they enjoy.
- ☐ be successful.
- ☐ be in a good relationship.
- ☐ have lots of friends.
- ☐ eat well.
- ☐ be open about his or her personal life.
- ☐ take care of other people.
- ☐ never reject other people.
- ☐ never make people feel bad.
- ☐ be very giving.
- ☐ always take care of him- or herself.
- ☐ have good taste.
- ☐ be in touch with feelings always.
- ☐ have control over feelings.
- ☐ never be angry.
- ☐ always be positive.
- ☐ use time well.
- ☐ be organized.
- ☐ be well groomed.
- ☐ be serious.
- ☐ have a good sense of humor.
- ☐ go with the flow.
- ☐ take control of the situation.
- ☐ have good judgment.
- ☐ not judge others.
- ☐ be sexually nonconflicted.
- ☐ be sensitive.
- ☐ stand up for his or her beliefs.
- ☐ keep physically fit.
- ☐ not have health problems.
- ☐ be well read.
- ☐ be uninhibited.
- ☐ be gracious.
- ☐ be compassionate.
- ☐ be charitable.
- ☐ have lots of energy.
- ☐ have good posture.
- ☐ be optimistic.
- ☐ be virtuous.
- ☐ be clean.
- ☐ take responsibility.
- ☐ not take life too seriously.
- ☐ talk about his or her personal process easily and openly.
- ☐ be in therapy or pursuing personal growth.
- ☐ not hold grudges.
- ☐ deal with issues immediately rather than storing them up.

Now take the ones you chose and put them together on a piece of paper. Feel free to add any others not on the list that come to mind. Look at them and see what model of health emerges. Then take another piece of paper and, using your list, write down your model of health as a statement.

Do you like your model? Can you live up to your model? What happens within yourself when you do not live up to this model? Would you apply this model to your clients? Does your model have "always" or "should" attached to all or part of it? Does your model attach these by implication or do so by other indirect ways?

Do you want to change your model? Try revising your model and see if you like your new version better.

Box 2.7

IDENTIFYING HOW YOU BELIEVE THERAPEUTIC OR PERSONAL CHANGE HAPPENS, WHAT CAUSES CHANGE, AND WHAT CAUSES RESISTANCE TO CHANGE

Consider these words carefully. First find out which words you use frequently with your clients or when thinking about your clients. Then look at them again and see which words most accurately describe how you really believe change happens. Place a checkmark next to all that you believe are true.

A. Change happens through or is caused by:

- ☐ Development
- ☐ Persuasion
- ☐ Transformation
- ☐ Evolution
- ☐ Facing adversity
- ☐ Rationality
- ☐ Transition
- ☐ Honesty
- ☐ Revelation
- ☐ Hard work
- ☐ Insight
- ☐ Choosing the best methods
- ☐ Learning
- ☐ Persistence
- ☐ Love
- ☐ Good morals
- ☐ Revolution
- ☐ Grace
- ☐ Crisis
- ☐ Self-analysis
- ☐ Good influences
- ☐ Faith
- ☐ Brainwashing
- ☐ Breakthrough
- ☐ Following an ethical code
- ☐ Awareness
- ☐ Transcendence
- ☐ Reorganization
- ☐ Unconditional positive regard
- ☐ Inspiration
- ☐ Epiphany
- ☐ Illusion
- ☐ Understanding
- ☐ Prayer
- ☐ Direction
- ☐ Environmental stress
- ☐ Reaching clarity
- ☐ Catharsis
- ☐ Surrender
- ☐ Synchronicity
- ☐ Eating properly
- ☐ Signs and portents
- ☐ Discovery

B. Here is another list of words about agents or causes of change. What words do you use with your clients? What do you believe causes change?

Change is caused or stimulated by:

- ☐ Necessity
- ☐ Pain
- ☐ Pleasure
- ☐ Awareness
- ☐ Opportunity
- ☐ Accident
- ☐ Effort
- ☐ Feeling
- ☐ Revelation
- ☐ Crisis
- ☐ Pushing
- ☐ Giving up
- ☐ Hitting bottom
- ☐ Confrontation
- ☐ Greed
- ☐ Love
- ☐ Support
- ☐ Failure
- ☐ Unhappiness
- ☐ Depression
- ☐ Anxiety
- ☐ Fear
- ☐ Desires
- ☐ Loneliness
- ☐ Anger
- ☐ Dissatisfaction
- ☐ Boredom
- ☐ Education

As a way of exploring your ideas about therapeutic and personal change, Box 2.7 lists words commonly associated with change. These words imply a model of how personal change happens.

Prejudices and Biases

Prejudices also have an impact on our models. Sometimes prejudice can be obvious, such as bigotry based on religion, race, creed, ethnic group, or sexual preference. Although we may think of ourselves as not being prejudiced because we are not bigoted, upon careful examination most of us will discover that we have many prejudices. The exercise in Box 2.8 helps you to examine your prejudices and biases. Some of these could have a significant influence on how you function as a therapist. Keep your list, because you will use it again when you read Chapter 3.

The list in Box 2.8 could probably go on and on. We all have our likes and dislikes. However, *we also tend to attach judgments to our likes and dislikes*, especially when we apply them to others. We unconsciously make the assumption that there is something wrong with them, that they have a problem that needs to be fixed. All such feelings and tensions can affect the massage therapist's work. For example, with shy clients, a judgmental therapist may become overly friendly to draw them out, minimize the person's need to be shy, feel impatient with their shyness, become irritated, imply that therapeutic intervention will "fix" the shyness, patronize them in some way, or feel ineffective or rejected when they do not open up easily.

Expectations

Expectations, such as fantasy, planning, and projection, are normal human functions that allow us to imagine and anticipate what will happen in the future. These expectations are also used to anticipate how a person will act or a situation will play out under certain circumstances. Expectations can serve the massage therapist well *if* he or she is conscious of them. However, when the massage therapist's expectations of what massage provides, the effect of his or her own work, or the client's responses to the work are unconscious, inner conflict can arise when these expectations are not met. For example, what happens to the massage therapist's feelings about his or her work when the technique that the therapist did well in in massage school gets a lukewarm reception from clients? What happens when the massage therapist who works at a health club that caters to athletic fitness enthusiasts uses subtle energy techniques to no avail? Expectations are formed largely from the therapist's personal and professional history, so we will discuss the influence of history next.

Personal and Professional History

The therapist's personal history deeply influences beliefs, values, and expectations about massage therapy and how he or she functions as a therapist. For example, his or her psychological history (primarily with his or her family) shapes how he or she feels and what he or she believes about touch, his or her relationship to his or her body and the bodies of others, his or her sense of how emotions and feelings should be experienced and expressed, his or her ideas about the role of the will, and his or her feelings about injury, illness, and the possibility of healing. Along with his or her mother, father, guardian, or siblings, other important institutions and individuals also help shape those feelings and attitudes—religious leaders and religion itself, schools and teachers, sports and coaches, physicians and nurses, clubs, peers, friends, favorite books and magazines, movies, television, and music. All these influences and ideas are at work from the very first day at massage school.

Massage training also creates expectations about massage. As discussed earlier in this chapter, the instructors' beliefs about massage are influential. The emotional atmosphere in the massage school also helps shape the student therapist's feelings about massage. The school's curriculum and teaching methods can say something about the school's philosophy of massage. This philosophy is passed onto the student in active and passive ways. How the student's instructors talk about different forms of massage, and what the student "picks up" about what methods the instructors approve of and what they do not, make an impression on his or her ideas and expectations.

The therapist's experience with receiving massage can mold his or her expectations of what will happen with clients. If, for example, the therapist has persisted in getting enough massage to create substantial change, he or she may expect that clients would be willing to expend the same kind of time, money, and energy to do

---

Box 2.7 (Continued)

C. Here is another list of words about what causes resistance to change. What words come to mind when you think about times when you have been in "stuck" situations with your clients? What do you believe causes resistance?

Resistance to change is caused by:

☐ Stubbornness	☐ Fear of loss
☐ Ignorance	☐ Homeostasis
☐ Anxiety	☐ Familiarity
☐ Comfort of the status quo	☐ Past lives
☐ Fear	☐ Survival instincts
☐ Anger	☐ Inertia
☐ Lack of moral fiber	☐ Laziness
☐ Defiance	☐ Religious beliefs
☐ Depression	☐ Neurosis
☐ Mistrust	☐ Dishonesty
☐ Lack of commitment	☐ Faithlessness
☐ Inconsistency	☐ Feeling overwhelmed
☐ Helplessness	☐ Too old, too late to change
☐ Circumstances	☐ Illusion, unrealistic expectation
☐ Pain	☐ Hopelessness

Now take the ones you chose in parts A, B, and C and put them together, grouped under the same three headings, on a piece of paper. Feel free to add any others that come to mind. Look at them and see what model of therapeutic or personal change emerges. Then, taking another piece of paper and, using your list, write down your model of change as a statement.

Do you like your model? Does it form a reasonable model for change? Would you apply this model to your clients? Does your model have any hidden "shoulds" implied? To what degree is your model compatible or not with how you practice?

Do you want to change your model? Try revising your model and see if you like your new version better.

Box 2.8

IDENTIFYING PREJUDICES

Think about each sort of person listed below. What assumptions do you make about them? Are they strongly positive or negative? Would you respond significantly differently to them than people you consider "normal?" How would you respond to them as clients? In the interest of self-discovery, be as honest as possible, even if you do not like or feel comfortable with you response. Jot down notes for each one.

Examine how you feel about:

► Women who wear makeup
► People who pierce their bodies
► Athletes
► People who do no physical activity
► People who wear perfume
► Old people
► People with blue, pink, or orange colored hair
► Atheists
► Intellectuals
► Uneducated people
► People driving beat up cars
► People who dress expensively
► People with tans
► Smokers
► People wearing odd clothing
► People who have a chronic illness
► People who have chronic pain
► People who have lots of accidents
► Sports fans
► People with tattoos
► People who shave their body hair

► Clumsy people
► Environmentally sensitive people
► Meat eaters
► Vegans
► Illiterate people
► People who drink alcohol
► People who use drugs
► People who watch television
► Conformists
► Nonconformists
► Survivalists
► Pet lovers
► Demonstrators
► Political people
► Sex workers
► Gamblers
► People on welfare
► People who do not work
► People with/without a computer
► People who drive slowly
► People who borrow things
► People who talk a lot
► People who are shy
► "New Agers"
► People who eat junk food

Now take another look at your notes. What prejudices and biases do you have? How could they affect your work?

the same. The therapist who had let fellow students or practitioners try new and different techniques on him or her might be surprised when clients want a routine and predictable massage.

The therapist's level of experience also affects expectations. The new student may have high expectations, lots of energy, and a willingness to experiment. A therapist with more experience might have lower expectations about what is possible with massage and a more realistic anticipation of how the client's personality sways the outcome.

Over time, the therapist's practice itself will affect his or her expectations. Both positive and negative experiences with clients, if dealt with consciously, can add knowledge to what to expect in the future. However, if the therapist does not work with these experiences, the expectations become automatic. The therapist may begin to make presumptions about how the client is responding that are based on his or her own personal experiences (i.e., project on the client, which is discussed in Chapter 3), rather than seeing whether previous experiences match what is happening with the client *now*.

THE CLIENT'S WORLD

Clients bring not only their physical body to the massage session, but also their beliefs, values, expectations, hopes, dreams, fantasies, and personal history. These may not be consciously acknowledged or verbally stated to the therapist, yet they can influence the progress of therapy as much as—or more than—the pain, injury, tension patterns, or other physical factors that the client usually does acknowledge. Dealing with unspoken psychological factors is a tall order for any massage therapist, and especially for the novice practitioner. The following discussions should help increase your awareness of these factors, and your ability to integrate them into your work.

Beliefs and Values

The client's beliefs and values also influence the work, particularly in the areas of roles and motivation. Each client has a belief or conception about what the role of a client should be. One of the more common examples is that the client plays a mostly passive role and receives the treatment the therapist chooses. In this sense, the client expects to be "fixed" by the therapist. In contrast, another example is that the client plays an active role and participates in the process. The client expects to be involved in deciding what to work on and accepts completing suggested therapeutic tasks between sessions, such as doing certain stretches.

Each client also has a belief or conception about what the role of the therapist should be. A client may believe the therapist is an expert and an authority who has complete control over the course of the therapy. Another client may believe the therapist is a facilitator who assists the client in meeting his or her therapeutic goals. The client's beliefs about the role of both client and therapist also are related to his or her conception of what massage therapy is. The client's conception of both roles will then vary accordingly if he or she believes massage is related to medical treatment, allied health, complementary and alternative medicine, wellness, personal growth, energetic balancing, or personal services, such as beauty or spa treatments.

What the therapist needs to be aware of regarding roles is to what degree the client's and therapist's beliefs about the roles of client and therapist converge with each other or diverge. The more the beliefs are divergent, the more likely the client and therapist may feel a certain dissonance or disharmony that may manifest in various ways, such as uncomfortable feelings about working with each other, dissatisfaction with results, or the client may have difficulty forming trust.

The client's motivation for receiving massage therapy is also affected by beliefs and values. Some examples of motivations for receiving massage therapy are being more relaxed, looking better, being in shape, being more functional and efficient, reducing aches and pains, maintaining health and wellness, and feeling more energized. Motivation underlies why a client is coming for massage therapy. It is what the client desires as his or her "pay-off" from being massaged. A client's motivation also can change over the course of the work. For example, a client may start massage therapy to feel less stressed, but later become more aware of what is causing his or her stress and want to use massage to affect those causes.

As with roles, what the therapist needs to be aware of is the degree to which the client's motivations and what the therapist believes he or she is offering converge or diverge. The more divergent these are, the greater the possibility that the client and therapist may work at cross-purposes. Also, divergence in the area of motivation may undermine the client's building of trust with the therapist.

Expectations

Massage therapy has gone through a remarkable evolution in the past 25 years. We rarely see now the stereotype from many years ago of the white-uniformed massage therapist pounding away on someone's back with karate-like chops. Contemporary massage has become more variegated, more complex, more powerful, and more wellness oriented. At the same time, the growing popularity of massage has resulted in increased attention from the media. People read, see, and hear more about what massage can do for them. It is understandable, therefore, that the public's expectations of massage have been shaped by this and have grown dramatically. These expectations can affect the outcome of the massage work. Therefore, finding out what the client's expectations are and how they developed is important.

As with beliefs and values about roles and motivations, the key is whether the client's expectations converge with or diverge from what the therapist expects will happen. The greater the divergence, the more likely the client is to become dissatisfied or the more difficult building trust may be. For example, the client's expectations may be unrealistic. He or she may expect tension to be released faster than is possible, or massage to be effective for a problem that it is not effective for, or work to be more or less painful than it actually is.

The client's expectations can also involve anticipation. The client may expect that he or she can or cannot speak during the massage or may not be sure what will happen when expected to disrobe. Previous experiences of massage shape another form of expectation. For example, if a previous therapist discouraged bringing up emotional content, the client may assume it is not okay to do so with you. The client may be influenced by friends' experiences of massage. The client may have friends who had great experiences and benefits from massage. In the same vein, he or she may know others who found it unhelpful or had certain complaints about the massage that they received. What these people say positively or negatively may create expectations about what will happen and how the client will feel.

Personal History

The client's psychological history has great potential to affect his or her response to massage. Because this factor is discussed extensively elsewhere in the book, we focus here primarily on the client's history of previous experiences of massage.

Previous experiences of massage may have given the client a wide or narrow set of expectations. He or she may have had a very positive and satisfying experience with massage with a particular massage therapist. This client may anticipate that other massage experiences will be just as satisfying and is not particularly wedded to the style of massage. Still other clients have had a positive experience and an enduring relationship with a therapist and may have difficulty in changing therapists or techniques. In the client's estimation, nothing else may match the experience with the previous therapist.

Clients can also have had negative encounters with massage that lead them to feel wary and mistrustful. They may have been injured or attributed an injury to the massage they received. They may have experienced their former therapist as having been unable to help them and are dubious whether massage can help at all no matter who is giving it. Some clients have experienced inappropriate behavior from previous therapists, such as the blurring or violation of sexual, social, financial, or personal boundaries. This kind of experience may place the client in a dilemma. The client may want to trust the therapist, but may be unable to do so because of the previous experience.

There are also clients who have had negative experiences because their own expectations were too great for the previous therapist to fulfill. They might have expected pain relief faster than was possible, or relaxation that lasts despite habits to the contrary. These clients might place the same outsized expectations on the subsequent therapist, hoping that this therapist is "the one."

Clients may have feelings about getting a massage that are influenced by how their family or spouse feels about their getting massage. The feelings can have to do with opinions about massage or how significant others feel about the client spending time and resources on such an activity. Others may feel that this is self-indulgent or a less than legitimate activity. Friends and family may have conscious and unconscious opinions about touch or being undressed that will influence the client.

Finding out as many of the client's expectations as possible is important for the therapist to do. The initial interview and first sessions are an advantageous time to discover clients' attitudes about massage. This also becomes an opportunity to address any inaccurate or distorted expectations that clients may have. Box 2.9 suggests questions that help you learn more about your clients' expectations.

INTERACTIVE FACTORS

The third "world" or sphere of the therapeutic relationship is formed from the interaction of the therapist and client. In addition to factors specific to the client or the therapist independently, psychological factors can emerge spontaneously from the interaction between these two individuals. The massage therapist and client, in particular, interact as the therapist touches the client's body and the client responds, discussing the terms and conditions for the massage sessions, talking about the client's history, inquiring into what is happening in the client's awareness during the massage, asking and responding to questions, asking for and giving advice related to the client's presenting problems, helping the client handle pain and pleasure, dealing with emotional release when it occurs, and offering and accepting a supportive presence.

Box 2.9

QUESTIONS TO ASK YOUR CLIENT THAT REVEAL EXPECTATIONS

Including these questions that you can integrate into the initial interview with a client will help you learn more about the client's expectations.

► Have you had massage before?
► Do you know what kind that might have been?
► Did you find it positive and helpful? What about it was positive and helpful?
► If you didn't find it helpful, what wasn't helpful?
► Did you work with the same person consistently? If so, did you find it a positive experience?
► If you didn't find it a positive experience, what was not positive?
► Besides your previous massage experience, what do you already know about massage?
► From what sources did you learn that?
► Why are you coming for massage?
► What results are you expecting or looking for from our work?
► Do you have any expectations about how long accomplishing those results would take and how often you would need to have sessions?
► Do you have any questions about the massage or what will happen?

These interactive factors influence the therapeutic relationship; therefore, you need to be consciously aware of them to the extent that it is possible. For example, what happens to your fantasies about a client when, in the initial phone call, he or she will not let you off the phone before telling you all of his or her physical history in detail? What happens in your imagination and even in your body when a client speaks to you in a whiny voice? What happens to your perceptions of the client if, as the first session has begun, he or she comes into your massage room before being invited in? All these interactions affect you psychologically, and those effects, if you keep conscious of them, will give you information with which to work.

The very beginning of the therapeutic relationship can have great influence on how well the relationship forms. The therapeutic relationship begins *before* the massage therapist even touches the client. It starts when the client makes the first appointment.

When a client calls to arrange the first session (we will assume that most first contacts are by phone), you are taking in much information. However, you may not be aware of it all. Box 2.10 suggests some questions to ask yourself that will help you become more aware of impressions about the client. Of course, the initial phone call also has the general purpose of providing information to prepare the client physically, mentally, and emotionally for the first session.

Here is another example of how paying attention to interactions and how interactions affect you can yield useful information. Returning to the client with the whiny voice previously mentioned, let's say you could not register the fact that your client even has a whiny voice. In not registering this, you could be throwing away valuable information, not only about your client physically, but how he or she will eventually behave with you if you are not able to satisfy the client's needs. If you really listen to a whiny voice, you can hear a great deal of constriction in the throat

Box 2.10

QUESTIONS TO ASK YOURSELF AFTER TAKING THE INITIAL PHONE CALL FROM A PROSPECTIVE CLIENT

Answering these questions will provide you with valuable analytical and sensory data you can use to keep interactive factors present in your conscious mind and improve your ability to do so.

▶ What do you hear in his or her voice?

▶ Do you hear fear, confidence, neediness, weakness, anticipation?

▶ As you talk to a new client on the telephone about the first massage, how do you find yourself interacting with the emotion you hear in the client's voice?

▶ Are you doing the same introductory routine you always do?

▶ Have you changed the routine consciously in order to respond to the tone your client is setting?

▶ Do you find yourself anxious to meet this client?

▶ Are you dreading it?

and chest. This can be an important guide to working with your client. The constriction of the whiny voice can tell you about the client's relationship to energy and expression. The whiny voice can tell you about how the client attempts to get needs met or fails to get these needs met. It may inspire fantasies about how this person relates to others.

The point is that whenever a client elicits a response from you in your role as therapist, being aware of such reactions is important. Be open to the possibility that *your response may have some significant relationship to the client's characteristic psychological patterns*. In turn, this may give you insight into what those characteristic patterns are (we discuss characteristic patterns in detail later in the book). We emphasize this here because we have observed that many therapists assume that their sense of obligation to focus on the needs of the client demands that they set their own felt responses and reactions aside and not pay attention to them. And especially when such feelings and reactions are uncomfortable, it can be all too easy and convenient to set them aside. However, doing this can come at the cost of missing valuable information and insight about your client.

Box 2.11 identifies several additional interactive factors. Consider these in the same manner you did for the previous box.

THE PARADOX OF THE HEALER

After having filled this chapter with much information and advice about ideas and methods for establishing, supporting, and guiding the therapeutic relationship, we have now arrived at perhaps the most important, yet elusive, quality for the massage therapist to embody psychologically—*the ability to be relatively inactive and simply be present with the client at the right moment*. The paradox of healing for the therapist is that despite all the therapist's expertise, authority, and wisdom, and counter to the common perception that a "good therapist" directs the client toward his or her goals, the key is achieving a studied state of "not-doing." We like to call this the **paradox of the healer**: that the healer heals *not by doing, but by not doing ... by being*.

The art of embodying the paradox of the healer—doing by not doing, by being—obviously involves more than doing absolutely nothing. It requires at least two crucial ingredients. First, *the therapist must be authentic*. Carl Rogers, in *On Becoming a Person*, and Jerome Frank, in *Persuasion and Healing*, both point out that the therapist should consistently reflect an interested respect and a desire to be benevolent and caring toward the client. The therapist must suspend moral judgment and be genuinely accepting and tolerant of a wide range of thoughts, feelings, and behaviors. The massage therapist needs a genuine concern and commitment to help another person within the confines and limitations of his or her role as massage therapist. Rogers termed this set of attitudes on the part of the therapist as *unconditional positive regard.*

The philosopher and theologian Martin Buber called this kind of authentic relating an "I-thou" connection. He believed the "I-thou" ideal is to place ourselves completely into a relationship, to truly understand and "be there" with another person, without masks, pretenses, even without words. Buber maintained that when the therapist truly, genuinely connects with the client with an "I-thou" relationship, rather than a less personal "I-you" relationship, or even worse, an impersonal "I-it" relationship, that something very special occurs. The client experiences new aspects of him- or herself and starts to open up more to him- or herself and therefore also more to other people. Hopefully, this experience of benign intimacy is carried from the therapy experience to the interpersonal world of the client.

> **Box 2.11**
>
> ### EXAMPLES OF MORE INTERACTIVE FACTORS
>
> A massage therapist may deal with other interactive factors, such as:
>
> ▶ How the client follows the therapist's directions
> ▶ The degree of intimacy implied in interactions by the client
> ▶ Relative talkativeness or unresponsiveness
> ▶ How the client relates to or treats the therapist's space and property
> ▶ How the client follows the therapeutic framework (discussed in Chapter 4), i.e., the agreement between the client and therapist about what the rules for the therapy are
> ▶ Nonverbal elements, such as how the client moves in relationship to the therapist, e.g., does the client leave the room before or after the therapist
> ▶ Eye contact
> ▶ Comments by the client about the therapist, e.g., the therapist's dress, appearance, etc.

The other key ingredient is that *the therapist's relative inactivity has to be a positive, benevolent, accepting inactivity.* D.W. Winnicott, an English psychoanalyst who was associated with what is named the "object relations school," called this being "good enough" (the main importance of object relations is its understanding of how infants relate to the important persons in their lives, and how these persons relate to them—the emphasis is on relating with others as the basic human motivation). On the first hand, the "good-enough" mother understands and responds to the child's spontaneous gestures. While, on the second hand, the "not good-enough mother," who cannot understand and react to such expressions, subjects the child to her own needs. A result is that the child is required to comply with the mother's needs and not the mother with the child's. If this statement is rephrased by substituting therapist and client for mother and child, an interesting adaptation is formed: The good-enough therapist understands and responds to the client's spontaneous gestures. The not good-enough therapist, who cannot understand and react to such expressions, subjects the client to his or her own needs. A result is that the client is required to comply with the therapist's needs and not the therapist with the client's.

This idea stemmed from Winnicott's recommendation that mothers (and fathers to a lesser extent) let their young child be "alone" with them. According to Winnicott, to be alone did not mean for either person to be literally alone. Winnicott maintained that children thrive when parents do not intrude too much on the child's emerging selfhood. He extended this idea to therapists and felt that the therapist should balance therapeutic techniques and interventions with a quiet, empathic, sympathetic acceptance. Put another way: an overabundance of objectivity, explanation, theory, analysis, or specific interventions spoils the quiet, gentle, humanistic connection between the therapist and the client that makes therapy a powerful endeavor.

The question then is how does one develop the ability to "be present?" We believe a key is *the massage therapist's willingness and ability to grow as a person.* This usually entails engaging in some kind of growth process. For this reason, we highly recommend that massage therapists who aspire to establish this kind of connection with their clients be involved in a therapeutic process of their choice that helps them develop the ability to "be present." Simply put, to be the therapist you want to be, start with your person—*you!*

Cultivating this quality in your work is in some ways even more challenging for a massage therapist than a psychotherapist because massage therapy by its nature is an active form of therapy. Massage therapists do not have the opportunity very often to just sit back and do and say nothing. However, the paradox of the healer informs the massage therapist about how the therapeutic relationship depends on more than technique.

In the next chapter, we discuss how the client protects him- or herself can affect the relationship between the client and therapist and the therapeutic process.

REFERENCES

Bohart, A. & Tallman, K. (1999). *How clients make therapy work: The process of active self-healing.* Washington, DC: APA Books.

Bolton, R. (1979). *People skills.* New York: Simon & Schuster.

Buber, M. & Smith, R. (2000). (trans.) *I and thou.* New York: Scribner.

DeJong, P. & Berg, I.K. (1998). *Interviewing for solutions.* Pacific Grove, CA: Brooks/Cole.

Egan, G. (1977). *You and me: The skills of communications and relating.* Pacific Grove, CA: Brooks/Cole.

Fanning, P., McKay, M. & Davis, M. (1995). *Messages: The communications skills book.* Oakland, CA: New Harbinger Publications.

Frank, J. (1991). *Persuasion and healing.* Baltimore: Johns Hopkins Press.

Heslin, R. & Alper, T. (1983). Touch: A bonding gesture. In: Weimann, J., and Harrison, R. (Eds.) *Sage 11th annual review of communication research: Nonverbal interaction.* Beverly Hills, CA: Sage.

Jung, C. (1965). *Memories, dreams, reflections.* New York: Vintage.

Jung, C. (1954–1979). Symbols of transformation. In: *The Collected works of C.G. Jung.* McGuire, W. et al., (Ed.). Vol. 5, 231. trans. R.F.C. Hull, Bollingen Series XX. Princeton, N.J.: Princeton University Press.

Kottler, J. (1994). *The heart of healing: Relationships in therapy.* San Francisco: Jossey Bass.

Martin, DG. (1999). *Counseling and therapy skills.* Prospect Heights, IL: Waveland Press. (See Chapters 2, Learning to Hear, and 3, Finding the Words.)

Murphy, B. & Dillon, C. (1998). *Interviewing in action.* Pacific Grove, CA: Brooks/Cole.

Perls, F., Hefferline, R. & Goodman, P. (1951). *Gestalt therapy.* New York: Dell.

Rivers, D. *The seven challenges: A workbook & reader about communicating more cooperatively.* http://www.coopcomm.org/workbook.htm.

Rogers, C. (1995). *On becoming a person.* Boston: Houghton Mifflin.

Teyber, E. (1996). *Interpersonal process in psychotherapy: A relational approach.* Pacific Grove, CA: Brooks/Cole.

Thompson, D. (2001). *Hands heal: Communication, documentation, and insurance billing for manual therapists.* Baltimore: Lippincott Williams & Wilkins.

West, W. (1994). Client's experience of bodywork psychotherapy. *Counseling Psychology Quarterly, 7*(3), 287–303.

Whiston, S. & Sexton, T. (1993). An overview of psychotherapy outcome research: implications for practice. *Professional Psychology: Research and Practice, 24* (1), 43–51.

Winnicott, DW. (1965). *The maturational processes and the facilitating environment.* Madison: IUP.

Psychological Defenses Affecting Massage Therapy

*B*ecause touch is so intimately connected with psychological and physical survival and development, and is also intimately involved in the emotional and feeling-centered life of the individual, touch plays a role in how a person protects or defends him- or herself. Touch is important in how we protect or defend ourselves psychologically, since the skin is the most concrete boundary of the physical self. Sigmund Freud, the father of psychoanalysis, stated in *The Ego and the Id*, "The ego is first and foremost a body-ego," contending that our first sense of self is as an *embodied* self.

Each person learns patterns of emotional protections that in psychology are called **defenses** (see the definition). These defenses are protective, but unconscious, mental processes. They help us to cope with our unwanted or unacceptable feelings or awarenesses. Because they act to shield us from something we feel unable to face or experience, they operate below the level of our awareness. Therefore, they are automatic and largely involuntary.

In this chapter, we expand the traditional understanding of defenses to include the physical implications of the bodymind connection. Thus, in describing each of the defenses we consider the added elements of touch and the body, focusing on how defenses affect the massage therapy relationship (please note that we will discuss what we consider the most relevant defenses, rather than every defense mentioned in the psychological literature).

Psychological Defense Mechanisms
Defense mechanisms (also known as ego defense mechanisms or mental mechanisms) are protective phenomena used to aid in the maintenance of repression. **Repression** is the *unconscious* prevention of a feeling or thought from becoming conscious. Therefore, we *are not* aware of repression within ourselves. The primary functions of these mechanisms are to minimize anxiety, protect the ego (sense of self), and maintain repression. Repression prevents discomfort and leads to some economy of time and effort, although it does so at the cost of awareness. *Repression is often thought of as serving as the basis for many defenses.* **Suppression** is the *conscious* prevention of a feeling or thought from being conscious. Therefore, in contrast to repression, we *are* or can be aware of suppression within ourselves because it is a deliberate act.

CLIENT DEFENSES

Both massage therapy clients and therapists themselves bring their unconscious defenses to the massage therapy relationship. However, in session it is the client's defenses that may be directly encountered and challenged. The defenses of the therapist may arise more subtly. Accordingly, we focus first on how they might be encountered in the client and provide some practical suggestions for the massage therapist's response. Later, we focus on the therapist's defenses. For a summary of the psychological defenses, see Table 3.1.

Denial

Denial attempts to erase an unpleasant or unwanted aspect of internal or external reality, usually replacing it with a wish-fulfilling fantasy or a more pleasant or acceptable behavior. Denial may also involve blocking certain sense impressions from the outside world. Even when clients are unable to completely deny an unwanted reality, they may be able to pay very little attention to it. In this way, denial serves the purpose of nullifying the painful consequences of the presence of unwanted pieces of reality. Put simply, *denial is used to make something literally not exist in a person's awareness* (Figure 3.1).

As a psychological defense, denial is inherently an *unconscious* process. Consciously denying something we know to be true, in effect, is lying or fooling ourselves. Consciously not feeling sad or angry, in effect, is making a choice not to feel. Denial draws its power from being an unconscious process, because this is how denial can effectively remove an unwanted reality or feeling from awareness (Box 3.1).

Table 3.1. Psychological Defenses

A simple way of understanding defenses is to see them as a way of getting rid of unwanted or unacceptable feelings or awarenesses. For each defense, this table shows how the defense disposes of the defended feeling or awareness and gives a simple example.

Defense	*How the Feeling Is Disposed*	*Example*
Denial	Making the feeling not exist or disappear	I'm angry, but don't know I'm angry; therefore I'm *not* angry.
Projection	Putting the feeling somewhere else	I'm angry, but I consciously perceive *you* as angry.
Introjection	Taking in the feeling whole, but not assimilating it	I believe I should work hard because my parents told me I should work hard.
Displacement	Putting the feeling on the wrong person or thing	I'm mad at my boss, so I'll kick the dog.
Deflection	Ignoring the feeling by changing the subject	I don't want to deal with feeling sad, so I'll talk about the weather.
Retroflection	Turning the feeling against oneself	I'm mad at myself; I shouldn't have let you hit me.
Reversal	Transforming the feeling into the opposite feeling	I can't say or show that I like that person, so I'll act like I dislike him/her.
Identification	Feeling what someone else would feel instead of one's own feeling	I admire/relate to you, so I feel what you would feel.
Resistance	"Refusing" to feel the feeling	I won't cooperate.
Transference	Putting the feeling about a powerful person onto another powerful person	To therapist: "You're kind and wise just like my mother."

Causative Factors in Denial

Often, denial occurs in clients who were raised by adults who frowned on the expression of feelings and emotions. Denial often develops from the following chain of events: (1) The feeling in question draws a negative response from the parent, which could be in the form of an angry criticism, a look of disgust, physical punishment, or a withdrawal of love and warmth. (2) The child begins to associate the particular feeling with the negative parental response. (3) When this association happens frequently enough, the particular feeling becomes regarded, usually unconsciously, as threatening to the child's well-being. (4) To defend him- or herself, the child obliterates the threatening feeling or emotion from awareness, thus denying its existence. A classic example of an origin of denial is when a boy cries and is admonished by his parent, "Big boys don't cry!" Eventually, he will not admit to or be aware of feeling sad or needing to cry. You may hear someone engaging in this kind of denial say, "I know I should feel sad and cry, but I can't."

A similar causative factor is in play behind one of the more common kinds of denial encountered by a massage therapist—the denial of pain—when the client has been raised in an atmosphere in which the expression of pain was frowned on or discounted. Nearly all massage therapists have encountered a client who is in pain, but asserts he or she is feeling fine or it is "not so bad." In other words, denial can physically manifest as numbness, not the kind of numbness associated with nerve-blocking drugs, but lack of feeling or response. In this case, denial can be so powerful that it leads to what is seemingly irrational behavior, such as denying discomfort in the office of the massage therapist, who is someone willing and able to help.

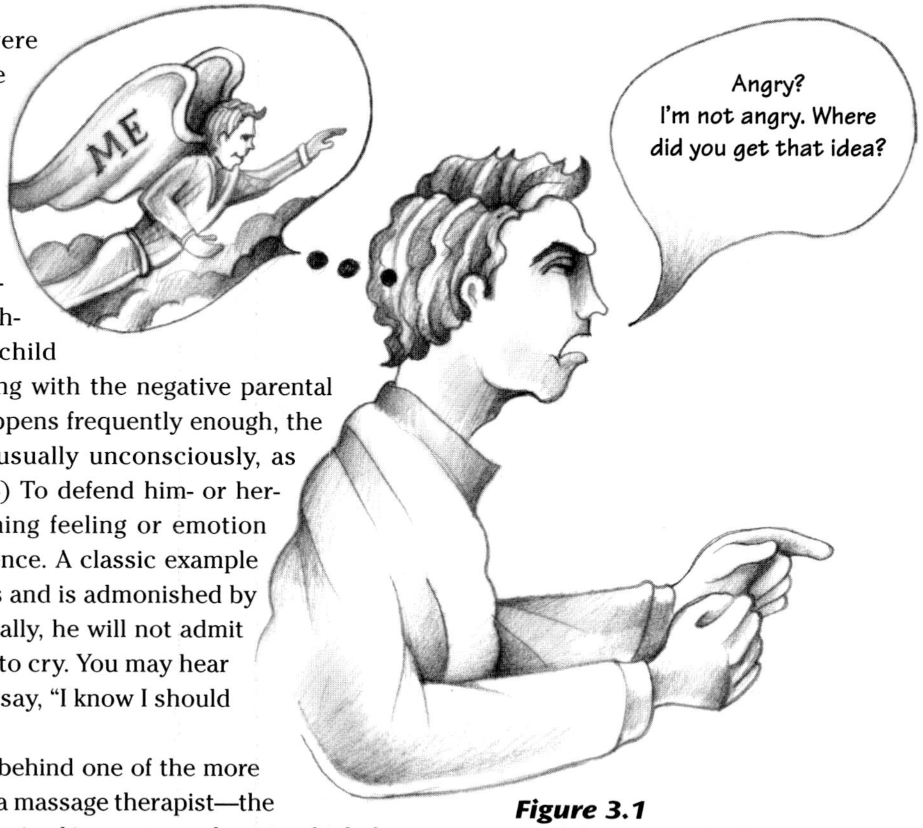

Another powerful motivation for denial is the sense of shame. The discomfort caused by shame can be even more powerful than the pain related to the original formative scene. The desire to avoid experiencing shame can lead people to deny what is perfectly obvious to almost any observer. For example, if a young boy expresses fear of the dark and is ridiculed by his parent(s) for his fear, he may grow to deny all fears, even those that are appropriate. The massage therapist needs to factor in the possibility that the client's denial may relate to feeling ashamed of the truth of whatever he or she is denying.

Another causative factor in denial is the motivation to avoid unpleasant realities or consequences. Massage therapists may see denial surface when the client feels unable to give up certain lifestyle choices that he or she

Figure 3.1
Denial. *An example of denial would be an angry person unable to experience both the feeling of anger and the expression of it. The person could also imagine himself as being different from how he is behaving in reality, such as thinking he is an innocent angel rather than an angry guy.*

Box 3.1

A HIERARCHY OF DEFENSES

Another way of looking at defenses is as a hierarchy based on degrees of forgetting. Denial is dense, primitive, and most unconscious. The object of denial may as well be in an alternate universe. It is as if there were no more memory of the object (a feeling or thought can be the object), and no amount of reminding will succeed. Repression is a bit less dense, since a direct reminder can breach it, but it still involves placing the object in a closed cupboard in another room and forgetting you put it there. Memory is stored normally, but retrieval is possible only with cueing. Suppression is even less dense, the object is placed on a shelf in the same room, but you are choosing not to look at it. Memory and retrieval function normally. The other defenses, such as projection, introjection, displacement, and so on involve partially obscuring the object and therefore are "next" in the hierarchy (adapted from e-mail correspondence with Dr. Michael Diamond).

knows are unhealthy. During the course of their career, therapists will probably hear clients deny—sometimes even vehemently—the negative effects of drugs, alcohol, poor nutrition, lack of exercise, extreme sports, abusive relationships, risky sex, overwork, family problems, chronic illness, financial problems, employment issues, loneliness, dishonesty, chronic stress, and more. Denial by the client may make the massage therapist feel confused or upset with the refusal to accept what seems to the therapist to be reality. The massage therapist may know that the choices that the client mentions are affecting him or her in a negative way, but may be unable to convince the client that this is so. It is important that the massage therapist stay centered with his or her own knowledge and not feel compelled to either join the client in denial *or* batter the client into admitting the truth.

Denial also maintains the emotional status quo. In massage, it commonly surfaces when the therapist affects a tension pattern that is acting to block emotions or personal issues. As is explored in Chapter 5, softening that physical area also softens the holding, and, as a result, unfamiliar or uncomfortable feelings may arise. As a response to the stirring of these feelings, the client may become anxious or overwhelmed. If the client does not know him- or herself well enough, he or she may not be aware of the relationship between that part of the body and his or her feelings. As a result, the client may attempt to get the therapist to work somewhere else, or change methods. The client may even stop coming. It is critical to understand that people use denial in such instances because they cannot handle being in touch with the feelings that were being blocked by their bodily tension.

Effects of Denial

Denial may literally numb the experience of physical and emotional pain. Often in massage therapy, feeling can begin to break through, leading the client to begin admitting to feeling pain and discomfort. When it occurs, this admission can be a huge step forward. However, *because the denial has been so effective as a defense, the client may experience it as originating from the massage therapy, rather than stemming from his or her own physical, emotional, and spiritual condition.* In such cases, the client may refuse to take ownership of it and may act out against the therapist.

As long as pain is numbed and denied, the client cannot work with the roots of either a physical or emotional problem. For example, a dancer we worked with had taken a fall and injured her back. To cope with the injury, she had numbed the tissue surrounding the injury itself. This numbing led to loss of flexibility and an inability to dance in the way she had before her injury. This, in turn, led her to a sense of defeat and depression, since dancing was the center of her life. As many of us do, she believed that by denying the pain of the injury and escaping the pain through stiffening, she would be in control and unaffected. Her denial, however, aggravated her pain and injury, since her stiffening led to increasing her vulnerability to further injury and prevented her from getting to the root of her problem. Body awareness is a critical component in preventing injury, because proprioceptive awareness allows one to maintain balance and mobilize the body so that it remains as close as possible to safe alignment while moving. Only by experiencing the pain—and therefore the reality—of her injury, and "listening" to it so the pain could guide her, could she avoid further injury and begin to heal.

Responding to Denial

Although the massage therapist may point out how various forms of denial have profound effects on the bodymind, avoiding a power struggle with the client is important. If the client says he/she is not in pain, not worried, not tense, or not angry, then insisting that the client appears to be can only disrupt the alliance formed by the therapeutic relationship and impede the progress of therapy. An exception to this might be if the issue involves a behavior that directly affects the work, such as coming to a session high on drugs. In this case, the client's denial makes the massage therapy ineffective and a waste of time and effort. It is important, even in this case, to not become self-righteous with the client. Whatever the client is denying is because he or she believes on an unconscious level that the denial is serving as a coping or survival skill.

Gary

Robert worked as a massage therapist at a fitness center. His client Gary came in each week with alcohol on his breath. Robert would smell the alcohol and become inwardly irritated. Robert took very good care of his body: he did not smoke, drink, or take drugs. Robert had to ask himself if he was being judgmental about Gary because he himself believed that alcohol was bad for the body and mind. Robert admitted to himself that his belief about alcohol might have some influence on his irritation, but even so, Gary's drinking concerned him in ways that could not be attributed solely to his own personal beliefs.

Robert decided to say something to Gary. At the next session, Robert said, "I've been noticing that you've been having a drink before you come in."

Gary tightened up and snuffed, "Well, not every time!"

Robert knew that it was, indeed, every time, but decided not to pursue that point. "Well," he explained, "I was concerned about the effect this might be having on the massage. Some of the physical effects of alcohol during massage are reduced sensitivity, dehydration of the tissues, and an increased load on the liver and kidneys as toxins are flushed out. The presence of alcohol in your bloodstream may prevent you from receiving the full benefit of the massage and may even contribute to your not feeling well after the massage."

"But a massage is to relax, isn't it?" Gary rationalized. "Well, having a few beers after my handball game lets me relax. That's what we want, isn't it? Besides, a little alcohol is good for you. They've done those studies. Good for your heart."

"Yes," Robert said, "alcohol can make you feel relaxed in a certain way, but it doesn't last. It lasts only as long as the alcohol is in your system. This massage is not only about relaxing you. It's about reeducating your body to relax. I think alcohol interferes with that."

"Well, I don't think it does," said Gary. "Are you one of those health nuts who doesn't want people to have any fun?"

Robert smiled. "You can call me that if you want to," he said, "but I do know about massage and how to get the absolute most out of it. I'd really like you to try experimenting to see what happens if you don't drink before a massage. You might experience something different."

"Oh, a little beer can't make that make that much of a difference," Gary argued.

"I'd like you to have the opportunity to find out," said Robert.

"OK, I'll try it . . . once," said Gary.

"No," Robert insisted, "One time is not enough to let you feel it. I'd like you to come in a few times with no alcohol in you to see what happens."

Gary accepted, saying, "Okay, but if I don't notice anything, I'm going to have my beers."

Robert said, "If you don't notice anything, we'll talk about it again."

Projection

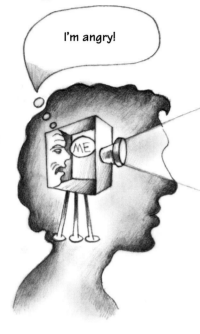

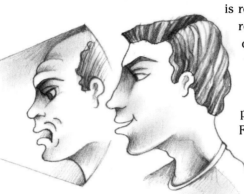

A **projection** is an attribute, impulse, feeling, or perception that actually belongs to an individual's personality, but is not experienced as such by the individual. Instead, it is attributed to objects or persons in the environment, that is, not oneself, and is then experienced as directed toward the individual by those objects or persons (Figure 3.2). For example, a woman who is the projector, unaware that she is rejecting others, believes that they are rejecting her; or, unaware of her tendencies to approach others sexually, the projector feels that they make sexual approaches toward her.

Projection is not necessarily pathological and can take many forms. For example: a plan is an organized fantasy projected into the future, an expectation is a projection of what is "supposed" to happen, an anxiety is a projection of what "might" happen, and a wish is a projection of a wanted event. Indeed, Carl Jung stated that projection is a natural function of all humans. In a sense, it is how we learn. It becomes a problem, however, when we cannot recognize projections as part of our own makeup. Box 3.2 lists some of the more common pathological projections.

The mechanism of projection acts to interrupt mounting excitement of a kind and degree that the person cannot accept. It typically functions in the following way:

1. A person becomes aware of an unacceptable attribute, impulse, feeling, or perception, but is not aware of its source.
2. The person then interrupts the approach to the environment that would be necessary for adequate expression of that attribute, impulse, feeling, or perception.
3. As a result, the person excludes it from being experienced as something that could come from him- or herself.
4. Therefore, the person concludes that it *must* come from an *external* source, that is, from someone else or from society at large.
5. In addition, it seems *forcibly* directed toward the person because, without being aware of it, the person is forcibly interrupting his or her own outwardly directed impulse. In this way, *projection allows a person to disown what is unacceptable or unwanted within or emanating from him- or herself.*

Unacceptable or unwanted feelings are not necessarily negative: we can also project onto others positive feelings or qualities that belong to ourselves. This commonly occurs when we believe that we are not allowed to have those positive feelings or own those positive qualities about ourselves. What is the difference between acknowledging a positive trait or quality in another person and projecting? A positive projection is usually accompanied, at some point, by a discounting of the same positive attributes in oneself. This can appear as a putting down of oneself while admiring the other person, or excessive admiration of the other person. Positive projections can form a component of positive transference, which will be discussed shortly.

Figure 3.2
Projection. *A projection is an attribute, impulse, feeling, or perception that actually belongs to a person's personality, but is not experienced as such. The person who is projecting attributes feelings or thoughts that belong to him- or herself as belonging to another person and then perceives the attributed feelings or thoughts as existing in external reality.*

How Projection Manifests

There are several ways projection can manifest in massage therapy. As we have seen, touch stimulates feelings. When feelings emerge during a massage therapy session, the client may not recognize that the source of the feelings is him- or herself. Instead, the client may believe that the therapist is the source. The client may think or even state openly, "You are making me feel this way," whether the feeling is positive or negative. In reality, the massage therapist cannot make any emotion or feeling occur, but can and does catalyze or stimulate emotion through touch. When the client believes that the massage therapist is "making me feel" something, the client disowns the feeling.

> **Box 3.2**
>
> ### SOME COMMON PROJECTIONS MANIFESTED AS BELIEFS
>
> I believe that you are "making" me feel something.
> I believe that you are feeling something I am actually feeling, but am unaware of.
> I believe that you have personal attributes that are actually attributes of my own.
> I believe that you are feeling something I want you to feel.
> I believe that you are feeling something I fear you will feel.
> (Please note that only the second and third examples strictly fit the *psychoanalytic* definition of projection)

Another way in which clients project during massage is by ascribing a feeling that they have to the therapist. Some examples are: "You must be feeling tired," or "Getting ready for one session right after another must be hard." This kind of projection prevents clients from being aware of—or taking ownership of—their own feelings. In the first example given, the client may be feeling tired. In the second, the client is probably assuming that the therapist feels the way the client would feel in the same situation. It also limits the client's awareness because the client may not experience that different people have different types of feeling responses to every situation.

Simultaneous levels of complexity also can be involved in a projection. Going back to the "You must be feeling tired" statement, the projection could also be blocking awareness of the client's concern that the therapist may be too tired to give full energy and attention to him- or herself.

A third way in which projection can manifest in massage therapy is within expectations about the future, whether catastrophic or wishful. Following is a case example.

Wanda

Wanda came to her first session with Nancy, her massage therapist, feeling very enthusiastic about the prospect of doing massage therapy. Wanda's friend Penny had told Wanda how much she was getting out of massage therapy. The first several sessions went well, and Nancy thought that Wanda was satisfied with their work. On the fourth session, Wanda did not get off the table with her usual, "I feel great!" In the fifth session, it became clear that Wanda was unhappy. Finally, at the start of the sixth session, Nancy decided to ask a clearly subdued Wanda what was wrong. "You don't seem as satisfied with our work," said Nancy. "What are you aware of about what is going on with you?"

Wanda sighed, "Well, I feel better right after the massage, but it doesn't last and my life hasn't changed like Penny's."

"Most people feel better over time," Nancy said.

"Well, I do feel better," said Wanda, "but not a lot better."

"How much better did you think you would feel?" Nancy asked.

Wanda

"A lot better!" Wanda realized that she had spoken quite loudly, "Sorry," she muttered.

Nancy asked, "Well, was there anything else that you thought would happen that hasn't happened?"

"As a matter of fact, " said Wanda, "I thought I would feel a lot better and that my life would begin going okay like Penny's does."

"Ohhh! Now I understand, " said Nancy. "You thought this would make everything better!"

"I guess I did," said Wanda. "But frankly, I didn't even know I was thinking that. I just felt disappointed."

"I think massage *can* help you feel better," said Nancy, "and that feeling can be a platform for making your life better. What I mean is, feeling better in your body can open up new channels in your thinking that can in turn help you to see new ways to act. But massage is only one piece in a whole process. You have to work in many ways to open those channels or get someone else to help you open those channels."

"Oh," said Wanda, "so maybe I've been wanting too much from this."

"This work can give you a lot," said Nancy, "but not what you were thinking it would."

Wanda's form of projection was an unrealistic and unspoken expectation. She thought massage therapy would change her life. This is a wish for a magical solution. Massage therapy *could* change her life for the better, but only as a support for Wanda actively changing her life.

A fourth common form of projection may be termed **parental projection**. *The vulnerability of the client lying unclothed or partially unclothed on the table (or massage chair sometimes) often stimulates projections, particularly parental projections.* The client comes to the massage therapist to be soothed or healed, as we did with our parents when we were children. Another similarity is that although one hopes the massage client will be actively receptive to the therapist's touch and care, the initial experience is a passive one. Being acted upon is also a condition we experience in childhood. For these reasons, *it is not unusual to experience the massage therapist at an unconscious level as a parental figure.*

Parents are powerful figures in a child's life. They not only soothe and heal, they also control, manage, support, judge, disapprove, guide, provide, discipline, reward, nurture, protect, punish, and educate. In childhood, as opposed to adulthood, our parents truly can "make us feel" good or bad. Consciously or unconsciously expecting the massage therapist to perform the parental actions mentioned above is not unusual. Consequently, the client will cast the massage therapist in any or all of these parental roles and, in turn, these become the basis of projections—*positive or negative*—onto the massage therapist.

Clients experiencing a parental projection may feel that the massage therapist is not satisfied with their progress or is disappointed with them in some way. Or, they may feel the massage therapist does not like them or that the therapist does not consider them a good client. In contrast, a client may feel as if he or she is a special client of the massage therapist. In some cases, of course, the client may perceive the massage therapist correctly; however, in most instances, these feelings are actually projections, often having their origins in childhood.

How we were seen and received by our parents and other important adult figures in the past plays a critical role in how we see ourselves and how our self-esteem was formed. Similarly, being touched and observed in massage can bring up issues related to how one feels about oneself. These issues then can become part of what is projected onto the massage therapist. This can account for some surprising statements that clients may make reflecting how they think the massage therapist is seeing them. For example, the massage therapist may make an observation, "You are having difficulty relaxing." The client hears it as a rebuke or an evaluation that he or she is not doing something right or good enough.

No matter what form the projection takes, a common response of the client to feeling or becoming aware of these issues is to become anxious or uncomfortable. In turn, the client may act out the discomfort. As explained in the definition, by **acting out**, we mean discharging a feeling by an action without examining rationally whether the action is appropriate to the situation. Acting out can range from the subtle to the dramatic. The client may become less open and honest with the therapist, be unwilling to relax, forget payments, or skip sessions. Verbal attacks by the client may accuse the therapist or the therapist's work of being inadequate in some way. In more extreme acting out, the client may shout at the therapist, make a threatening gesture at the therapist, or push the therapist away.

Dealing with projection and acting out can be uncomfortable and confusing for both the client and the massage therapist. Neither party may know what is actually causing the distress and subsequent behavior: is something wrong with the work, or has something surfaced because of the effect of the work? What makes projection even more difficult is a failure to recognize it as such. In other words, the client or the therapist may believe that the client's projection *actually is* an accurate perception based in present reality. The next two discussions provide some suggestions for responding to projection and telling the difference between projection and "accurate" perception.

Responding to Projection

It can be challenging for the massage therapist to respond to projection without stepping into the role of psychotherapist. We discuss several strategies for maintaining your professional boundaries in Chapter 4. A way to do this is to *"hand back" the projection* to the client. For example, if the client says, "You're making me feel really jumpy today," the therapist could say, "Are you feeling jumpy today?" If the client says, "You must be feeling really tired after doing so many massages," the therapist can ask the client, "How are you feeling? Are you feeling tired?" If the client seems to be anticipating the future, the therapist can ask, "Is this what you are expecting will happen?" These responses must be made in a casual and nonchallenging manner. Asking in a manner that is too penetrating makes the client feel self-conscious and possibly judged. Handing back a projection is a good strategy because projections are a way a person puts, displaces, gets rid of, or abandons something of him- or herself into the environment and away. By handing it back, the therapist gives the client an opportunity to become more aware of it as belonging to him- or herself. This way of dealing with projection is free of psychological interpretation to the client. For example, saying, "Are you feeling tired?" is much different from saying, "It is you who must be tired," or, "You are projecting that you are tired onto me."

Another way of dealing with projections into the future is to **ground** the client in the present (see the definition). This can be accomplished by talking with the client at length when beginning massage therapy to find out what the client's fears and

Acting Out

Acting out occurs when a feeling is expressed or extended into action without first being examined as to whether it is appropriate to the situation. It is a way of discharging a feeling without being aware of it. Acting out can accompany many of the defenses included in this chapter, such as projection, deflection, and denial, and can be verbal or physical. The most common verbal forms are snapping, criticizing, and accusing.

Grounding

Grounding means that the client is in the "here-and-now," in reality, and in his or her body. Grounding is experienced particularly in the legs and feet as a sense of "having one's feet on the ground." It is also experienced in the eyes, hands, and arms, which are parts of the body used to contact reality.

fantasies are about the process. This will not prevent all projections, but it will give an initial foundation to the process. The massage therapist can then use this as a reference point when a client begins to project. For example, if the massage therapist has grounded the client about how long it may take to work out a chronic pain, the therapist can refer back to the delivery of this information if the client gets upset that his or her pain has not disappeared in only a few sessions.

Distinguishing Projection From Perception

It is possible that neither the client nor the massage therapist may ever become aware of all the projections that are occurring during the course of massage therapy. Projections might emerge in extremely subtle comments such as, "Do you have many clients as messed up as I am," or "You must get frustrated when you keep finding that knot in my neck," or even, "I can tell you are not feeling well today." Whether projections are subtle or obvious, distinguishing them from client insights based in reality is often difficult for therapists. The therapist may be thrown off guard and wonder, for example, "Is it true that I'm not feeling well?"

Massage therapists can be particularly vulnerable to confusion triggered by projection. Many massage therapists have a high degree of empathy, which usually is a very good quality in a therapist. However, because empathy involves being open and receptive to the feelings of others, sometimes the therapist "feels what the other person is feeling," sometimes even when the *client* does not know he or she is feeling it. For a variety of reasons, the therapist may have difficulty recognizing who is the source. Finding the source of projected attributes, impulses, feelings, and perceptions can be tricky, causing the therapist to continually need to assess, asking him- or herself, "With whom does this originate—with me, or with my client?"

One essential factor in being able to distinguish projections from true perceptions is to clarify what we ourselves are feeling. This means that we must be clear and honest with ourselves about our beliefs, feelings, and agendas. A therapist who does not understand him- or herself is far more likely to take on the projection of a client. The therapist might accept the projection as real because understanding of his or her own emotional organization is not firm enough. This is problematic for both therapist and client. The therapist's understanding of the client becomes confused and distorted, and the therapist's self-perception or perception of his or her work can be inaccurately altered. The client loses an opportunity to become aware that the feelings, originating within him- or herself, are being blocked by the projection. For example, if a projecting client says, "You are angry with me," and the therapist, who is not actually angry, accepts the projection as valid or does not question it, the client likely will not have the opportunity to discover his or her own anger.

Thus, *the most important tool for distinguishing between projection and true perception is self-knowledge.* This is no easy task: it requires that you pause daily and sometimes even hourly to evaluate honestly your feelings about your work, your clients, and yourself. As difficult as it is, self-knowledge is the best way to avoid taking on a projection.

Self-knowledge is also the best way to avoid placing the projecting client into a therapeutic bind. The therapist may place a client in a bind by taking anything the client says or feels and labeling it projection. For example, a client may comment that the therapist is treating him or her in an authoritarian manner, but the therapist may refuse to consider the validity of the observation and instead see the client as projecting a hidden desire for control upon him or her. The therapist who had done personal work would likely know whether he or she behaved in that way characteristically. The therapist would then be able to affirm the client's perception, if true, or help the client expand in a limited way on how he or she might feel about being in control, if the therapist knows that this is a projection. Without a foundation of self-knowledge, distinguishing projections from true perceptions can be very difficult and can strain the therapeutic relationship. Therefore, it is important that therapists engage in activities that build self-knowledge.

Roxy

June's client, Roxy, groaned as she climbed onto the table. "I know you're tired of hearing this," Roxy said, "but that point on my sacrum is acting up again."

June internally began to consider the validity of Roxy's perception that she was tired of hearing about Roxy's sacrum problem. She asked herself if she *was* actually tired of hearing about it. Did she secretly believe that Roxy was causing her own pain? The answer came up, "No!" She quickly reviewed her recent interactions with Roxy. Had she said something to Roxy that might indicate that she was tired of working with Roxy or tired of giving massage at all? Had she sighed when Roxy talked about the pain or given some other nonverbal signal that Roxy had taken for impatience with her problem? June's internal checklist again came up with a "No!" This led June to think that Roxy's comment might have something to do with how Roxy might feel about her own pain in her sacrum, how Roxy's partner might feel about her complaints, or how Roxy's parents might feel about her ongoing problems.

June said to Roxy, "That's interesting. What's going on that you would think I was tired of the pain in your sacrum?"

"I feel I'm being a pain in the butt," said Roxy.

"Now that's really interesting!" said June with a smile on her face. At that moment, Roxy heard what she had said, and they both laughed.

"Sounds as though being a 'pain in the butt' might have some significance for you," June said. "Now, I know that the pain in your sacrum is taking a lot of time to heal. I understand that and I am fine with it. The question is how *you* might feel about it."

"Wow," said Roxy, struck by the accuracy of the analogy, "I'll have to think about that."

June said, "Okay, just put it in your internal tape recorder, and play it back when you want. I thought I could start with your neck today, and then work on your lower back, okay?"

Introjection

Introjection is the act of attributing to oneself a trait, attitude, feeling, or behavior that actually belongs to one's environment, usually an influential person, such as a parent or teacher (Figure 3.3). As such, it can be seen as the reverse of projection. A key characteristic of introjection is that it is usually activated through the will of another person and causes the introjecting person to adopt *unquestioningly* the trait, attitude, feeling, or behavior *as if it originates from within*. For example, a child might adopt an attitude from parents—such as that science is more important than art—well before the child would be able to come to such a conclusion on his or her own.

Introjection can have a healthy purpose. For example, as a process for learning, babies take everything in *en bloc* until much later in life. Introjections can be benign

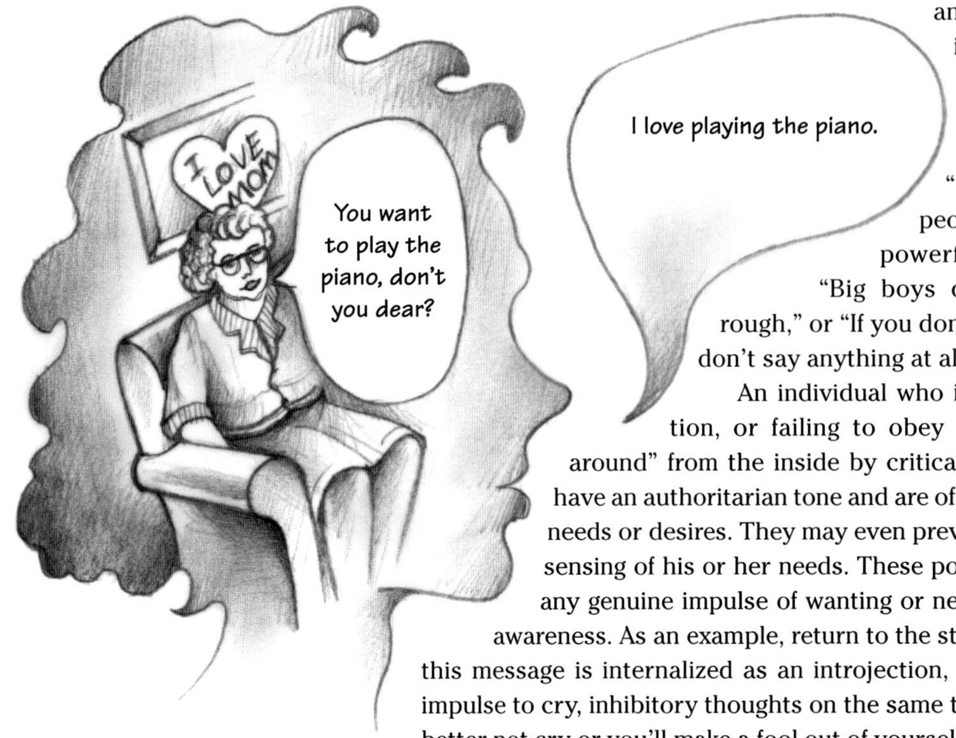

Figure 3.3
Introjection. In introjection, a person takes something in "lock, stock, and barrel." He or she mistakes the will or desires of another person for his/her own.

and even protective, as when a child internalizes a message from parents such as, "Don't go anywhere with strangers." However, introjections are often not benign, such as, "Don't talk to black/white/yellow people." Introjections can also contain powerful emotional messages, such as, "Big boys don't cry," "Girls shouldn't play rough," or "If you don't have something nice to say, then don't say anything at all."

An individual who is experiencing a negative introjection, or failing to obey one, often literally feels "pushed around" from the inside by critical thoughts. These critical thoughts have an authoritarian tone and are often contradictory to the individual's needs or desires. They may even prevent the individual from any internal sensing of his or her needs. These powerful thoughts may steal or crush any genuine impulse of wanting or needing totally out of the individual's awareness. As an example, return to the statement, "Big boys don't cry." Once this message is internalized as an introjection, whenever the boy or man has the impulse to cry, inhibitory thoughts on the same theme arise: "You big baby!" or "You better not cry or you'll make a fool out of yourself!" or, "Be a man! Stop whining!"

Introjection first occurs in childhood. Children have no choice but to give over their autonomy to their parents. In a healthy situation, parents use their authority to set realistic limits for the child and occasionally to win a conflict for the good of the child. Nevertheless, most parents recognize and respect the fact that the child has an independent will. In an unhealthy situation, parents do not acknowledge any legitimate authority in their child. They view the child's expressions of preferences as episodes of willfulness that need to be stamped out.

How Introjection Manifests

Digestion provides body-oriented metaphors for introjection. In *Gestalt Therapy*, Fritz Perls said, "To compare the acquisition of habits, attitudes, beliefs, or ideals to the process of taking physical food into the organism strikes one at first as merely a crude analogy, but the more one examines the detailed sequence of each, the more one realizes their functional identity. Physical food, properly digested and assimilated, becomes part of the organism, but food which 'rests heavy on the stomach' is an introject (p. 189)." An introjection is not "digested" and assimilated, nor is it "thrown up," rejected, and eliminated. Instead, it is "swallowed whole," uncritically accepted as one's own—"keeping it down" instead of "getting it out of your system."

On the bodily level, tension resulting from introjections may settle in the throat, stomach, or gut. In terms of body language, this is related to distress over difficulty swallowing, stomaching, or digesting something noxious. In this sense, introjections can be toxic. Sometimes work on these areas causes release of intensely uncomfortable feelings, such as nausea, gagging, or disgust. Disgust is an instinct that stimulates the elimination of or repulsion from what is harmful to us. It allows us to discriminate the good from the bad in our environment. Although disgust is often an unwanted or unpleasant kind of response, it serves a positive purpose if it properly guides us to reject or eliminate what is harmful or toxic to us. Consequently, these kinds of reactions—nausea, gagging, disgust, and so on—may be not only physical reactions, but forms of emotional release.

Introjections may also manifest as body postures or gestures that duplicate or nearly duplicate someone else's. For example, a parent may have a "stiff upper-lipped poker face" and the client may unconsciously emulate that expression under certain circumstances. A part of a person that such an introjection affects may be resistant to change until the client makes a psychological connection between that part of the body and the person from whom he or she has taken the introjection.

Introjection also frequently dampens our sense of taste, which in turn diminishes our ability to discriminate. If we perceive something as tasting bad or harmful, we spit it out. The term "in bad taste" is a metaphor for something that merits rejection or elimination. Someone with bad taste is someone who seems to have failed to realize the noxiousness of something they are doing, saying, or wearing. If working with a client on the areas of the body used for or related to taste discrimination—such as the jaw, mouth, tongue, throat, or abdominal area—brings up such discomfort, the client may be experiencing a psychological reaction to introjection.

Responding to Introjection

An appropriate way for a massage therapist to work with introjection is to help the client to allow or tolerate the conflict felt in the body. When someone feels the discomfort caused by an introjection, it is a sign that it is starting to bubble up to awareness. In this way, for example, nausea or feelings of disgust are not a bad thing, although feeling such may not be pleasant. The conflict is a way for the person to begin to deal with the introjection; that is, it provides an impetus to deal with it. This is most evident when the introjection involves something that contradicts what a person really needs or feels. Then the "true feeling" must inevitably run into or clash with the introjection, with the result being some type of feeling of upset. If the upset grows strong enough, then the introjection can be "thrown up" and rejected. Rather than hurry to make such feelings go away, the massage therapist can instead work with the client to accept these feelings by such ways as maintaining breathing, offering support for feeling the difficult feelings, accepting the client's reaction, and being present. The following case study is an example of dealing with introjection in a massage session.

Yvette

Yvette came to massage therapy because she was experiencing moderate to severe pain in her jaw and throat area. She had been raised in a family in which the children were expected to be extremely obedient and not express negative feelings. If Yvette said anything in opposition to her mother's wishes, her mother would say, "Young ladies do not speak like that to their mother. You need to show respect and keep your mouth shut."

After several months of massage therapy, she had gotten to feel fairly comfortable with her massage therapist and developed a sense of trust in his skills and abilities. The tension around Yvette's jaw and throat had started to soften at a faster pace. After a particularly good session, Yvette reported she had started experiencing more tightness in her throat and feelings of nausea. The pattern continued for the next two sessions.

In the next session, Yvette's massage therapist suggested that she allow the feelings of nausea to surface while he worked on her jaw, rather than trying to push the nausea back down. After a few minutes, Yvette started to murmur a few times in a low voice, "You make me sick."

Yvette

Then her jaw started to lock up and she apologized for making so much noise. Her massage therapist did some more work to soften the holding and told her, "No need to apologize. I don't mind you speaking up and saying what you are feeling."

Within a few moments, Yvette began to say, "Shut up! I can say what I want!," increasing the volume with each utterance. After a few minutes of this, a big smile broke out on Yvette's face. "I'm not so nice, am I," said Yvette, with a laugh, "What a relief . . . and guess what, my nausea is gone." She also shared what her childhood experiences of her mother's strict rules had been like (which were briefly summarized at the beginning of this case study).

Over the next several sessions, whenever Yvette's jaw muscles would soften and she felt nausea, she would allow herself to say whatever came up. As she and her massage therapist repeated this process, the nausea and tension began to lessen until it was no longer present. Yvette learned that whenever the nausea and tension happened again, it was a cue from her body reminding her that there was something she needed to express.

Displacement

Displacement is the substitution of one person or object for another as the target of feeling, that is, the process of switching feeling from one person or object to another. This is the classic "kick the dog" defense (Figure 3.4). For example, if a person has a frustrating day at work, she may come home and get angry with her spouse. The frustration with work is displaced onto the spouse. Another common example is when someone has feelings about one person, but rather than approach that person, unconsciously chooses another who is perceived as safer or more socially appropriate. A target for displacement may be safer because she is perceived as sympathetic and accepting, and thereby nonthreatening, or weaker or will not resist as much as another person would, or is stronger and can take it.

A massage therapist's tendency to be nonjudgmental makes him or her a good displacement target for the client. For example, a client who has had a bad day may direct negativity toward the therapist or the process. In such situations, the massage therapist should encourage the client to discover whom or what the feelings are really about. However, this needs to be done properly and nonjudgmentally. Simply suggesting to the client that his or her feelings are invalid or misdirected tends to either aggravate the situation or shut the client down. Instead, allow the client enough space to release the emotion in a safe way, listen carefully to what is being said, and see if it is possible to identify what the client is actually having feelings about. For example, if the client is angry and gives some clues that the anger has something to do with an incident at work, you could say, "It sounds as if being criticized at work was difficult for you." If the client is angry, but gives no clues about what it is connected to, then you can say, "What happened today or recently that may have left you feeling upset or angry?" The main idea here is to encourage the client to express him- or herself enough to let the incident surface, connect, and pass.

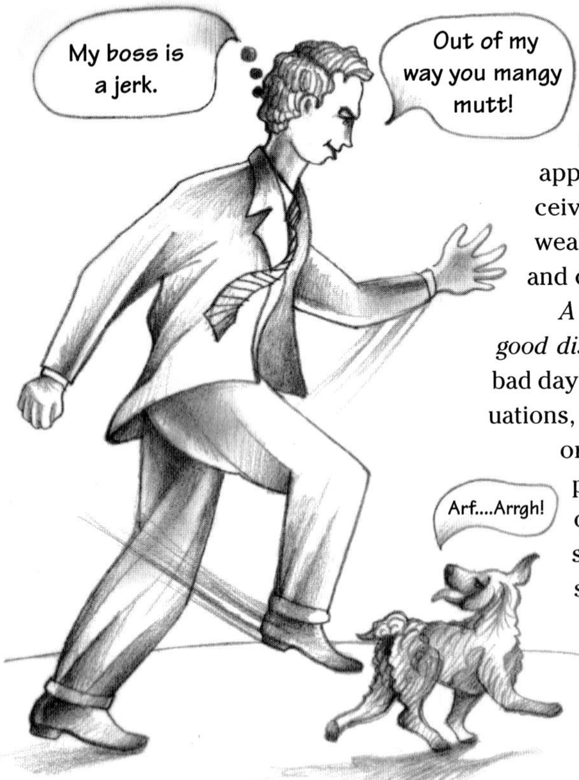

Figure 3.4
Displacement. *Displacement involves "dumping" feelings onto somebody or something else.*

If you are the target of a displacement, it is very important not to become defensive, because doing so tends to increase the client's effort to get you to accept or admit to it. Think how you would feel or react if someone, in response to your feelings, told you it had nothing to do with him or her. It is also important for you not to dig for more psychological material, but simply focus the displaced feelings back onto whom or where they belong. Doing more than this goes beyond the scope of massage practice.

Deflection

Deflection occurs when a person unconsciously diverts the attention or action of another person away from a psychological or physical area that feels threatening (Figure 3.5). A key quality of deflection is that it is meant to occur without the other person noticing. It is often done so pleasantly or innocuously that the other person may not even notice that his or her attention has been diverted. A simple way in which deflection may manifest in a massage session is that each time the therapist begins to approach a psychologically "loaded" area, such as the belly, the client may complain of a headache or tension in the foot, gently deflecting the therapist's intent. Verbally, the client may deflect feedback. The simplest deflection is to change the subject. For example, if the therapist observes, "You are not breathing much," the client then responds, "Can I turn my head?"

A form of deflection that appears particularly in body-oriented work such as massage therapy is shifting body awareness. In this case, the client reports sensations surfacing in various areas of the body, movement of energy, or profound shifts in tension. For example, the massage therapist may be working on the chest, and the client may say, "Wow, I just felt something really open up in my right calf," or "I'm feeling rushes of energy around my face." The therapist, eager to pursue this opening, stops working on the chest and moves to the new area. The therapist's challenge is to figure out if the lead is true or false. When it is a false lead, then it may be a deflection.

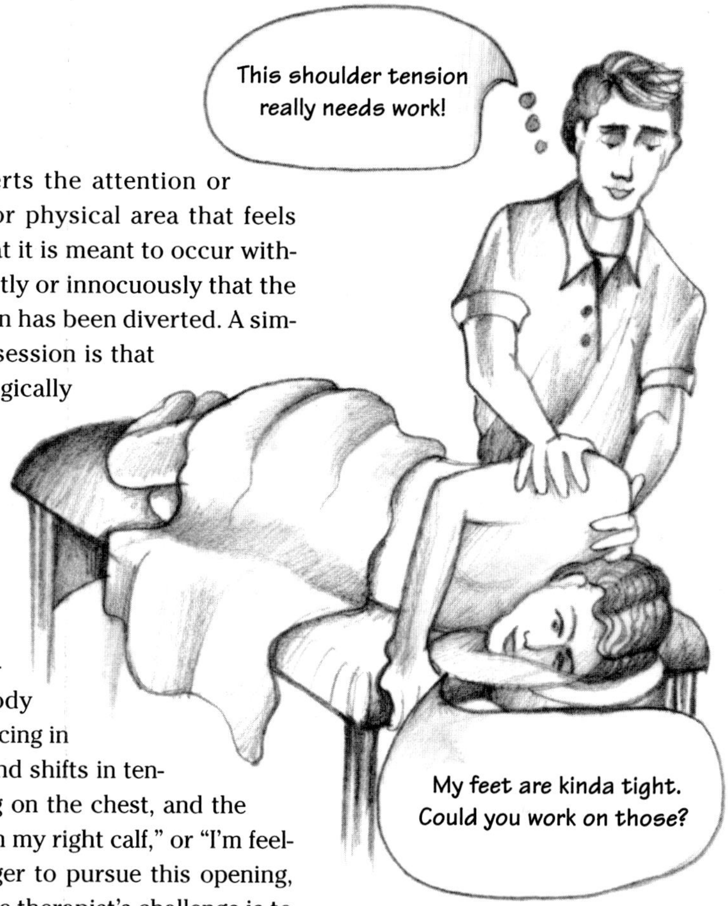

Instead of overlooking and excusing these deflections as accidents, as the client not hearing, or as some perceptual mistake by the therapist or the client, the therapist can use these deflections as clues to what might threaten the client. The therapist does not necessarily have to tell the client about this, but can note and gently approach those areas of which the client is unconsciously fearful or blocked. The simplest and least confrontational way to do this is to return the client's awareness to what was deflected. For example, after the client says, "Can I turn my head?" the therapist can say, "Yes, if you want to, then go back to observing your breathing and see what you are aware of about that."

A massage therapist does not need to analyze or interpret the meaning of the deflection to the client, which is something a psychotherapist might do. For example, let us go back to the instance of a client bringing up how his or her foot feels soon after abdominal work begins. Avoid saying, "You were deflecting by talking about your foot, which means there must be something about having your abdomen worked on that disturbs you." Instead, acknowledge what the client said about the foot and then say, "See if you can bring your attention back to your abdomen."

Deflection may leave you feeling ignored, manipulated, or confused. It helps to bear in mind that clients are deflecting primarily from *themselves*; that is, they are

Figure 3.5
Deflection. *Deflection is a diversion. As the therapist hones in on the source of tension, the client unconsciously attempts to shift the therapist's attention elsewhere.*

attempting to reduce their *own* awareness. Deflecting the therapist's awareness is only one of many actions that clients take to maintain their own self-deflecting behavior. It is not an intentional attempt to deceive the therapist.

Retroflection

Retroflection is the unconscious act of turning something sharply back against oneself rather than against someone or something in the environment (Figure 3.6). For example, if a person feels angry with others for not being responsible, retroflection may prevent him or her from feeling any anger at other people. Instead, the person may castigate *him- or herself* for not being responsible enough. Essentially, retroflection serves as a defense against feelings or actions that one cannot direct toward the outside world. The motto of retroflection would be, "Do unto oneself rather than doing unto others." Therefore, retroflection, like all defenses, serves the purpose of reducing or avoiding risk. The retroflecting person cannot risk interacting with the environment in an aggressive way. When aggression is unexpressed or unresolved, sooner or later it turns back against the person feeling it.

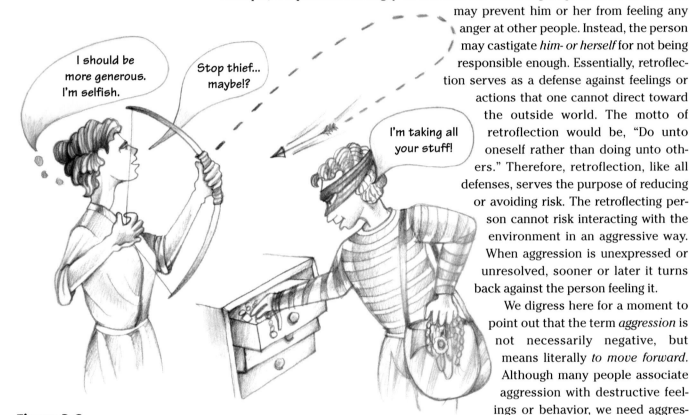

Figure 3.6
Retroflection. *In retroflection, a person turns his responses against himself.*

We digress here for a moment to point out that the term *aggression* is not necessarily negative, but means literally *to move forward.* Although many people associate aggression with destructive feelings or behavior, we need aggression to feed ourselves, construct or seek shelter, find suitable companionship, or find and get whatever it is we need to survive and flourish. In this sense, unless a person is entirely self-sufficient, aggression is necessary. Therefore, psychologically a person's level of aggression has something to do with the degree to which the person moves out into the environment to meet his or her needs.

When a person retroflects behavior, she does to herself what originally she wanted to do to or with other persons or objects. She stops directing energy outward in attempts to positively manipulate the environment in ways that will satisfy her needs; instead, she redirects her activity inward and substitutes herself as the target of her behavior. In a sense, a person who uses retroflection is attempting to supply all of her own needs, rather than find them in the environment. This usually leaves the person feeling frustrated and stuck. To the extent that a person retroflects, she internally splits her personality into "do-er" and "done to."

Because retroflection disowns aggression, when the massage therapist begins to intervene with a part of the body that expresses or holds aggression, such as the jaw or shoulders, he or she may encounter resistance. Usually, the resistance manifests as the person "just not getting it"—the involved tension pattern keeps reasserting itself.

Someone who retroflects often needs permission and support to feel what is for him or her quite forbidden. For example, retroflection may be involved during a massage session when the client exhibits or reports self-critical behavior during or after work done on a target area such as the jaw or shoulders and when the tension in those areas resists release. A sign that the retroflection is beginning to weaken is if the client exhibits or expresses any aggression in response to being touched in that area. The therapist should appropriately support such expressions. The therapist can model for the client a sense of acceptance of such feelings, replacing the harsh, internal critical thoughts that block those feelings. Again, the massage therapist can do this without acting as a psychotherapist by offering analysis or interpretations. For example, if a retroflecting client curses and then apologizes, the massage therapist can simply say, "That's okay. I'm not offended. Sometimes it can feel good to say that."

Reversal and Reaction Formation

Reversal is defending against a feeling or thought that is too threatening to be felt or expressed by transforming it to its *opposite* feeling or thought. Through this mechanism, hate may change to love, assertion to passivity, longing for an object to rejection of that object. For example, reversal is at work when a schoolboy who is infatuated with a girl goes to great lengths to show her and everyone else how much he dislikes her or has no interest in her (Figure 3.7).

In massage therapy, you may hear clients talk about situations that involve reversal; however, to respect scope of practice boundaries, you should not pursue these discussions through analyzing or interpreting them. When reversal involves the massage work itself, it usually manifests as the client reporting the opposite of what he or she is actually feeling. A classic example of reversal is when the client says the massage work is not affecting him or her and so is not coming back (which the client may or may not tell the therapist), but what the client is really feeling is that the work is getting to him/her too much. In this instance, the client may not be able to tolerate getting a certain need fulfilled, or the work is touching something with which the client cannot deal. This can be a very frustrating situation for the massage therapist, because often he or she can do very little, since the issue is not out in the open.

Closely related to reversal is a defense called **reaction formation**. In reaction formation, people take on characteristics that are the opposite of what they actually feel. For example, a person may take on the attributes of a prudish person as a reac-

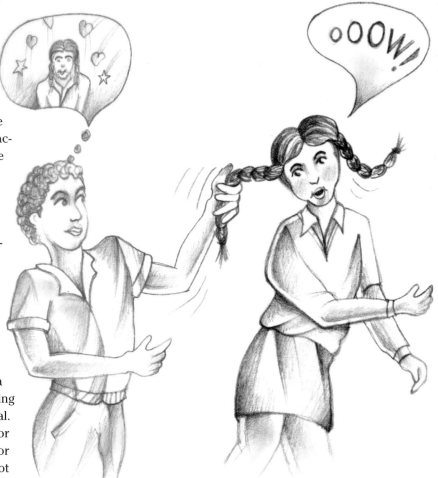

Figure 3.7
Reversal. *In reversal, a person expresses a feeling that is the opposite of one that cannot be expressed.*

tion formation in defense against his or her sexuality. Please note that the psycho-analytic literature uses reaction formation instead of reversal.

Identification

Identification is the process by which a person either blurs or eliminates the distinction between self and others, thereby extending his or her identity, borrowing identity from another person, or fusing identity with another person (Figure 3.8). Put simply, in identification, a person copies traits of another person or even a fictional character.

In a healthy sense, identification is a way in which we practice new ideas or behaviors. In this healthy way, identification involves a person learning from another trusted or admired person who serves as a model. We do this naturally with our parents and heroes when we are children. For example, children around the world admire Michael Jordan and want to "be like Mike," so when they play basketball they protrude their tongue while driving toward the basket just like their hero. Over time, we may keep some of these models or drop them; in this way, identification allows us to "try out" different ways of being.

As a defense, identification may involve some loss of a person's sense of self, which is exchanged for protection through adopting the traits of more powerful people. In this way, identification is a form of hiding or compensation for a sense of inadequacy or a weak sense of self. For example, a young man who has never formed a secure sense of himself may adopt his father's career, mode of dress, mannerisms, and political views to protect himself from his own sense of emptiness or asserting his own style.

In massage, identification may manifest as a client becoming interested in being a massage therapist, dressing like the therapist, copying the therapist's lifestyle, adopting the massage therapist's mannerisms in speech or other areas, taking on the therapist's attitudes or beliefs, or—if the client knows other clients in the therapist's practice—even taking on characteristics of other clients. This can suggest to the therapist that the client *may* have weak psychological boundaries and, subsequently, weak body boundaries. While psychotherapy may be needed to strengthen the client's psychological boundaries, massage therapy can be used to strengthen the client's body boundaries. For example, the skin is a body boundary that has psychological significance. For some people, the stimulation that massage gives to the skin can help the client feel separateness from his or her environment. The musculature also provides a boundary. Enlivening a person's sense of the musculature can give a client a sense of solidity and ability to defend boundaries in a positive manner.

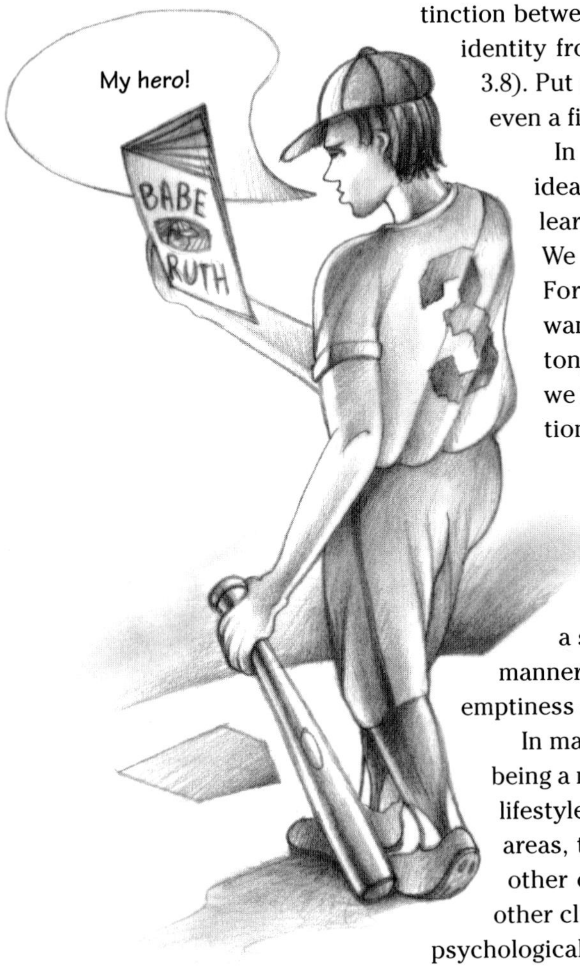

Figure 3.8
Identification. *Identification causes a person to take on the traits or characteristics of an admired person, perhaps even appearance.*

Resistance

Resistance is a failure of or refusal by the client to cooperate with the therapeutic process. When resistance manifests as a psychological defense, it is usually unconscious (Figure 3.9).

The basic purpose of resistance as a defense is survival. The object of the resistance is perceived as threatening harm in some way, although the object may also be desired or objectively helpful. Thus, the paradox of resistance is that the unconsciously perceived threat from what is desired is greater than the consciously perceived benefit.

In adults, resistance is usually a contemporary response to a situation from the past. Very often, the resistance is opposite in form to how a person behaved in past situations in which she felt threatened. Thus, a woman who felt overwhelmed as a child by domineering parents may resist similar experiences that cause her to feel overwhelmed now. She may describe herself as feeling taken over, controlled, invaded, swallowed up, oppressed, pressured, or annihilated. Other clients may resist feeling abandoned, seduced, humiliated, shamed, or otherwise hurt. Resistance can be directed outward toward another person or situation, or inward toward a feeling or thought.

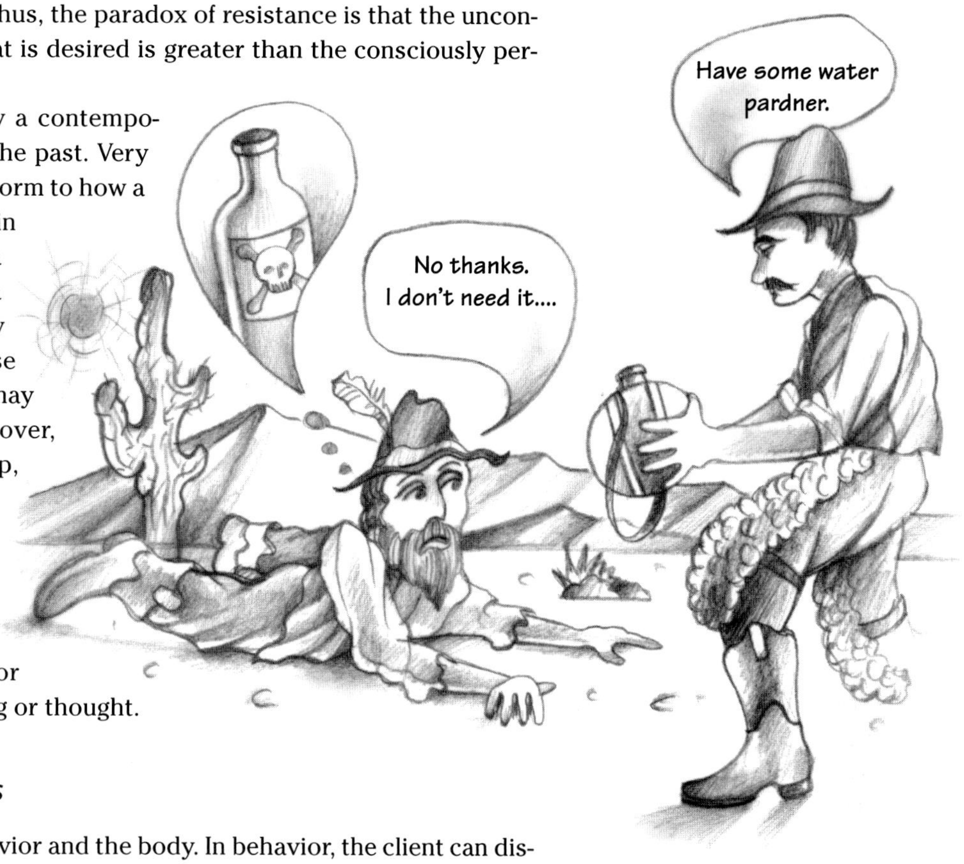

How Resistance Manifests

Resistance can appear in both behavior and the body. In behavior, the client can display resistance by not showing up to sessions, being late, canceling frequently, delaying ending the session, not doing recommended exercises, or forgetting to pay. During the massage, the client may not give verbal feedback about how he or she is feeling, restrict breathing, fall asleep, talk incessantly, cut off or numb bodily feelings, or stiffen or brace a part of the body.

In massage therapy, resistance tends to appear in the body as the recurrence of tension patterns cleared in the previous session, just at a time when certain psychologically critical junctures are reached during the work. The person may *unconsciously equate maintaining tension patterns with psychological survival* and therefore *need to maintain the tension*. Although the client may be coming for massage therapy to change a pattern or feel better, the resistance undermines the work of the therapist, frustrating both when the work does not seem to be succeeding. The following case study illustrates the manifestation of resistance in massage therapy.

Figure 3.9
Resistance. *The object of the resistance is perceived as threatening harm in some way, although the object may also be desired or objectively helpful. The perceived threat is greater than the perceived benefit.*

Scott

Scott sought out massage therapy because he experienced a lot of tension around his shoulders and neck. He decided to do something about it after his friends remarked about how "uptight" he appeared and one of his golf buddies suggested his swing looked stiff and awkward. Indeed, Scott's tension patterns caused him to move very stiffly and deliberately. When his massage therapist worked more deeply into certain spots on his left trapezius and rhomboid, Scott would tense his shoulder and his arm would stiffen. Even though his massage therapist pointed out the holding pattern, Scott continued to stiffen and resist the work. His massage therapist switched to a nonverbal communication by

Scott

tapping Scott on the arm lightly whenever his arm stiffened. Scott would respond to the signal by relaxing his arm somewhat, but would stiffen again moments later. After a while, Scott gradually was able to sustain the relaxation increasingly longer.

After the fifth massage session, Scott suddenly exulted, "I get it! On a deeper level I feel you are going to harm me in some way—even though intellectually I know you're not—and it's like I'm flinching whenever you touch me there. I'm using my shoulder and arm like a shield and I'm cowering under it. I wonder why I'm doing that."

His therapist said, "Feel free to share with me what it is, if you connect with what it's about, or that could be a good question to take up with your psychotherapist. I recall you mentioned in our initial interview that you are working with one. In the meantime, see if you can let go of the fear and anticipation by breathing into the spots I'm working on when I touch them and focusing your awareness on your body."

Resistance is commonly accompanied by acting out, often in ways that are difficult to read. The actions themselves serve to keep the feelings unconscious and unfelt. For example, a man who is desperately afraid of losing his girlfriend, but is unaware of these feelings, may become extremely angry with her when something she does irritates him. Rather than becoming aware of his fear of loss, which would be a highly charged emotional situation, he discharges his fear through his anger and does not question its source. Acting out may take place in a massage situation when the work starts to unblock feelings that were previously blocked. The predicament with acting out is that rather than really satisfying a need or leading to resolution, the problem is pushed back down by the acting out. For example, work on the chest may release feelings about deprivation or loss and sometime afterward the client spends a large amount of money shopping or eats large quantities of a favorite snack. The shopping or eating satisfies the deprivation only superficially. Making the problem less irritating or painful in the moment allows it to be pushed back down.

One problem with the classic definition of resistance is that it is often used as a therapist-centered term, in which it is assumed the therapeutic procedure is always good for the client, or the therapist is always correct. *Sometimes a client may have a good reason to resist.* As Carl Jung wrote, "The cure may be a poison" (1965, p. 141). The techniques being used may not be what the client needs or may reinforce the tension pattern. For example, some people have negative responses to light touch and friction. These strokes actually make them more tense. They might have trouble telling you this, but their body will. Therefore, it is very important that the therapist distinguish whether there is a legitimate reason for the client to resist, because some circumstances may actually be harmful to the client. We prefer to think of resistance as *negative or positive resistance.* Negative resistance takes place when the resistance undermines the client's progress, whereas positive resistance protects the client from harm.

Responding to Resistance

A key to understanding resistance, and the nature of psychological defenses in general, is *that it is not necessarily based on rational perceptions.* In massage therapy, resistance typically forms against the therapy itself for the very same reason a person seeks it out in the first place, which is that it brings about *change*. When a client is responding from the part of him- or herself that is survival oriented (we *all* have a part of us that is survival oriented), anything that may change the status quo could be perceived as a threat. The following is a simplified resistance scenario that illustrates the paradoxical nature of resistance.

Lyle

Lyle came for massage therapy because of chronic back and neck pain. Lyle is a workaholic whose pain is forcing him to work less. Lyle had been able to ignore his pain while it gradually got worse through using his well-developed will power. Lyle viewed having to seek massage therapy as an act of weakness on his part, feeling that he should have been able to tough it out. As the massage therapy loosened his neck and back tension, Lyle also began to experience feelings of relief, accompanied by feelings of exhaustion. Lyle was no longer able to stay up as late as he did and slept later, missing his usual 5:00 A.M. start of his daily routine. Although the pain was being relieved, Lyle became upset with his inability to treat his body like a machine as he once did. This loss of control was threatening for Lyle, and he stopped coming for massage therapy, figuring he had made enough improvement to get back to work. In Lyle's case, while the massage therapy was loosening his back and neck muscles, on the level of the bodymind those very same muscles were part of Lyle's ability to control his feelings and needs. Psychologically, Lyle had been taught that spontaneous expression of feelings and needs were not acceptable and could get a person into trouble (an introjection!). As a result, the therapeutic goal of relieving his back and neck tension conflicted with his unconscious need to maintain control, so the therapy was a threat to be resisted.

Besides being aware of resistance, you can make some suggestions *and* stay within the boundaries of scope of practice by prompting the client to deal with his or her resistance. For example, you can make nonpsychotherapeutic statements like, "You may feel that you want to relieve this tension, but another part of you may feel the tension is needed and is protecting you in some way. Has the tension served any positive purpose for you?" It is possible that a suggestion like this may uncover a deep-seated problem of the client's and may bring up the need to refer the client to a mental health professional so she can work through the problem. For example, a client may have tension around the diaphragm that the massage work is not resolving, and it becomes clear that the client feels she needs the tension to keep from crying and expressing neediness. As long as these issues remain unresolved, the client's diaphragm will resist change and remain tight despite what the massage therapist does. Such issues would best be worked through in psychotherapy, so a referral is called for.

People who are on the receiving end of resistant behavior often see it as stubbornness, willfulness, or even spite. There may even be a defiant edge to the resistance. This perception often stirs up power struggles between the resisting client and the therapist. When confronted by resistance, remaining centered and not being engaged or manipulated by it are important. Avoid allowing the behavior to damage your self-confidence or to make you feel hurt or angry. Such a reaction on the therapist's part could be called countertransference, which is discussed later in this chapter. Understanding the dynamics of resistance gives you some perspective on the client's behavior, which can decrease the countertransference reaction.

Transference

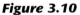

Transference is the displacement or transfer of feelings, thoughts, and behaviors originally related to a significant person, such as a parent, onto someone else, such as the massage therapist (Figure 3.10). It is a common reaction of clients to their therapists. A bit of transference happens in most relationships in which there is feeling present. Usually, transference-related feelings were formed in the past, so it could also be said these feelings transfer from the past to the present. In transference then, the client relates to the therapist and the present moment as if the therapist *were* the significant person. In this sense, transference is a projection of the internal drama of the client, and the therapist is assigned a particularly important role and script. Clients may verbalize transference feelings quite openly, with such remarks as, "When you smile, you look just like my father." Or, they may be unspoken and very diffuse, such as the client "looking up to" the therapist.

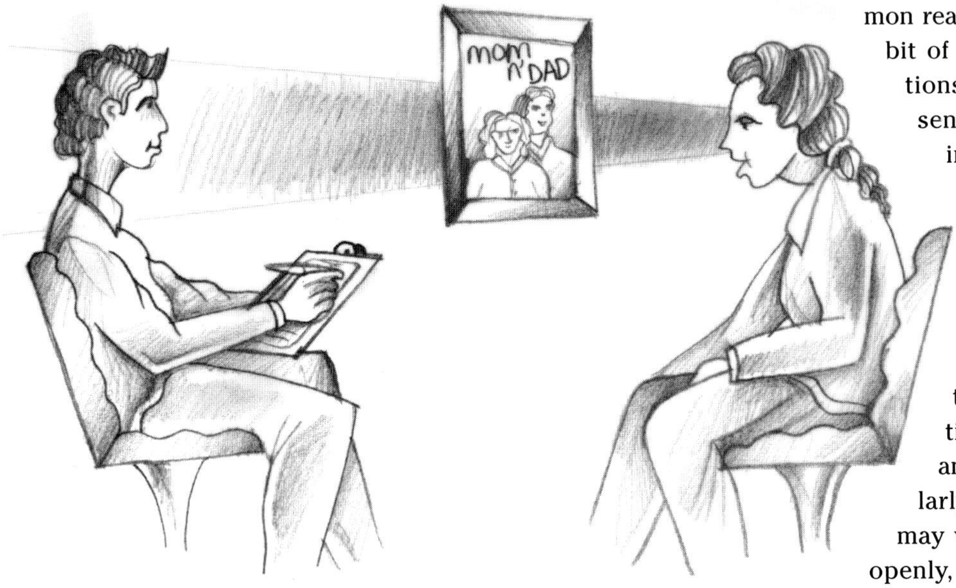

Figure 3.10
Transference. In transference, the client transfers feelings, thoughts, and perceptions about someone from his or her personal history onto the therapist.

Transference can be attributed to the nature of the role the therapist plays. The therapist on a certain level *is* knowledgeable, powerful, helpful, and accepting. The client *is* coming to the therapist for some form of help and care. These attributes are similar to that of the parent-child relationship or other relationships that involve interaction with an authority or caregiver, such as a teacher, physician, or religious advisor. Although transference is often a central component in psychotherapy, it has the potential to appear in nonpsychotherapeutic encounters that have similar attributes. Massage therapy is included because it *does have* many of these attributes. In addition, by removing some or all of one's clothing and lying on a table for a massage, the client has placed him- or herself in a vulnerable position. *Vulnerability by itself can be enough to stimulate transference.*

Transference "happens by itself," which is to say that *it does not require any effort by the therapist to stimulate it.* The therapist also cannot prevent or stop transference from happening. However, after transference has occurred, the therapist must learn how to handle it and manage it. Often unknowingly, and especially if the massage therapist is unaware of transference issues, a female therapist can encourage an unhealthy expansion of the transference by her response to the client. For example, the client may begin complimenting the work of the therapist. The therapist may become visibly pleased, and because a male client is in a transference in which he would like to please his mother, the client gives even more compliments, to which the therapist continues to respond with great pleasure. The client begins to feel special and even begins to believe he is indispensable to the self-esteem of the massage therapist. The client then is surprised and somewhat disappointed to not receive special favors in return, such as not being charged when he misses an appointment or not being given extra time if another client is not in the waiting room. After all, is he not Mommy's favorite? Without the skills to handle this, in this example, the massage therapist may foster a relationship that is too dependent and may create overly high expectations for the client.

Positive Versus Negative Transference

One way of seeing transference is that it is a kind of spell generated by one's own psyche. When a person is under the spell of transference, he or she can see the therapist only in the way that the spell dictates. The person cannot see the therapist and/or the therapy as they actually are. **Positive transference** occurs when the client projects positive feelings or "good" attributes onto the therapist. In a **negative transference**, the client projects negative feelings or "bad" attributes onto the therapist. In either case, the projections are usually based on the relationship that the client had with significant caretakers during the formative years.

Positive transference is usually based on a fantasy of what a "good parent" would be like; this usually involves something along the lines of being all knowing, all powerful, and totally accepting and loving. One has to admit that these are very outstanding and attractive attributes! Who would not want parents like that? Positive transference becomes part of the foundation for therapy, because it inspires the client with the belief that the therapist is able and willing to help him or her.

At first glance, positive transference seems like a good thing. As previously mentioned, it is the foundation for the healing relationship. However, positive transference also can be a trap for both client and therapist. The client may reenact all of the ways he or she attempted to garner love from the parent. These can include giving gifts, making compliments, referring clients, doing favors, being seductive, becoming sick, needing extra time, trying to pay more than the agreed upon fee, trying to establish a social friendship with the therapist, not being "much of a bother," borrowing things from the therapist, being a "good" client, emulating the therapist, being overly submissive or agreeable, or buying products the therapist may be selling. The therapist, who is the recipient or subject of all these actions, may be influenced by the client's positive transference-inspired behavior. After all, such deference can be attractive. Buying into the positive transference helps keep it unconscious to the client. In fact, any such client behavior that the therapist colludes with is likely to remain unconscious. Being involved in the transaction tends to render the therapist less effective, if effective at all, in making the client aware of the behavior, its meaning, and any attendant tension patterns.

Another problem with positive transference is that it can increase the likelihood of the therapist to collude with the client in boundary violations (discussed in Chapter 4). We may be a little more willing to bend the rules for someone who admires us or seems easy to deal with. For these reasons, *maintain your objectivity when confronted with positive transference.*

In massage therapy, negative transference is more problematic. Since most clients come to massage therapy to feel "good," the appearance of negative feelings is disconcerting and may drive the client away from the therapist or from massage therapy. Also, in many instances, massage therapy clients are not expecting to experience discomforting feelings, nor are they necessarily committed to working through them. In addition, the massage therapist is much more limited than a psychotherapist in dealing with transference. Thus, when negative transference arises, you should avoid purposely stimulating it or attempting to work through it.

Responding to Transference

Some form of transference occurs in massage relationships, whether or not the massage therapist is psychologically minded and whether the client is coming in for emotional work or physical relief. Consequently, the therapist needs to be prepared to be aware of transference and to handle it appropriately.

First, learn to recognize transference and to avoid unconsciously being drawn into playing a role in the client's drama. Being drawn in may only reinforce old patterns or lead to confusing interactions with the client. Simply understanding what is happening and taking some fairly simple measures—to be described shortly—can be very effective.

What the massage therapist *should not do* with transference is try to resolve it psychotherapeutically. This means the massage therapist should not interact with the client by encouraging the client to imagine the massage therapist as being a parent or authority figure and by examining how their interactions are similar. Such *interpretation* is within the realm of psychotherapy, not massage therapy. Indeed, many schools of thought in psychology hold that working with transference is the *core* of psychotherapeutic treatment. Sigmund Freud once asked Carl Jung what he thought of transference. When Jung replied, "It is the alpha and omega in treatment," Freud said, "You have understood." (Bennet, 1961, p. 34).

Since the massage therapist does not have the skills to work through and resolve transference, building up the transference through actions and interpretations can lead to an extremely uncomfortable and potentially harmful situation for the client. For example, the client may see the therapist as extremely powerful and all-knowing, yet also fear the therapist. Perhaps the client is coming for massage therapy to deal with a specific injury and accidentally aggravates the injury by doing something the therapist suggested to avoid. Such a client may be afraid to discuss this with the massage therapist for fear the therapist will be upset. The fear may originate from the client's past in which his parents were upset whenever he made a mistake. Although many people may feel sheepish in admitting to a mistake, transference may make a mistake so shameful or onerous that the client conceals it. Each time the client sees the therapist, the impact of the transference can build up until the client reacts or responds to the therapist in an ungrounded manner.

The therapist may not understand how much power the client is actually attributing to him/her. For example, even the most casual statements, such as, "You must be having a bad day," can appear to a client in the throes of a powerful transference to be highly enlightened and almost psychic on the part of the therapist. The client may fantasize that the therapist not only knows his or her emotional experience, but also knows why he or she is having a bad emotional experience *and* has the solution to it.

This kind of transference makes the client vulnerable to the actions of unethical, or untrained, massage therapists, since someone in a deep transference relationship is likely to follow the therapist's suggestions or recommendations without question. The client in the grasp of positive transference may defer judgment to the therapist not only in bodily matters, but also in psychological health, spiritual, and even financial matters. For example, consider the medicine cabinets of certain massage clients that are filled with a variety of partially, but not recently used pills, lotions, herbs, and the like, which were sold or recommended to them by someone who convinced them the products would do something special for them. The therapist who promotes products is not necessarily a swindler, but even the most benign and well-meaning therapist can unintentionally take advantage of the transference situation.

The massage therapist who is probably more at risk of mishandling these issues is someone who has taken some workshops in which emotional release has taken place during a demonstration or where students were practicing on each other. He or she wants to recreate the same results in his or her massage practice. When witnessing such a powerful event, the combination of emotional release and transference makes the massage therapist appear very potent. For some people, this kind of power is very attractive and may draw them to trying to get the same effects, despite the likelihood they do not have training about transference or emotional release nor counseling skills.

Although massage therapists must be careful about transference issues, it is also important not to go to the other extreme. Having discussed how transference issues are complex and challenging, it is understandable that a massage therapist may not want to deal with them. However, they "come with the territory" of the therapeutic process and cannot be ignored if the therapist is committed to the well-being of the client. We realize that this leaves a massage therapist with a very fine line to walk in regard to transference. On the one hand, the massage therapist needs to be aware of transference and how to deal with it. On the other hand, training, ethical, and legal standards limit the massage therapist in how he or she can handle transference.

In our opinion, what is appropriate for a massage therapist to do regarding transference is the following:

▶ to understand and be aware of transference
▶ to understand how transference affects the client
▶ to understand how the therapist's behavior may affect transference
▶ to modify that behavior accordingly
▶ to avoid building or intensifying the transference

Summary of Client Defenses

All emotions and defenses manifest in the body through energy flow, tension patterns, and differing sensations. This includes the feelings that clients have toward their massage therapist. For example, if a client is afraid of displeasing the therapist, this shows up in the body as tension. Relaxing under such conditions may be difficult for the client even if the therapist is doing excellent work. As another example, a client who is defensively angry may project that the therapist is like his or her mother or father, who always wanted him or her to be nice. In this case, the client may unconsciously feel that the therapist's efforts to induce relaxation are really efforts to subdue or defeat his or her anger. While the therapist is working, the client may be holding out and simmering underneath.

As a massage therapist, don't expect to be able to divine all of this psychological material at all times. Whenever you feel daunted by this task, keep in mind that Carl Rogers' (a psychologist and originator of client-centered therapy) highly regarded and influential list of conditions for therapeutic success—unconditional positive regard, empathy, and genuineness—emphasizes qualities of the therapist over mastery of theory and technique. Nevertheless, careful listening to and observation of your clients' behavior, as well as their bodies, will yield clues to any underlying dynamics. Although we urge you to avoid directly confronting these dynamics, you can create an atmosphere in which your clients can grow. For instance, with a client who wants desperately to please you and therefore maintains control to prevent "messing up," a simple statement such as "You can't do anything wrong" as the client begins to relax may reduce performance anxiety and help him/her let go. To an angry client, you could say, "Sometimes when you relax, you may not always have mellow feelings come up, and that's okay." This gives the client permission to experience anger. To the client who is excessively complimentary about the work, you might say, "Thank you. You are making it possible to make progress because you are playing an active role here." This returns the power given to the therapist back to the client. Again, Table 3.1 on page 34 summarizes the psychological defenses.

THERAPIST DEFENSES

Even though the therapist's defenses are not being challenged in the same way as the client's, many aspects of the work, particularly the emotional challenges that may be presented by the client's transference, can summon up the therapist's own defenses. The therapist brings particular sets of preexistent defensive strategies into the therapy room. These may be active or lie dormant unless triggered.

Countertransference

We rarely approach a new client as if he or she were completely unknown, regardless of how objective we think we are. The more we are interested in a new person, as a therapist is bound to be, the more we begin to "size him up." People—including massage therapists—have a natural tendency to "fill in the blanks" about another person. More often than not, we draw from our previous experiences. When a therapist does this, the process is known as countertransference.

Countertransference describes a system of projections by the therapist onto the client (Figure 3.11). This includes the therapist's reaction to the client's transference onto the therapist. In its widest sense, countertransference is formed from the therapist's emotional attitudes toward the client. The problem with countertransference is that it may blind the therapist to the client's actual psychological and physical situation. When not examined, such attitudes and feelings may be mistaken for perception, intuition, or even fact. As a result, countertransference prevents the client from being seen as who he/she actually is as a person and influences the choices the therapist makes in working with the client.

One way in which countertransference manifests is by identification. In the service of countertransference, identification is akin to empathy gone wrong. A therapist may identify so intensely with a client, may put him/herself in the client's shoes so well, that the therapist loses the objectivity needed to see the client clearly. This makes it difficult to see the client's role in his or her own problems—for example, to see how the client contributes to remaining stuck. Ironically, the more a therapist likes a client,

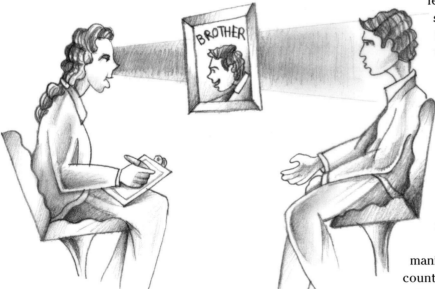

Figure 3.11
Countertransference. *In countertransference, the therapist transfers feelings, thoughts, perceptions about someone from his or her personal history onto the client.*

the more possible it is that this situation could happen. As shown in the following case study, identification driven by countertransference can also lead a therapist to unwittingly exploit a client.

Petra

Petra is a massage therapist who came to us for supervision. She had a client who came for treatment of a knee injury and lower back pain. The physical problems were aggravated by an overweight problem complicated by poor muscle tone in the lower body and back. The client had a history of deep-seated emotional neediness. Petra found herself having deep sympathy for her client, who shared many stories of being neglected and abandoned in relationships. Whenever Petra would try to initiate deeper work, her client would cry and tell Petra that she could not take it, then provide an explanation that would include another sad story demonstrating her inability to get what she wanted. Petra always backed off, even though she knew the deeper work needed to be done to effectively deal with her client's physical problems. The same thing would happen whenever the subject of the client's weight came up. The client would get upset, claiming all her attempts to reduce her weight had been miserable failures and she was not ready to try again. If Petra made any suggestions, there would always be something wrong with them, so Petra gave up making such suggestions and instead simply acknowledged how hard things were.

In supervision, Petra explained that she could not bear her client's tears and could not bring herself to cause her client more pain. Instead, she listened intently to her client's complaints and troubles, offering much sympathy. Petra often found herself giving extras to this client, such as running overtime in her sessions and letting her owe her money for sessions. Although the client was not making much progress with her physical maladies, she seemed very content with coming each week.

What came out in supervision is that Petra had a deep-seated need to make people feel better and ignore their problems. Both of Petra's parents were alcoholics and Petra, being the oldest child in a family with four kids, not only often took care of the other kids, but also dealt with the aftermath of her parents' drinking episodes. She learned never to confront her parents about any problems, but to hold things together by being strong. Petra identified strongly with her client as someone who needed her help.

Through her countertransference with this particular client, Petra was actually satisfying her own need to play that role through her behavior with her client. As a result, Petra was not able to see ways in which her client was contributing to her predicaments, and was also unintentionally colluding in the replaying of her client's destructive patterns. Petra's feelings about her client and her passionate desire to help emotionally rendered her ineffective therapeutically.

A client's similarity to the therapist can also set off countertransference. The therapist is more likely to feel greater empathy for and identification with the client who psychologically more closely resembles the therapist. If someone appears to be *similar* to the therapist, he or she may tend to see the client as the *same*. Then the therapist may also perceive the client's needs as being the same and believe that the client will benefit from the same solutions that worked for the therapist. A comparable situation can occur when a client appears to be similar to another client with whom the therapist has successfully worked, leading to an assumption that the same approach will work. *Mistaking similarity for sameness is a hallmark of countertransference.*

Countertransference can also occur when the therapist accepts positive projections from the client. Having our work appreciated feels wonderful, but it becomes countertransference when it creates a relationship in which the client feels special, and the therapist feels exceptionally powerful and talented in an ungrounded manner. The therapist who encourages the client to continue with this behavior reinforces the client's psychological defenses and character structure (character structure is discussed in Chapter 8).

Similarly, accepting negative projections can also form countertransference. The therapist may develop such a poor image of him- or herself and the work, or may reexperience such painful feelings from the past that have been stirred up by the negativity that he or she may be discouraged from working in areas that the client is afraid of, but needs work.

Countertransference can also stir up *negative* feelings toward a client. Usually, this happens when a client displays some similarity to another person in the therapist's life toward whom the therapist harbors negative feelings. Not only does this cloud the therapist's perceptions of the client, it also can compromise the therapist's ability to act in a therapeutically effective manner. For example, if you have negative feelings toward a client owing to negative countertransference, then maintaining a nonjudgmental and accepting stance toward him or her may not be possible. Such a situation is bound to have an effect on the work. This form of countertransference occurred in the following case.

Sheila and Juanita

Sheila, a massage therapist, began to dread sessions with her client Juanita. Juanita had a little girl's voice. She frequently came in with a "little something" as a gift, such as a bag of herbs, an inspirational booklet, a tiny dreamcatcher for her window. Whenever Sheila asked how Juanita was, Juanita would tear up and look at Sheila appealingly. Sheila's abdominal area would tighten up. She felt resentful. She felt Juanita wanted her to do something. She heard all kinds of negative comments in her head about Juanita, such as "Juanita is too needy," or "Why doesn't Juanita take care of herself?"

Sheila's mother had been needy, too. When Sheila was little, her mother would confide in her with tears in her eyes. Sheila felt sorry for her mother. When Sheila became a little older, she realized that her mother was leaning on her; that her mother really could take steps to stand on her own feet, but did not. Sheila became very angry with her mother, but never said anything. She listened and silently seethed. This was a lot like what she did with Juanita.

Then the situation took a turn for the worse. During a session, Sheila's response to one of Juanita's stories was a little more curt than usual. Juanita burst into tears, but all she said to Sheila was, "I'm sorry," repeatedly. The next session, Juanita noticed the dreamcatcher she had given Sheila wasn't in the window and suddenly demanded that Sheila return it. At the end of the session, Juanita declined to set up another appointment because she "needed some time off." Shaken by the turn of events, Sheila sought out supervision.

Sheila and Juanita

It took many sessions of supervision for Sheila to begin to understand that Juanita was having transferential feelings that she was placing on Sheila. Juanita wanted maternal caring just as Sheila's mother had. In addition, she was unknowingly trying to cope with Sheila's countertransference. Though never verbalized, Sheila's anger was nevertheless perceptible, and it only increased Juanita's feelings of neediness. Both the therapist and the client were playing out their childhood feelings in this situation—Juanita as the abandoned child and Sheila as the burdened child. Sheila began to understand that all she had to give Juanita, indeed *could* give Juanita, was a massage. It took a while, but Sheila stopped dreading Juanita's sessions.

Finally, countertransference can cause the therapist to misperceive and misunderstand the client. This can lead to errors, as shown in the following case.

Marissa

Marissa, a massage therapist, discussed in supervision some work she had done with a couple of clients that involved emotional release. During these sessions, Marissa was drawn into trying to solve certain emotional problems that these clients were having by using some techniques she had learned in her own psychotherapy work. She was beginning to overstep her professional boundaries into the realm of psychotherapy.

During supervision, Marissa came to see that countertransference issues were a cause. These particular clients reminded Marissa of someone close to her, whom Marissa identified with and felt a great need to help. Unconsciously motivated to satisfy her desire to make things turn out better for these clients than they had for the person Marissa was close to, she made two mistakes. She wrongly determined the solution to these clients' problems was what Marissa imagined the person she was close to needed. She also assumed she could apply what had worked for her in her own psychotherapy and, spurred on by her need to solve the problem and use what seemed to be more powerful techniques, chose to work more like a psychotherapist would.

As Marissa became aware of the countertransference dynamics involved, she took steps to correct the situation. She stopped using the techniques in question, repaired the relationship with the clients involved by using some suggestions given during supervision, and referred the clients to a qualified counselor. Marissa also learned to be especially careful with clients who fit the profile of her loved one.

Countertransference issues not only involve misperceptions, but also can lead the therapist to seek emotional gratification through the relationship with the clients. Such behavior can risk damaging the therapeutic process. The familiarity that can develop between the client and therapist can have the attributes of a friendship. As the client reveals personal information about him- or herself, the therapist may want or feel obliged to reciprocate. The therapist may even believe

Box 3.3

WARNING SIGNS OF POSSIBLE COUNTERTRANSFERENCE

Unreasonable dislike
Inability to feel with the client
Overemotional reaction or involvement to the client's troubles
Excessive liking of the client
Dreading the session with the client
Undue concern about the client between sessions
Defensiveness on the part of the therapist
Being argumentative with the client
Indifference
Inattentiveness
Provocativeness
Impatience
Feeling angrily sympathetic with the client

that this is for the client's benefit, subtly turning the principle that a good bond between therapist and client strengthens the therapeutic alliance into a rationalization for the therapist's behavior. When the therapist goes too far in revealing him- or herself to the client, the therapeutic relationship can transform into an ordinary mutual exchange. This provides the therapist with the same sort of gratification that occurs between friends. However, the therapist's job is to understand the client, not to gain understanding *from* the client nor get social needs met. The therapist is an agent acting for the client, serving the client. The therapist's gratification legitimately comes from using special skills, earning a living, and feeling he or she is doing a good job.

Since countertransference comes from attitudes about clients, working on your self-awareness is important. Keeping aware of what you think and feel about your clients and examining those thoughts and feelings closely will help you to bring unconscious or unarticulated attitudes to the surface. Knowing yourself also enables you to understand how your own psychological dynamics may influence how you interact with your client. Self-knowledge also helps you to be better able to differentiate between accurate perception of the client and countertransference. Knowing yourself also helps you to notice whether you are feeling something unusual in your emotional flow. Noticing such unusual ripples identifies countertransference reactions. Box 3.3 can help you identify these reactions.

Self-Awareness and Supervision

While we have been discussing countertransference in this section, have you considered prejudices or biases as related or involved? We may not realize it, but prejudice acted out within a therapeutic setting can be a form of countertransference.

If we agree that dealing with countertransference is critically important for the therapist, then it follows that being more aware of our prejudices, both large and small, is also important. Return to the list you made for the exercise on prejudices in Chapter 2. Follow this with several days of observation of how these prejudices affect your practice. If you find these prejudices coming up in your work, then we suggest you either bring them up with a supervisor, or work on them with a counselor or psychotherapist. If you are not currently in supervision, this can be a time to seek it out. If there is no formal supervision available to you, try selecting an experienced and trusted colleague. Ask if he or she would be willing to help you deal with this.

Depending on where you have trained, you may be unfamiliar with the concept of supervision. **Supervision** consists of formally meeting with someone significantly more experienced with appropriate skills to discuss and work out problems arising in practice. Supervision is *not* a form of psychotherapy. Rather than focusing on the reorganization of one's whole personality through analyzing and working through problems rooted in the personality of the individual as psychotherapy does, supervision assists the therapist in understanding his or her dynamics as these relate to his or her professional self and work. The focus may be on problems arising from clients, from what the therapist is experiencing internally, or from the interaction between therapist and client. The focus may shift from time to time during supervision.

Some examples of reasons for seeking supervision include:

- ▶ Knowing you have countertransference issues or being aware of warning signs of them
- ▶ Having disproportionately strong positive or negative feelings toward a client
- ▶ Needing help when "stuck" with a client
- ▶ Feeling burned-out or bored
- ▶ Feeling ineffective
- ▶ Feeling burdened by confidentiality
- ▶ Being aware of boundary violations or being tempted to bend the frame
- ▶ Having an unusually large number of dependent clients
- ▶ Behaving negatively toward a client (e.g., impatiently, judgmentally, unkindly, temperamentally)
- ▶ Needing help with psychological issues presented by a client, needing modeling of boundaries
- ▶ Seeking support
- ▶ Getting a better understanding of how your personal dynamics affect the work and vice versa
- ▶ Sorting out beliefs and prejudices

Depending on the supervisor's experience and training, the supervisor may ask the therapist to present a case or describe the client and the work being done; ask questions; provide information; give homework assignments; make suggestions about how to handle situations and issues; ask the therapist to examine feelings about the work and the client; and bring in the therapist's personal history and background as part of looking at what is happening. If the supervisor also has training as a counselor or psychotherapist, he or she may work with the supervisee's personal psychological issues, particularly to understand and resolve countertransference issues.

Supervision can take place in a one-on-one situation, group setting, leaderless peer group, or mentoring relationship. To find a supervisor, you can check with the massage school at which you studied or one in your area to see whom the faculty would recommend. You can also check with colleagues with whom you network. A supervisor should have substantial experience (preferably at least 5 years), advanced training (preferably more than 1000 hours), experience working with a variety of clients, and have at least a basic understanding of transference, countertransference, and psychodynamics. Counseling, psychotherapy, or psychology training may be a plus if you need to discuss psychological issues related to your work as a massage therapist. However, if not a massage therapist, the supervisor should comprehend and value the therapeutic dynamics of touch and massage. A supervisor preferably is not a friend or colleague whom you consider a peer, because such a dual relationship may subvert the person's ability to critique your work and behavior or otherwise bring up sensitive material. A solid frame (discussed in the next chapter) is important for supervision, too.

Discussing your prejudices and negative feelings in supervision may initially be awkward. They may even seem trivial or silly. You may feel ashamed of having any prejudice and feel uncomfortable dealing with it. You may tend to censor such thoughts or feelings or want to deny that you have them. But being human means having some prejudices, and being more tolerant and nonjudgmental means admitting it.

Letting go of having to be perfect and without flaws makes it possible to admit imperfections, which in turn makes it possible to deal with them and become a better massage therapist. Softening attitudes toward oneself also has a way of making it more possible to do the same with others. Such reactions and feelings confirm needing to work on them. Supervision is an effective method to do this. Being open to being supervised and honestly looking at where one may be stuck or have difficulty are marks of maturity and commitment for a therapist.

Struggling with these issues is what makes psychotherapists, counselors, and social workers better at dealing with psychological problems, which is why supervision is given great importance in these professional fields. Similarly, dealing with beliefs and prejudices, as in a process such as supervision, helps massage therapists learn how to better deal with such issues and become more adept as therapists and more open as people. Most important, *supervision can provide a supportive space for you to examine your emotional attitudes toward clients.*

Other Therapist Defenses

In our discussion of countertransference, we mentioned projection and identification. How would the other defenses manifest in the therapist?

Denial can function in two ways: we can deny feelings, thoughts, or attributes about ourselves; or we can deny them about others. A therapist, for instance, can deny almost anything about herself to maintain the status quo unconsciously. The therapist could, for example, deny a mounting feeling of dislike for a client because he or she believes that therapists are not supposed to have negative feelings about clients. The denial can undermine the therapist's awareness that he or she is slightly curt with his or her client, cannot manage to find the client the appointments he or she wants, or cuts the session short by 1 or 2 minutes each time. All these are forms of acting out. His or her denial can lead him or her to say sincerely "nothing's wrong" when his or her client asks if something is wrong between them. This can confuse the client, undermining his or her capacity to relax—a major purpose of massage therapy. The massage therapist may also deny that he or she is burned out, attracted to a client, feels ill, or has other feelings, attitudes, and attributes that might not fit him or her idealized self-image of a massage therapist.

The therapist might also deny characteristics and behaviors of a client. The therapist, for example, might deny that he or she sees signs of anorexia, addiction, or severe illness. He or she might deny the extent of an injury or that him or her client is acting out. He or she might ignore him or her client's seductive behavior because it is too frightening or uncomfortable to confront. Almost any uncomfortable situation or aspect can be denied, particularly if the therapist does not feel emotionally and intellectually equipped to handle it.

If the therapist is particularly vulnerable to introjecting, he or she can take in the client's needs and demands as if they were his or hers. He or she will anticipate what the client needs almost too much and feel obliged to take care of everything the client wants, without discriminating whether it is good for the client or the therapist. A signal that introjection is at work is when the therapist feels an oppressive and heavy feeling of "no choice." This is a different feeling from that of being overly responsible, although it can be mistaken for it. Introjections tend to push therapists to overwork, overextend, and take too much emotional responsibility for their clients.

Retroflection is also marked by an exaggerated sense of responsibility. When the therapist is captured by a retroflection dynamic, he or she may not question how his or her client is behaving or what his or her client's resistances may be. Retroflection is a psychological anti-aggression device. It may lead the therapist to hang back from challenging certain kinds of tension patterns or dealing directly with certain kinds of behavior patterns on the part of the client. By taking responsibility for everything, the therapist *deprives* the client from taking responsibility for anything, thereby *disempowering the client.*

Deflection by the therapist can prevent him or her from picking up important information that the client is trying to deliver to him or her. If the therapist deflects either positive or negative statements that the client says by making a joke, changing the subject, or starting an interesting story, he or she may miss an opportunity to better know his or her client.

Resistance can also show up in the therapist. Again, this usually happens in the context of countertransference. The therapist may develop feelings of resistance and dread toward working with specific clients. These feelings are alarms and great opportunities to explore exactly what it is about the client that he or she is resisting. He or she may have feelings arising from his or her own background, such as not wanting to work with people who are overweight because his or her mother was overweight, or he or she may have a form of resistance that we previously termed positive resistance. He or she may be resisting dealing more directly with a certain behavior or dynamic in the client. For example, if the therapist resists making appointments for a client who always tries to extend the session, the therapist needs to determine that it is this particular behavior—extending the session—that he or she is resisting. He or she then either needs to find a way to deal with the client more directly so that the sessions are not extended, or refer the client on. The therapist's resistance is not only unpleasant to experience, it does not allow him or her to open up and give what might be needed to the client.

In summary, defenses are inherent to being human. Consequently, our relationships can be curious mixes of connections *to* each other and defenses *against* each other. In massage therapy, sometimes the defenses of the client come into the foreground. The massage therapist then must try to understand these defenses and help support the client through them without too much intervention. The therapist, however, has his or her own set of defenses that are *not* the focus of the therapy. He or she must learn to bring them into focus *within him- or herself* to understand how they might interact with those of the client. In this way, the client can come more deeply into somatic and psychological awareness without being "pathologized."

We have discussed the importance of the therapeutic relationship in the previous chapter, and in this chapter we have seen how psychological defenses and transference and countertransference issues point out the complexities that can develop in the therapeutic relationship. To support and protect this vital relationship, it needs special structuring, as discussed in the next chapter.

REFERENCES

Bennet, E.A. (1961). *CG Jung*. London: Barrie and Rockcliffe.

Carlino, L. (2002). The therapist's use of self in the therapeutic process: Countertransference and ethical implications. In: *Proceedings of the third national conference of the United States Association for Body Psychotherapy*. 154–157. Bethesda, MD: USABP.

Freud, S. (1912). *The dynamics of transference*. London: Hogarth Press.

Jung, C. (1965). *Memories, dreams, reflections*. New York: Vintage.

Jung, C. (1985). *The practice of psychotherapy: essays on the psychology of the transference and other subjects*, trans. R.F.C. Hull. Princeton, NJ: Princeton University Press.

Keleman, S. (1996). *Bonding*. Berkeley, CA: Center Press.

May, J. (2002). Perspectives on the therapeutic relationship and a matrix of therapeutic attention. In: *Proceedings of the Third National Conference of the United States Association for Body Psychotherapy,* 195–206. Bethesda, MD: USABP.

McWilliams, N. (1994). *Psychoanalytic diagnosis.* New York: Guilford Press. (See Chapters 5, Primary Defensive Processes; and 6, Secondary Defensive Processes.)

Menninger, K. (1958). Transference and counter-transference. In: *Theory of psychoanalytic techniques.* New York: Basic Books, pp. 77–98.

Perls, F., Hefferline, R. & Goodman, P. (1951). *Gestalt therapy.* New York: Dell.

Reich, W. (1933). *Character analysis.* New York: Farrar, Straus, and Giroux, 1949.

Rogers, C. (1965). *Client centered therapy.* Boston: Houghton Mifflin.

Zois, C. (1992). *Think like a shrink.* New York: Warner Books.

Boundaries and Limits in Massage Therapy

*I*n this chapter, we describe the scope of practice boundaries—particularly the dividing line between massage therapy and psychotherapy—and boundaries of behavior you need to be aware of and consistently maintain throughout your career. We conclude with a discussion of how to use a therapeutic frame to help you maintain these essential boundaries and provide a "safe space" for your clients.

SCOPE OF PRACTICE BOUNDARIES

Scope of practice boundaries, explained in the definition, identify what is included in the practice of massage therapy and what is excluded. They also help distinguish what is performing massage therapy from what is performing psychotherapy. We also will characterize psychotherapy and contrast it with massage therapy so that the differences between them become clear. This will help you to maintain appropriate scope of practice boundaries, but at the same time to work on a more sophisticated psychological level. We begin by exploring what psychotherapy is.

Defining Psychotherapy

According to Lewis Wolberg in his influential text, *The Technique of Psychotherapy*, **psychotherapy** is "The treatment, by psychological means, of problems of an emotional nature in which a trained person deliberately establishes a professional relationship with the [client] with the object of (1) removing, modifying, or retarding

Scope of Practice

Strictly speaking, a scope of practice delineates which regulated practices, services, actions, or procedures that a duly licensed, certified, or registered practitioner may or may not perform legally. Therefore, a scope of practice defines primarily: (1) what a qualified practitioner of a particular profession may or may not do, and (2) what a person who is *not* a qualified practitioner may not do. A regulatory law is based on a scope of practice. In legal statutes, a scope of practice sometimes appears as a definition and is sometimes followed by statements describing what is not included in the scope.

Nongovernmental organizations, typically a professional association, may also establish a scope of practice that may be influential, but may not have legal status and may also communicate an idea of the competencies and professional accountability required to perform the particular practice. Therefore, a scope of practice also serves to define what a profession is.

An example of a legal scope of practice for massage therapy is this one currently in effect in Maryland (USA): "Massage therapy means the use of manual techniques on soft tissues of the human body including effleurage (stroking), petrissage (kneading), tapotement (tapping), stretching, compression, vibration, and friction, with or without the aid of heat limited to hot packs and heating pads, cold water, or nonlegend topical applications, for the purpose of improving circulation, enhancing muscle relaxation, relieving muscular pain, reducing stress, or promoting health and well-being." This statement is followed by several clauses that state what massage therapy does not include, such as, "The adjustment, manipulation, or mobilization of any of the articulations of the osseous structures of the body or spine." The practical effect of this scope of practice is fourfold. First, someone who is licensed may perform what is included within the scope. Second, someone who is licensed may not perform what is specifically not included within the scope and/or is included in *another* legal scope of practice for another profession (e.g., the exclusion stated above about osseous structures falls within the scope of chiropractic). Third, someone who is not licensed may not perform what is included within the scope (unless the law specifically exempts him or her). Fourth, anyone may perform what is not included within the scope and also is not included within any other legal scope of practice (i.e., it is unregulated).

existing symptoms, (2) mediating disturbed patterns of behavior, and (3) promoting positive personality growth and development." Although Wolberg's definition is perhaps one of the more frequently referenced, definitions of psychotherapy differ broadly enough to justify concluding that there is no universal definition. If this seems odd, there are other psychological phenomena such as resistance, which nearly everyone agrees exist, but for which there is no widely agreed-upon definition. Perhaps a simpler alternative to Wolberg's definition of psychotherapy is "a service provided by a qualified support person to help clients with their emotional/social/mental processes." Much psychotherapy is not limited to a particular school, and many psychotherapists are trained in several different approaches. As many massage therapists do, psychotherapists take techniques from the approaches that fit their own style and personality.

Usually, a psychotherapist has a master's level degree or higher and is generally licensed by a state licensing board for psychologists, social workers, counselors, or marriage and family therapists, although certain licensed physicians or nurses (e.g., psychiatrists and psychiatric nurses) may also perform psychotherapy. However, as with massage therapy, state laws regarding psychotherapy vary, so we can make only general statements about them here. In some states, regulatory statutes do not control the terms psychotherapy or psychotherapist; that is, they may not require a license to use the terms, but may restrict certain practices associated commonly with psychotherapy. If you have any questions about this, check the laws in your state to be sure which titles and practices are regulated.

Psychotherapy is similar to counseling, and the two terms are often used interchangeably. When a distinction is made, it is often based on the severity or nature of the client's problems rather than the methods. However, over the past 25 years, even this distinction has blurred as psychotherapy and counseling have become accepted processes for personal growth as well as treatments for psychopathology. We present a more extensive discussion of psychotherapy and counseling, and the possible differences between them, in Chapter 11. Throughout this book, we use the term psychotherapy as an inclusive term encompassing *all* other related forms such as counseling, clinical psychology, clinical social work, psychoanalysis, psychiatry, and so on. Since the definition of psychotherapy has limited usefulness in determining the boundary line between massage therapy and psychotherapy, we turn to identifying its characteristics.

Recognizing the Dividing Line Between Massage Therapy and Psychotherapy

Jenna and Rachel

Jenna was going over the forms a new client, Rachel, had just filled out. One of Rachel's responses caught Jenna's attention.

"Oh," said Jenna, "I see you've been in massage therapy before. How was it for you?"

Rachel appeared to be choosing her words carefully. "The body part of it was great," she said, "It was a real revelation for me. Besides feeling less stressed, I had memories of my childhood I never had before."

"And—," asked Jenna, encouragingly, sensing Rachel had more to say about her previous massage experience.

Jenna and Rachel

"Well," said Rachel, "My massage therapist was just too *talky*."

"What do you mean?" asked Jenna.

"Well, after I told my massage therapist that I had memories that I never had before, she just couldn't get off of it. She kept talking about it, saying that because I had new memories that there must be a terrible memory way back there. She kept pushing. It made me nervous and uncomfortable."

"What do you think about that?" asked Jenna.

"Frankly, I think she didn't quite know what she was talking about," said Rachel. "I *have* a psychotherapist, and I took what came up in massage to her and we talked about it. We're still working on it, but it turns out the memories weren't about what the massage person thought. I liked the massage part of it, but her digging into my personal stuff made me so frustrated, I left."

The dividing line between massage therapy and psychotherapy is difficult to draw because there is no physical or mental "border" between mind and body, psyche and soma. It would be convenient, in a schematic sort of way, to echo the mind-body split and insist on a clear distinction between massage and psychotherapy. However, insisting that massage should never involve psychological issues or emotional responses or that a massage therapist should never encounter or stimulate psychological material in the course of massage therapy would be too dogmatic and unrealistic and would deny the unity of the bodymind—to the detriment of the client. *Working with the body, the therapist encounters the whole person.*

As discussed in Chapter 1, massage may indeed evoke, as a bodily experience that stimulates interaction between body and mind, elements of the psychological life of the client. However, these elements are *byproducts* of the massage, rather than the central purpose or focus. Once these byproducts become the central purpose or focus of the massage therapist, it is likely that *the line has been crossed,* and the massage therapist is acting in a psychotherapeutic capacity. Unless the therapist has proper training to do so, this is not acceptable. Furthermore, this risks ethical and legal breaches, exposing the massage therapist to professional disciplinary action, legal action for working outside the scope of practice of massage therapy, legal action for working within the scope of practice of a mental health profession, or all of the above.

Box 4.1 identifies characteristics of psychotherapy, which will help you in making a distinction between massage therapy and psychotherapy. If in the spontaneity of a massage session a therapist finds that he or she reasonably uses one or two of

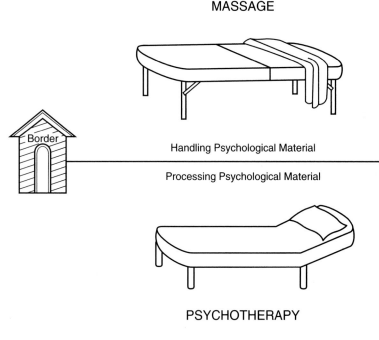

MASSAGE

Border

Handling Psychological Material

Processing Psychological Material

PSYCHOTHERAPY

Figure 4.1
The boundary line between psychotherapy and massage therapy.
The line between processing and handling psychological material can often appear to be a thin one.

Box 4.1

EXAMPLES OF TYPICAL PSYCHOTHERAPY TECHNIQUES

The following are psychotherapeutic techniques that are not within the scope of practice of massage therapy:

► Attempting to deepen or intensify the psychological aspects of an experience
► Initiating a verbal exploration of, or otherwise working with, transference issues
► Placing a greater emphasis and taking more time on psychological aspects during sessions
► Making a psychological diagnosis
► Giving advice about psychological or emotional issues
► Making psychological interpretations, i.e., giving a psychologically based analysis or explanation of the client's words or actions
► Having an intent about what the outcome of an emotional release should be
► Directing or encouraging the client to deepen or intensify an emotional response
► Eliciting information that goes beyond or deeper than the material that has come up spontaneously
► Becoming more involved in the client's life than in the massage work itself

these techniques in the course of tending to the client, this may not be a problem. However, problems begin when the therapist *intentionally* and *regularly* does this. In this case, the massage therapist who engages in these practices is likely engaging in psychotherapy, which, we restate for emphasis, would also be *unethical, outside the scope of practice of massage therapy, and/or possibly within the scope(s) of practice of the mental health professions.*

If there were one single practice that characterizes psychotherapy and the dividing line between massage therapy and psychotherapy, we would say it is working through transference. Many methods of psychotherapy place working through the transference at the core of the process. Therefore, *if a massage therapist deliberately works through transference, this would be a strong indication that he or she has crossed over the line and is doing psychotherapy.*

Mistaking your own psychotherapy, reading, or workshop experience as the equivalent of professional training is very easy, which can tempt a massage therapist over the line. Although any of these experiences may make you more aware, more psychologically sophisticated, and even wiser, they do not train you to work psychotherapeutically with others. Being psychologically insightful, sensitive, or intuitive also is not enough. In fact, sometimes having enhanced personal psychological knowledge may even increase a person's tendency to project his or her own experiences because it provides more material upon which to draw. It takes training to learn how not to do this.

Handling Versus Processing Psychological Material

Rather than avoid psychological material, the massage therapist must recognize its importance, but at the same time limit his or her involvement with it to the degree that is appropriate. An example of this in ordinary life is how you view your boss (if you have never had one, substitute someone similar to a boss). You might consider how your body reacts to seeing your boss, and you might experience your feelings about your boss. However, if you verbalize these feelings you might act inappropriately, even lose your job. Another example that might help is that of an operating room nurse, who must know a great deal about surgery, yet cannot perform it. Similarly, the massage therapist must know a great deal about the psychological aspects of the body and the process of massage therapy, but not deliberately elicit psychological material nor induce psychological reactions. Essentially, the massage therapist must learn to *handle* psychological material, but not *process* it. Box 4.2 helps you see the difference between these two very different responses.

It is imperative that a massage therapist knows *when* and *why* he or she is stepping over the line between massage and psychotherapy. Recognizing the warning signs in advance can reduce your risk of violating this boundary. The warning signs include:

▶ Feeling a sense of discomfort with what you are doing or saying; that is, things feel "shaky" or "murky"

▶ Finding you are giving psychological advice or using psychological terms

▶ Noticing that the session time has become mostly verbal

▶ Observing that you are becoming more involved in the client's life than in the condition of the client's body

▶ Realizing emotional release is or has become the focal point of your sessions

▶ Seeing the client become so overwhelmed by emotional release or become so emotionally flooded that he or she is unable to do anything else, such as being unable to: stop emoting, to come back to the here-and-now, or to talk about what he or she is experiencing or has been experiencing

▶ Seeing the client become unstable

Consequences of Violating Scope of Practice Boundaries

A variety of consequences can result from a massage therapist crossing the line between massage therapy and psychotherapy. All of these consequences are substantial and, in some cases, can be severe. For example, the therapist may:

▶ Create a relationship that is not appropriate for either the client or the therapist

▶ Misdirect the client, such as (incorrectly) telling someone who is dissociated (emotionally disconnected from the body) that dissociation always originates from being sexually abused

▶ Prevent the client from receiving treatment from someone more qualified or from receiving any treatment at all

▶ Be in a situation that is beyond the therapist's ability to deal with, causing him or her to underestimate the depth or tenacity of a client's psychological problem, become entangled in a client's life, or receive a great deal of negativity from people with certain types of character disorders

▶ Lose the client because the client feels invaded, intruded upon, or overpowered

▶ Encourage the client to make explorations that are contraindicated for the actual problem, such as inappropriate treatment or suggestions, for example, to encourage someone with a dissociative disorder to emote more

▶ Open up an issue with a client, but not be able to resolve it, which leaves the client psychologically and emotionally "stuck" or in an uncompleted condition that could subject him or her to greater stress and suffering

▶ Otherwise harm the client

▶ Be exposed to professional sanctions and legal actions

Box 4.2

DIFFERENTIATING BETWEEN HANDLING AND PROCESSING PSYCHOLOGICAL MATERIAL

The massage therapist is *not* trained to *process* psychological material. This work falls within the domain of psychotherapy and involves the following:

▶ Eliciting or encouraging the client to give more information

▶ Encouraging stronger emotional release

▶ Suggesting what the emotional material might be related to

▶ Focusing on emotional problems

▶ Interpreting either verbal information or emotional expression

▶ Talking about transference issues

▶ Deepening transference by encouraging exploration of whom the therapist represents and how the client feels about that person

The massage therapist may *handle* psychological material. Handling psychological material involves the following:

▶ Acknowledging the presence of psychological material when it appears

▶ Using active listening and reflection

▶ Providing nonjudgmental support

▶ Being present and centered

▶ Creating a safe environment

▶ Helping the client ground him or herself through the body

▶ Making an appropriate referral if needed

Box 4.3

CORRECTING VIOLATIONS OF THE LINE BETWEEN MASSAGE AND PSYCHOTHERAPY

To correct scope of practice boundary violations between massage therapy and psychotherapy, the massage therapist:

▶ Identifies the problem
▶ Identifies behaviors on his/her part that evoke, elicit, or expand psychological reactions and material
▶ Makes decisions about how to alter these behaviors
▶ Identifies the problem to the client and proposes clearer boundaries
▶ Reviews the contract, i.e., the explicit or implicit agreements about the goals of the massage therapy, and practice policies, and possibly revises them.
▶ Looks at his/her motivations in pursuing psychological interventions
▶ Gets supervision and more training

Correcting Violations of Scope of Practice Boundaries

Sometimes, massage therapists realize too late that they are in over their heads. It takes courage to admit that you have gone beyond your scope of practice, extent of training, or abilities. Furthermore, it can be embarrassing or humiliating to face your client or professional colleagues while dealing with such a situation. But the first essential step toward correcting scope of practice violations is to take responsibility for the problem.

Next, the massage therapist should seek supervision. Having help with such a dilemma can aid the massage therapist in deciding whether the damage can be repaired and the massage therapy process can be put back on track. See Chapter 3 for an explanation and discussion of supervision.

Sometimes, the situation has gone too far, and even supervision cannot restore the therapeutic relationship. *As tough as it might seem in such situations, the best action is to end the massage therapy and refer the client to another massage therapist. The reason for such a strong action is to terminate the inappropriate relationship that has been created.* This is in the best interest of the client because it allows him or her to move on freely to continue with either massage therapy or psychotherapy or both, based on the client's needs.

It takes compassion, courage, and a deft touch to be able to do this in a way that is supportive of the client. If the massage therapist has encouraged a psychotherapeutic relationship and then drops the client improperly when realizing the mistake, this can be damaging to the client. The client may even resist attempts to terminate. This resistance needs to be handled, but not given in to. The massage therapist must first take full responsibility for the situation. This means he or she must be the one to initiate and carry out whatever needs to be done to correct the situation. In terminating, the massage therapist needs to affirm the validity of the client's psychological process and emphasize that he or she is not responsible for the problems stemming from the therapy or the termination of the work. The massage therapist must also consider referring the client to a new massage therapist, a psychotherapist, or both.

Sometimes, however, the massage therapy can be salvaged. Again, we urge a massage therapist to seek supervision for guidance on how to go about this. Some steps to salvage or repair the therapy are suggested in Box 4.3. However, keep in mind that violations of the boundary between massage therapy and counseling and psychotherapy vary in severity. Minor violations are more likely to be helped by these suggestions, but they may not be adequate for more severe violations.

We want to state again how easy crossing the line can be because the line between massage therapy and psychotherapy is indistinct in many ways. Managing to not cross the line and maintain boundaries can call for very keen judgment and perception. Few therapists who cross the line do so on purpose or with malicious intent. Guilt and blame do not solve such situations, but awareness and appropriate action can.

BOUNDARIES CONCERNING LIMITS OF BEHAVIOR

This section focuses on the particular concept of boundaries concerning behavior that define our personal physical and emotional space. Boundaries of behavior serve to facilitate the therapeutic process, create safety, and protect the integrity of the client *and* therapist.

Therapists must maintain certain boundaries of behavior first and foremost because the client and therapist are in an unequal power equation in their relationship. This often goes unrecognized by many massage therapists, probably because they focus on the caring and concern massage involves, rather than on the dynamics of power. Low self-esteem, minimizing the power of touch, not seeing oneself as powerful, and countertransference are other reasons the therapist may not recognize or understand the power that the client and the process have invested in them. But as discussed in Chapter 2, any kind of healing constellates power issues because we give power to someone we expect to heal or otherwise help us. We also grant a great measure of authority, trust, and dependence to those whom we perceive as having the knowledge, ability, or spiritual connection to help us. This is an essential ingredient in the healing process. Furthermore, it is a psychological likelihood that we perceive healers as parental or authority figures on some level, which sets into play any number of positive and negative forces.

The therapist also needs to define and uphold boundaries of behavior that apply to the client, because such boundaries for the client serve to keep both therapist and client safe and emotionally comfortable. Boundaries also protect the therapist from overextending, from being emotionally or financially used, and from being manipulated concerning the rules the therapist makes about conducting his or her practice.

Clients have boundaries to abide by which keep the client safe, centered, and realistic about the nature of the relationship and the process. These same boundaries also help the therapist keep the client on purpose and on track in the process.

Boundaries are also related to the "frame" the therapist creates by means of rules regarding time, payment, telephoning, types of touch, outside contact, cancellations and setting appointments. We discuss the maintenance of a therapeutic frame fully later in this chapter.

In the context of the therapeutic process, boundaries involve a number of issues. A discussion of boundaries concerning limits in several domains of behavior follows.

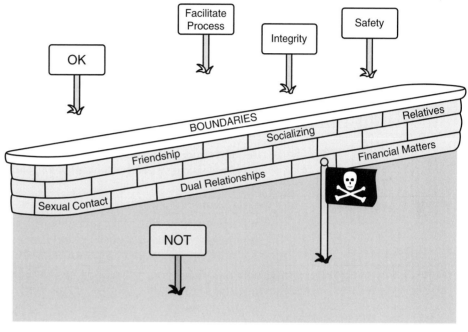

Figure 4.2
Boundaries place limits on behavior. *Boundaries serve to facilitate and protect the therapeutic process and relationship, create safety, and protect the integrity of the client and therapist by setting limits on sexual contact, friendships, dual relationships, financial matters, and other relational issues. Violating boundaries can put the therapy at risk.*

Sexual Boundaries

Sexual contact with a client is *unequivocally forbidden* and *wrong* either in or out of the therapy room. Overwhelming evidence exists that sexual contact between a therapist and client is harmful. In most jurisdictions, it is also illegal. Any romantic fantasy that love somehow justifies an exception to this rule or sexual contact is in any way helpful to the client is an illusion. This boundary is the first one we discuss because it exists to *prevent certain emotional harm* to the client and therapist. The boundary concerning sexual contact also applies to dating or any relationship with a client that has romantic significance and applies to *anyone* with whom a massage therapist is currently working. The unequal power relationship between therapist and client taints the dynamics of an intimate social relationship, which requires a more equal status of power. Because massage therapy also involves varying amounts of exposure of the body and varying degrees of intimate personal interaction between client and therapist, the ingredients of attraction are inherently present. Nevertheless, learning to deal with and contain sexual attraction between therapist and client, when it exists, is one of the responsibilities that a therapist must undertake. Massage therapists *must not* allow themselves to act upon such an attraction.

How do you apply this in the real life situations encountered by a massage therapist? Sometimes a massage therapist works only once with a client. Does this mean a massage therapist cannot have any further contact with this person? Obviously not, but the therapist must formally terminate the massage relationship with that person if they want to begin dating—*whether or not* the therapist anticipates that sexual contact will occur.

To determine whether a massage therapist and *former* client should be able to date, some factors to consider are:

▶ The ethical guidelines established by regulatory boards, certification agencies, and professional associations that you are obligated to follow.
▶ The nature of the professional relationship: number and frequency of sessions, types of issues dealt with in massage, and intensity of issues dealt with; generally, the greater the factors, the greater the potential problem.
▶ Time lapsed since ending the professional relationship: generally, the more significant the factors, the longer the elapsed time period needed. (Professional ethical guidelines may specify the time period; see the paragraph that follows this list.).
▶ Emotional maturity and stability of the client: To what degree is the client able to relate to the former therapist as an equal? Does the client have any emotional conflicts that would interfere with making a successful transition to a different type of relationship? Does the client have any emotional conflicts that would be worsened by being in a social relationship with the former therapist? Is the client acting out by seeking this relationship? Does the client have sufficient emotional resources available, other than the former therapist?
▶ Emotional maturity and stability of the former therapist: To what degree is the former therapist able to relate to the client as an equal? Is the former therapist trying to meet unsatisfied social needs or resolve a personal problem by forming this relationship? Is the former therapist acting out by seeking this relationship? Does the former therapist have sufficient emotional and professional support, such as supervision?
▶ Status of transference and countertransference issues: Did transference and countertransference issues form? If so, to what degree and intensity? To what

degree are the transference and countertransference issues still existing or resolved? Will either the client or former therapist be harmed by entering into this relationship?

Because these factors are often not easy to evaluate, we can look to the psychotherapy profession for guidance. Psychotherapy standards state unequivocally that it is unethical to date any *current* client. The rules about whether a therapist can date a *former* client vary among the professional associations and certification agencies for psychotherapists, psychologists, psychiatrists, counselors, and massage therapists. The National Certification Board for Therapeutic Massage and Bodywork has established an ethical standard of not dating for 6 months after terminating massage therapy. The ethical standards for the American Psychological Association and the United States Association for Body Psychotherapy are stricter, requiring a 2-year waiting period. However, some professional groups take the ethical position that having a sexual relationship of any kind with a former client is never acceptable.

Massage therapy is not psychotherapy and the relationship between client and massage therapist may not be as involved or complex, but some of the transference-countertransference issues are similar. Consequently, problems associated with dating clients also exist for massage therapists. These boundaries limiting relationships exist for the emotional safety of *both* client and therapist.

In the eyes of the client, transference often makes the therapist appear more wonderful, attractive, confident, powerful, and wise than a person could reasonably be. The client may not be attracted to the therapist's actual personality, but rather to a fantasy spun from the threads of the transference. If a therapist and client were to date, transference may also set the therapist up to disappoint the client, because the therapist cannot live up to the client's fantastic expectations. In the end, both parties can be enormously hurt and disappointed.

It is important for the therapist to keep in mind that, even if the romantic or sexual contact is initiated or otherwise encouraged by the client, it is the *therapist's* responsibility to hold the boundary. This is true no matter how emotionally or sexually seductive or persuasive the client may be. The therapist cannot make an exception to this boundary based on the client's behavior.

In contrast, if the therapist initiates the romantic or sexual contact, it can be extremely difficult for the client either to consent or to resist. In fact, *legal theorists regard the therapeutic relationship as having such a strong effect on a person that a client in a therapeutic relationship is considered unable to give informed consent*, in much the same way that a child cannot do so. The unequal power differential between therapist and client places the client in a weaker position. The client is apt to believe that the therapist is an "expert" acting in the client's best interest and thus to go along with the therapist's suggestions. The saying "doctor knows best" reflects the unquestioning trust a client can have. The client may also feel confused, may want to say no but cannot, or may be amenable when it happens but have a negative reaction later.

Some guidelines can be offered to help massage therapists determine how to maintain sexual boundaries and limits. Look at the level of dependency that has developed between you and your client, and try to understand how your client sees you. For example, if a client sees you as a savior, magician, or all-giving maternal figure (this can include male therapists), then quite obviously the client is not seeing you as you are in reality. While being seen as such a great person can be very flattering and can feel good, it is likely to lead to an unsuccessful sexual, romantic, or social relationship. Healthy relationships are, in most cases, based on each partner being reasonably and equally able to give and receive. Dependency that developed during therapy can distort social relationships. The adulation received in the therapy room can become burdensome outside it. The magic that goes on in the therapy room happens because it *is* the therapy room, which is a safe space with well-formed, clear boundaries that allow emotion and sensation to arise. Outside that room, which is where your social life occurs, the boundaries dissolve, leaving you and your client unprotected, uncontained, and potentially in psychological danger. Sexual or romantic relationships also have a social aspect, so we will discuss social boundaries next.

Social Boundaries

Knowing where the boundaries are in nonromantic *socializing* can be equally or even more difficult than in romantic and sexual relationships, since there are many variations in types of social relationships as well as in degrees of intimacy. Although the psychotherapy profession has very clear guidelines about socializing with clients, these rules do not always transfer to massage therapy. As the massage therapy profession continues to develop, consensus is emerging that there needs to be some limitations on socializing with clients. However, until these are more fully developed, you need to form your own policy concerning socializing. Your decision about socializing depends on variables such as how long you have been working with the client, the focus and intent of the work, what your understanding is of how the client sees you, and the precise nature of the relationship.

Friendships

We define *friendships* as nonromantic, nonsexual relationships with varying degrees of intimacy between two consenting adults not related by blood. While engaging in friendships with clients may at first seem unproblematic, the following are some examples of decisions you may need to make concerning friendships with clients:

▶ You give massages to your best friend as part of your practice session for a training program. Your friend then asks you to be his or her massage therapist. What do you do?

▶ You give one massage to a person at a health club. You feel you would like to form a friendship with this person. Do you go ahead with the friendship, do you say you cannot be the person's massage therapist any longer, or do you tell the person he or she can be either your client or your friend, but not both? Next, consider how you would deal with the situation if it involved a client with whom you have worked with for 10 sessions.

▶ You have been working for 2 years with a client whom you really like. There has been no emotional work connected with the massage, and there seems to be no transference issues to be concerned about. Your client invites you to go to a ball game. What do you do?

▶ You have a client who has had an emotional release on your table. You attend a workshop and discover that this client is also attending. You go out to lunch with a group, which includes this client. You find out that you and your client have much in common. Do you proceed with the budding friendship?

▶ A client sees you for a sore shoulder. After six sessions, the work is successful and the massage therapy ends. A couple months later you join a book discussion group and find that this client also belongs. The former client invites you to his or her house for a dinner party. Do you accept or decline?

If your client sees you as a hero, guru, or healer, there is already an inherent inequity in the balance of power in the relationship. As the therapist, you need to be prepared to discover that the nature of your interaction with that person is affected when you interact with them in a social setting. For example, what if your client idealizes you as a paragon of healthy habits and at a restaurant or a dinner party the client sees you having two glasses of wine and a steak smothered in cream sauce, or sees empty potato chip and doughnut bags in your car? We have actually had clients see junk food wrappers in the trash basket in our offices and then earnestly want to know if we had eaten such unworthy substances, as if it could not and should not be possible for us to do it (though in truth previous clients left the wrappers, not us . . . of course!) (Figures 4.3A & B).

The intimacy a person may find in the therapeutic situation often is not reproduced in friendship outside of therapy because of the special nature of the therapeutic relationship. Both therapy and friendship can include warmth and connection, but in the massage therapy situation the client is the center of attention, whereas the therapist reveals much less personal information. However, a friendship depends on a relatively equal exchange of personal information and feeling. In a friendship, the type of restraint used professionally by the therapist would probably come across as withholding, patronizing, rude, or otherwise inappropriate. *In deciding whether to socialize with a client, you need to consider what kinds of restrictions you may put on yourself to maintain your role, fulfill your client's expectations, or deal with a client's particular character.* You may find yourself feeling resentful and otherwise more negative than positive about the socializing. For example, you may feel you need to accept invitations to socialize to avoid an angry or hurt response from your client.

It is common knowledge that people in the helping professions have the tendency to devote themselves to their work to the point of sacrificing a personal life. In doing this, they end up not taking care of their needs in a natural way. It can become dangerously convenient to rely on those who are the most present and available to you for contact—your clients, *especially* those you really like. It can be tempting to fill a personal void by socializing with clients. The exercise in Box 4.4 may help you to confront this if it is happening to you.

Sometimes taking care of others becomes more comfortable than having a personal life. This dynamic is difficult to confront within oneself, since the idealized self-image of being good, caring, and self-sacrificing to the point of not having a social life can be easy to rationalize. American culture reinforces this attitude. For example, television shows depict physicians, nurses, police, and attorneys who apparently do not keep regular office hours and have no personal lives. After all, it can become rather pleasant to always be in control of the situation and play the role of the superior person, but you may also impair your own growth by surrounding yourself with an entourage of people who look up to you. It may not do your clients much good either. They may be simply reenacting behavior patterns with you through this social entrainment. Such patterns are often the very ones that they need to change before they can progress in their own growth process. Then

Box 4.4

FRIENDSHIP LIMITS EXERCISE

Here is an exercise to try. First, write down a list of your friends. Then list anyone with whom you have interactions in which you talk about your personal life. Now see how many are your clients. Can you identify why it is important for both you and your clients that you expand your social circle? What steps can you take to do so?

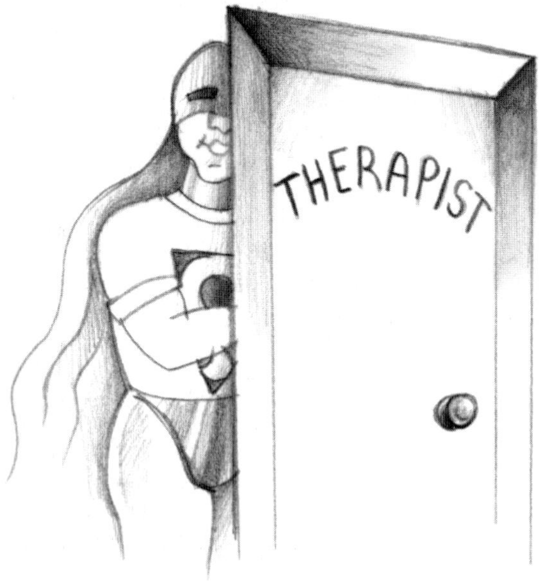

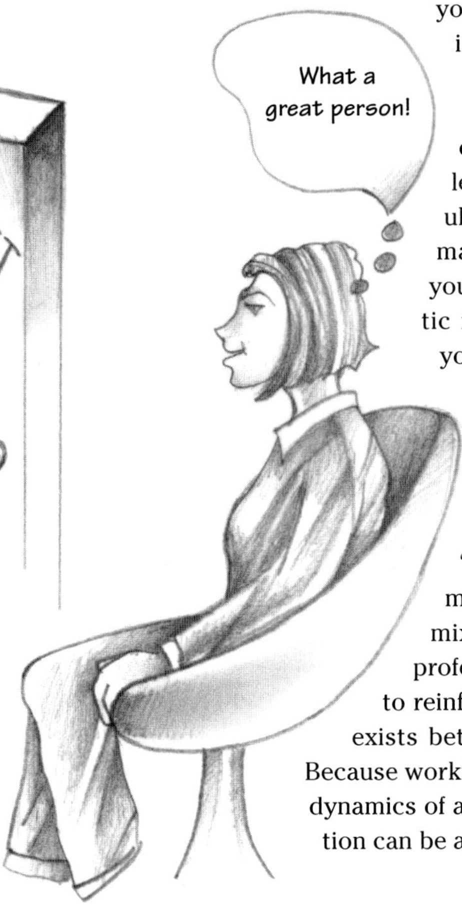

What a great person!

Figure 4.3A
Man of Steel. *Within the therapeutic environment, the therapist may take on heroic qualities for the client. But . . . (see Figure 4.3B)*

your relationship with them can end up impairing their growth, too.

Besides the situation of clients becoming friends, friends becoming clients can also bring up issues and problems. While working with a friend, particularly one with whom you have an informal, relaxed relationship, do not loosen your professional boundaries and therapeutic framework with them when you are in your role of massage therapist—no matter how easy and tempting it can be. With friends, you must redouble your efforts to maintain confidentiality. Since the social worlds of you and your friend are bound to intersect, any "leaking" of confidentiality can leave much damage in its wake. Similarly, do not mix social conversation while acting in a professional mode with a friend. The idea is to reinforce the understanding that a boundary exists between the therapeutic and social roles. Because working on a friend also presents many of the dynamics of a dual relationship, much of the next section can be applied to friendships.

Dual Relationships

A ***dual relationship*** is a situation in which multiple roles exist between a therapist and a client. Examples of dual relationships are when the client is also a student, friend, family member, employee, business associate, teacher, or health care provider of the therapist. The problem with dual relationships is the difficulty of maintaining a continual awareness of what belongs in one relationship and what belongs in the other. The nature of one relationship often colors the other. Another way of putting this is that dual relationships can be "sticky," meaning that aspects of one relationship can transfer over or "stick" to the other relationship, or they become entangled (just as adhesions can cause soft tissue fibers to get entangled). For example, if your physician comes to you for massage, you might become anxious about displaying your knowledge of anatomy or concerned that your massage work may affect his or her attitude toward complementary care. Massaging a client with whom you also have any kind of business relationship may draw you into giving too much extra time to that client so that your client will like you more and be more likely to buy your product or service, or otherwise do business with you. Or, you may need to criticize an employee or assistant, but if that person is also your therapy client, your criticism may damage your therapeutic relationship. Conversely, you may withhold needed criticism because you feel obligated to protect or always be positive toward your client. On the other side, the party in a dual relationship with you also may feel constrained or otherwise affected. As another example of problems that can arise with them, dual relationships make maintaining confidentiality even more important (Figure 4.4).

You are the gatekeeper to your massage practice, especially if you are in private practice. You decide whom you take as a client. When you already know someone who wants a massage from you, consider whether this is going to create a dual relationship that will cause you to alter your behavior inappropriately or lead to other problems. Doing so would be against your best interests and the best interests of your client. It may also be harmful to either or both of you. This calls for careful consideration of whether to accept as a client a person with whom you have an existing relationship. Many of these dual relationships can be very flattering, and this may lead you to set aside the cautions evident in the situation. If you are not in private practice, you need to find out from your employer or supervisor what latitude you have regarding declining to work with someone and, if necessary, negotiate the right to do so. You may need to explain the ethical issues presented by dual relationships and other social boundaries.

Limits concerning dual relationships are not absolute, and avoiding them may not be possible, so each situation must be evaluated on its own merits. Indeed, psychotherapists Lazarus and Zur (2002) argue that under certain circumstances not all dual relationships are harmful. Generally, the greater the power differential or degree of contact, the more likely a dual relationship may be a problem and should be declined. Some dual relationships that should be avoided are with your family members, co-workers, spouses/boyfriends/girlfriends, roommates, and health care providers. In tight-knit communities, avoiding dual relationships may be difficult. In the event that you do choose to enter into or stay in a dual relationship, primary critical considerations are the welfare of the client, avoidance of harm and exploitation, conflict of interest, effect on the massage therapy, and possible impairment of clinical judgment. The existence of the dual relationship should be acknowledged and time provided to discuss it if either party wishes to do so. Establish an understanding at the outset that if either party finds it difficult to handle, then terminating the therapy will be okay. Box 4.5 helps you to identify, consider, and reflect on your own dual relationships.

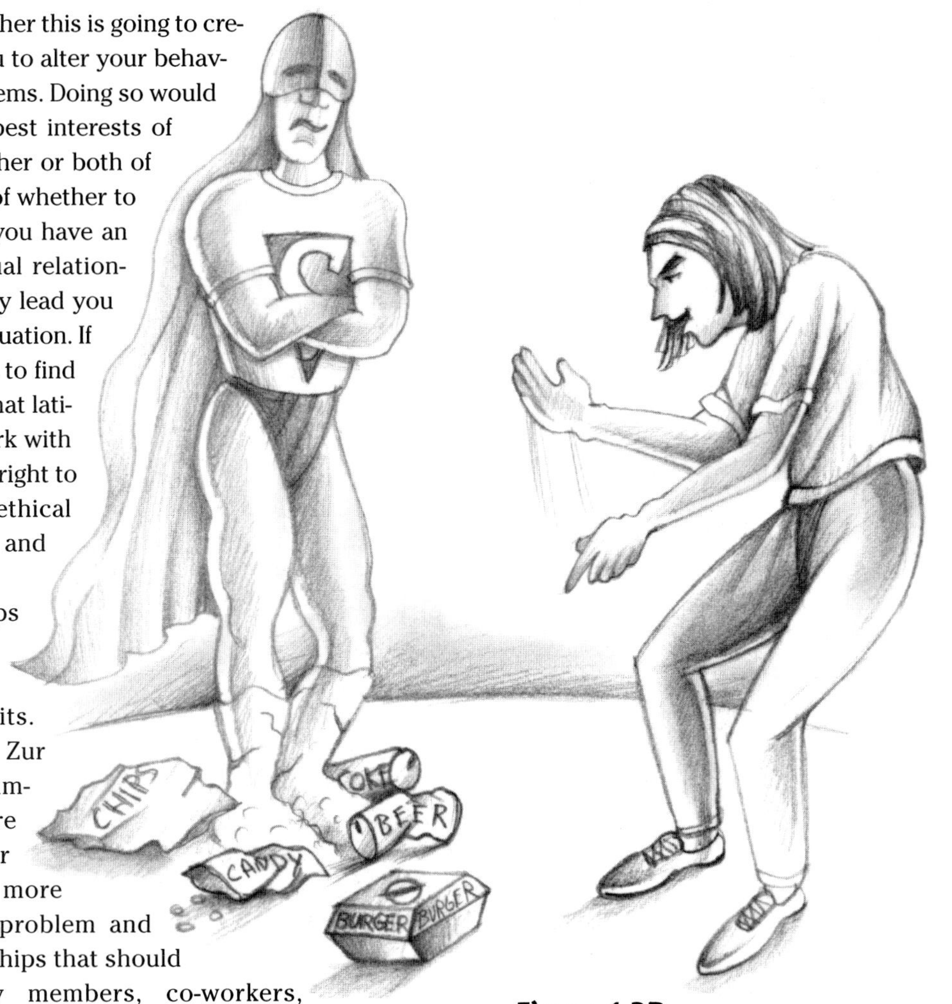

Figure 4.3B
Feet of clay. *Interaction with a client outside the therapy setting runs the risk of affecting the client's idealized view of the therapist. The hero can end up with feet of clay. Boundaries that limit socializing help preserve the therapist's potential to fulfill a role for the client because they limit familiarity.*

Family Relationships

It is not unusual for a relative to ask you to give a massage or for you to feel the need to give a massage to a relative who is suffering or is otherwise in need. Very often a massage therapist is confronted with this situation for the first time while a student, because students need to practice on many different people as a part of their training program. Recruiting your spouse, parent, sibling, or some other relative is convenient, but whether it is a good idea to work on a relative depends on the nature of the relationship. If the relationship is good and open, it can be a joy. However, your views of family members are bound to be colored in powerful ways. If there are underlying problems in the relationship, these likely will surface in the massage situation. This is because the skills needed to function as an effective therapist, such as appropriate detachment and objectivity, are nearly impossible for a therapist to apply to family members. For example, if you have trouble saying no to your mother, you will have trouble saying no to giving her a massage when you may not want to do it. If your sense of self-esteem revolves around praise from your older sibling, then receiving constructive feedback from him or her may be difficult. Family members may not be willing to accept the same conditions and policies you apply to your clients. They may expect to not have to pay you for your services, or they may be unusually cooperative or uncooperative. As with other kinds of social relationships, the external and internal pressures to relax and bend your professional boundaries and the therapeutic framework can be considerable. As with these other social relationships, not maintaining your boundaries and the frame with family members presents certain risks. Not being able to maintain the frame can be a good reason to turn down a relative or to keep the massage work relatively very limited in time and scope.

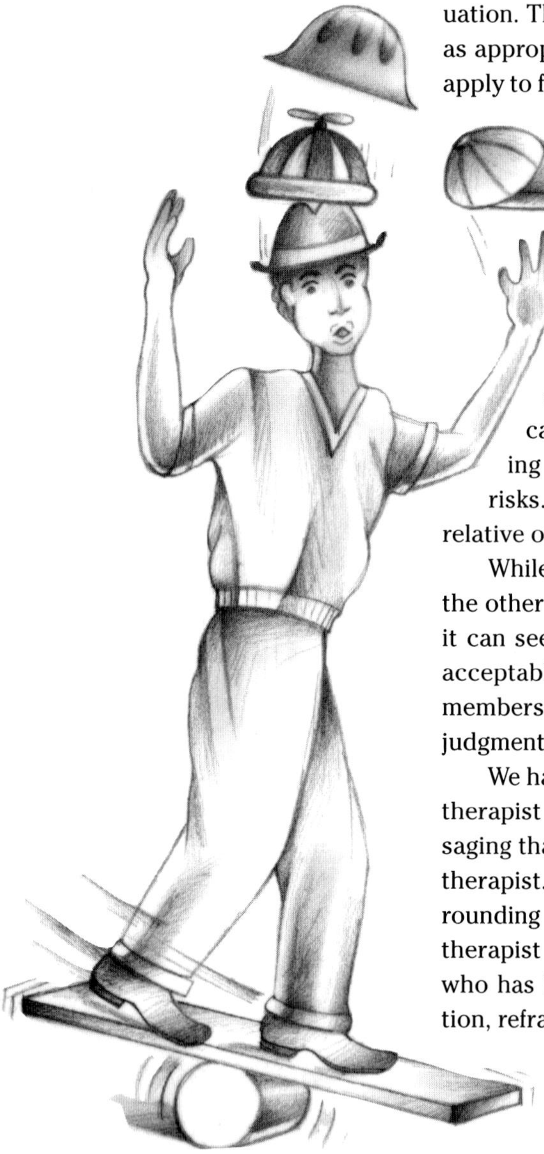

While saying no to a family member can be difficult for a massage therapist, on the other hand massage is such a strong agent for change and healing, withholding it can seem neglectful or even cruel. Wanting to help via massage is natural, and acceptable, as long as the therapist is not attempting to save or impress family members. Such powerful countertransference situations can cloud the therapist's judgment.

We have one caveat to add concerning limits with family members. If a massage therapist has been abused—sexually or otherwise—by any family member, not massaging that person or anyone else associated with such abuse is important for that therapist. Persons who have been sexually abused often deny the implications surrounding their abuse. Particularly with those who have abused them, the massage therapist may not understand the potential implications of touch. Even if the person who has been abused and the abuser both feel that they have resolved the situation, refraining from a massage relationship is still important.

Financial Boundaries

As we have emphasized before, giving massage places the therapist in a position of power and trust in a relationship. For example, if the massage therapist recommends that the client put ice on a sprain, the client is likely to do it because he or she believes the therapist is both knowledgeable and committed to helping. Similarly, a client may be more disposed to accept a financial recommendation or offer from the therapist based on this heightened sense of trust. Furthermore, certain character types (discussed in Chapters 8 and 9) may be especially disposed to following a therapist's suggestions and are particularly vulnerable.

For example, a therapist may be involved in a multilevel marketing business that encourages participants to recruit people they know. The marketing company may put forth the idea that participants are doing a good thing for people by encourag-

Figure 4.4
Dual relationships. *Wearing too many hats. Playing too many roles in a relationship, especially when one of them is the therapeutic relationship,*

Box 4.5

DUAL RELATIONSHIPS EXERCISE

Write down a list of your clients and then put down every relationship you have with each one. See if there are clients with whom you have more than one type of relationship. Then see if each of these relationships constrains or otherwise affects the other. If they do, how and to what extent do they?

ing them to also belong. Since therapists usually see clients regularly, they are available for a sales pitch. Furthermore, if a therapist does not interact with many people outside the therapy setting because of a busy practice crowding out free time for a social life or some other reason, the clientele presents a tempting "captive audience." Even if the therapist is being completely honorable, if such a deal goes bad, the therapist runs the risk of damaging the therapeutic relationship, along with the risk of damaging his or her professional reputation.

Furthermore, the deal does not have to go bad for it to be a problem. The therapeutic relationship also depends on one level on belief—the belief that the process will help the client. Any other belief that gets interjected into the therapeutic relationship runs the risk of spoiling it.

Financial involvement with a client may also be a conflict of interest. The therapist clearly may stand to profit from selling products and other such financial dealings. This runs counter to the professional and ethical principle that the therapist is dedicated to the interests of the client and is the client's agent. Staying out of positions in which you have a conflict of interest ensures that you will not be tempted to act against your client's welfare or be unable to take actions that may advance your client's welfare. Even if you have nothing to gain, you need to be circumspect about suggestions you make to a client, because the client may follow your suggestion without thinking it through as clearly as if it came from another source. For example, a therapist might mention to a client that an investment in certain stocks will pay off big. If the client subsequently makes such an investment, then it raises the question of whether the client acted according to an informed decision based on extensive research ("due diligence") or simply because the therapist suggested it. If you find that you have made such a suggestion, perhaps inadvertently, you can always say to the client that he or she needs to think it through independently and not follow the suggestion simply because you made it.

The precariousness of the situation is magnified if the therapist stands to benefit. *The question that the therapist must be able to answer is whether he or she acted in the best interest of the client or in his/her own financial interest, thus presenting a conflict of interest.* Let's say the therapist sells over-the-counter nutritional supplements to a client. The therapist may believe with complete sincerity that the supplements will be beneficial to the client, the supplements complement the emphasis on health and self-empowerment the therapist has in his or her work, or selling products is a generally accepted business practice. However, another critical question is the following: Is this objective truth, or is this a rationalization by the therapist? Sometimes, it can be very hard to tell. Therefore, it is important for a therapist who decides to have any financial transactions with clients, other than receiving a fee for service, to carefully think through how to conduct this activity appropriately. Our opinion is that if there is any doubt, do not engage in the activity. Selling products is not worth the possibility of risking harm to or otherwise compromising your client's welfare, your professional integrity, or the integrity of your relationship with your client.

Before we close our discussion of financial boundaries, let's revisit the issue of consent. The dynamics of the therapeutic relationship make the therapist potentially so influential to the client that the client is much more likely to follow the therapist's suggestion, rather than make his or her own decision. This raises a question: If the client agrees to buy something from the therapist, has the client actually consented, or is the client assuming that he or she is dutifully following a therapeutic suggestion . . . or even being overpowered by the therapist?

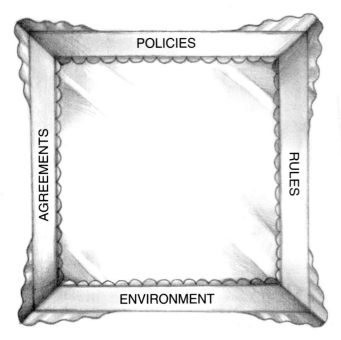

POLICIES

AGREEMENTS

RULES

ENVIRONMENT

Figure 4.5
The therapeutic frame acts as a
container. *The elements of the thera-*
peutic frame, such as policies, rules,
environment, and agreements form a
structure that protects and contains
the therapeutic process.

THE THERAPEUTIC FRAME

In the therapeutic relationship, the therapist is responsible for deciding and communicating what the "game rules" are for the process. We call these rules or boundaries collectively the **therapeutic frame** or *framework*. Smith and Fitzpatrick (1995) state that a therapeutic frame "defines a set of roles for the participants in the therapeutic process" and includes structural elements of the therapeutic work. This means that the therapeutic frame includes rules or policies for a variety of circumstances that one encounters while doing therapy, including all of the business and logistical issues such as payment, making appointments, cancellation policy, and responsibility for missed sessions; time issues such as being on time for sessions, lateness, ending on time; the environment of the working space; socializing with clients; telephone calls from the client to the therapist; the agreed-upon goals of the therapy; and the type or styles of massage therapy used. What constitutes the therapeutic frame profoundly influences the work that occurs because the therapeutic frame allows you to identify and deal with acting out and boundary issues in a forthright manner and also sets the tone for how boundary issues are dealt with.

Although establishing, supporting, and maintaining healthy boundaries are part of the frame, the frame is more than boundary policies and issues. If you think about a frame, it is a structure or border into which something—a door, a picture, or, in the case of therapy, a process—is set. In this sense, the therapeutic frame lays out a structure that contains and defines the therapeutic process. It delineates what will and what will not take place between client and therapist. By doing this, a well-defined and clear framework also provides security for the therapeutic process to unfold.

We live within frames more than we realize. Being part of a civil society, we tend to regulate our ways of living together with the help of a societal frame formed from laws, orders, and regulations. We also manage our interpersonal lives with a social frame formed from myriad cultural norms about social behavior. Such social frames are a vital function of cultural development. Considering the relevance of the frame in everyday life, we can see that frame components, such as recommendations, expectations, agreements, rules, and logistical management, would be a crucial part of any therapeutic management of relationships. *Managing the frame thereby becomes the crucial work of any therapy that involves relationship.*

Many massage therapists tend to resist creating a clear therapeutic frame, associating it or its components with being overly rigid, unkind, or burdensome. They also may want to avoid confrontation. If there are few or no rules, then confronting another person about a breach is less likely to become necessary. Creating a frame may also bring up self-esteem issues for the therapist. To create and enforce the rules that are part of the frame means that one is worth paying attention to, that one's time is valuable, and that one has authority. If a therapist does not believe these are true about him- or herself, or if the therapist has a personality or character structure that does not tolerate confrontation very well, he or she may be unwilling or afraid to hold the frame.

But the necessity of having a frame goes beyond providing rules, policies, or boundaries. It is absolutely *psychologically essential* for *both* client and therapist, especially when psychological issues come into the forefront. If there is no frame, there is no *containment* for the process; that is, there is no structure for keeping whatever happens in both the client's process and in therapy within the therapeutic process, rather than outside the therapeutic arena where it may be acted out without examination. Furthermore, by holding the frame, the therapist really is being considerate of the client by proactively preventing possible problems; this leads to a *better* therapeutic environment, *not* a harsher one. The frame ensures a safe therapeutic environment; that the environment is predictable, consistent, and focused on the client's process and needs; and that it is free from judgment, criticism, and physical and emotional harm and serving anyone else's needs other than the client's. Setting up a "tight" frame at the outset *prevents* future problems.

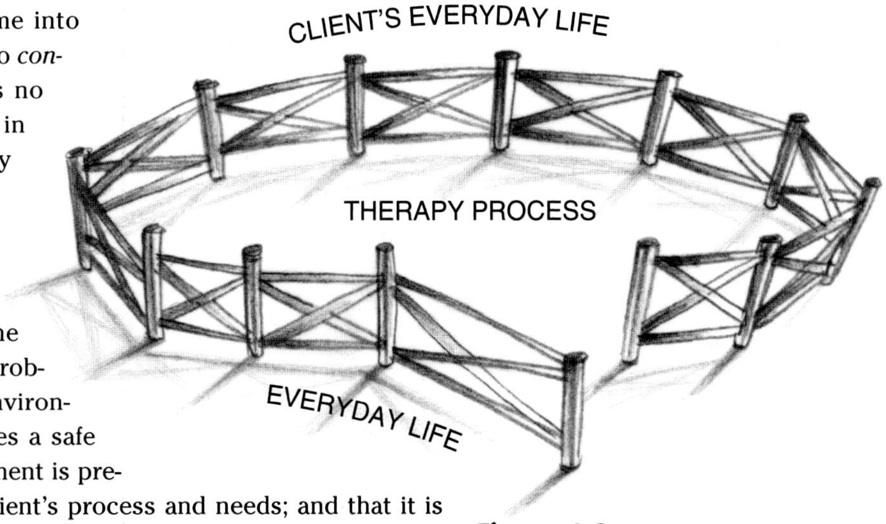

Figure 4.6
The therapeutic process. *In a sense, the therapeutic frame corrals what the therapy stirs up, so that it stays within the therapy process rather than acted out in the client's everyday life.*

Lack of a frame affects clients in different ways, depending on their character and personality. Some clients perceive unclear or unstated limits as permission. For example, when the massage therapist keeps allowing the massage session to extend beyond the time limit or has not included time issues in the frame, the client is going to assume this is normal and okay to do.

Other clients test unstated limits. For example, a massage therapist who sees us for supervision gave both her office and home telephone numbers to her clients. One Sunday morning she heard her phone ringing at 7 A.M. Thinking it was an emergency, she jumped out of bed and raced to the phone to pick it up. It was one of her clients wanting to clarify how to do an exercise the therapist had suggested to her a month ago. The therapist, who was speechless at first, politely gave the clarification and hung up. However, she was furious. The client had gone over a limit that the therapist did not anticipate she would need to state explicitly, assuming common social norms would be sufficient. She learned (the hard way, unfortunately) that whatever she did not state was part of her frame was open to being tested by a client. Each test from a client can be an opportunity to learn more about what might need to be framed therapeutically. For example, this therapist needed to state explicitly what hours she accepted calls, both at home and at the office, despite any assumptions about social norms.

Other clients expend energy trying to guess what the limits are, not knowing whether or not they have crossed them. In contrast, some clients do not ask for anything for fear that any request is too much. For this type of client, the frame is very important because it tells them how much they *can* ask for. This points out that the frame is not only about what one cannot do, but also what one *can* do. Without a frame established, it is difficult for clients to understand and respect your expectations for their behavior and for you to identify or contain it. This kind of misunderstanding about frames and enforcing them can bring to the surface the therapist's issues about consideration (you ought to know that going overtime is inconvenient to me); explicitly stating needs (we need to end now); and taking a stand (we must end now). Because many people entering the massage therapy profession are intuitive and can sense someone's needs before they are stated, they often expect this in return.

The framework also creates healthy limits for the therapist, thereby facilitating the process. The more clear the therapist is about the framing issues, the less likely the therapist will be to act out and meet his or her needs in an inappropriate manner. For example, if the therapist creates weak limits around money issues, he or she may be more likely to compensate for the financial lack of clarity by gaining remuneration by other means, such as selling clients unrelated products or involving them in pyramid schemes. Since the therapist subconsciously feels he or she is giving something away to clients, he or she may also feel entitled to a reward or self-compensation in some way. In a sense, the frame takes the guesswork out of what is okay or not okay and helps guard against acting out countertransference.

Here are some specific framework issues that you should clarify for yourself and your clients related to money, time, telephone calls, appointments, office environment, and process issues. We have purposely put these points in the form of questions, rather than statements, so that you can explore and think through each one, and then use your responses to form your own policies. You also may want to use the following as a checklist or to create one.

Money issues:

- ▶ How much do you charge as your fee?
- ▶ Do you feel you are charging what your services are worth?
- ▶ What are you basing the worth of your service on?
- ▶ Are you willing to take an IOU if your client cannot pay?
- ▶ How do you feel about a sliding scale in which some clients pay you less?
- ▶ How do you feel if someone says they cannot afford you? What do you do about such a situation?
- ▶ Do you feel you should subsidize someone else's health care by lowering your own fees?
- ▶ What is your policy on payment being made on time? What if a payment is late?
- ▶ Are you willing to make payment plans or arrangements?
- ▶ Would you make a verbal agreement regarding payment or would you make an agreement as a written contract?
- ▶ Do you accept checks or credit cards?
- ▶ What is your policy on bounced checks?
- ▶ What is your policy when someone forgets to bring cash or a check?
- ▶ How do you feel about bartering?
- ▶ When do you want to be paid? At the beginning of a session? At the end of a session? Upon presentation of an invoice?
- ▶ If you travel to your client's location, do you include your travel time and expenses in your fee?
- ▶ Do you accept gifts?

Time issues:

- ▶ Do you have a policy on starting the session time at the beginning of the hour whether or not the client is present or do you "start the clock" when the client arrives?
- ▶ Do you end sessions on time?
- ▶ If you allow sessions to run over, do you charge for the extra time? If so, do you ask the client if it is okay to run over?
- ▶ How far would you allow the session to run over?
- ▶ Does your hour include or not include the time your client uses to discuss anything at the beginning of the session, undressing, dressing, paying, making another appointment, or leaving?
- ▶ How do you feel about your client hanging around the waiting room after the session?

Telephone call issues:

▶ Do you accept calls without limits? If you do have some limitations, what are they?

▶ Do you accept phone calls only within certain hours?

▶ Do you limit what the subject or content of telephone calls can be on either your part or the client's?

▶ How do you deal with initial phone calls? Do you mainly stick to determining a mutually workable time, giving directions to your location, and basic information or do you engage in longer discussion? What would you discuss and not discuss?

▶ Do you charge for telephone consultation time? If you do, are there any conditions, such as you charge only if phone calls are over a certain length, or if they are on a subject other than appointment logistics?

Appointment issues:

▶ Do you require advance notice for cancellations? How far ahead?

▶ What happens if someone cancels without adequate notice?

▶ Do you charge for missed appointments?

▶ Do you make any accommodation for emergencies in your cancellation policy?

▶ Do you make any other exceptions to your cancellation policies? If yes, how do you determine whether an excuse is acceptable?

▶ How much notice do you give to regular clients if you are going to be out of town?

▶ What happens if *you* miss an appointment?

▶ Are there times of the day or week that you will not make appointments? Do you make exceptions?

▶ Do you try to provide regular times for your clients to the extent possible—for example, 2 P.M. every Tuesday—or do you set up appointments on different days of the week or times of the day?

Office environment issues:

▶ If you work in an office in your home, how do you feel about working out of your home? Is there a room in your home dedicated to your practice (which is used exclusively for massage)? Does your office area have any separate facilities, such as an entrance or a bathroom? Do you have any policies specifically for your home office, such as where a client may or may not enter, or may or may not park?

▶ Have you given any thought to how your office is arranged in terms of how it affects the therapeutic situation?

▶ Do you do outcalls, that is, come to the client's location?

▶ If you do outcalls, what do you ask of your client about the conditions of the working space?

▶ How far would you be willing to go to accommodate a client's request to change your office environment because of a special need? For example, would you not wear perfume, remove or change certain items that a client considers unhealthful, or buy certain items a client says he or she needs?

▶ How do you dress while you are working?

▶ Do you display your license, diploma(s), national certification certificate, association membership certificate, training certificates of completion, or awards?

▶ Do you display personal objects in your office, such as family photos, or do you refrain from doing so out of concern for stimulating clients' projections about you?

Process issues:

▶ Do you allow sessions to be interrupted by anything, such as phone calls, a client in the waiting room, a salesperson knocking on the door?

▶ Do you have a confidentiality policy? Do you mention it to clients? Do you explain it? How strictly do you maintain it? Have you ever said anything outside of a session about something said or done during a session? Do you have a permission form for clients to sign if you need to release information to another party?

▶ Do you have a policy about clients in your practice being aware of each other? Do you make an effort to control contact between clients in your waiting room and treatment room? How would you respond to one client asking you about another client in your practice, for example, if a client asks the name or occupation of the previous client whom he has seen leaving as he entered?

▶ Do you stay within the scope of practice of your work and your ability?

▶ Do you or did you have any dual relationships with clients in your practice? What policies do you have to avoid entangling relationships?

▶ How often do you refer to yourself (self-referencing) during your sessions? Whom are your self-references intended to benefit?

▶ Are there circumstances that would cause you to terminate a session? If so, which ones? Do you inform clients in advance about these, or do so when they occur?

▶ What is your philosophy or policy about selling products or services (other than massage) to your clients?

▶ What is your philosophy or policy about working on relatives?

Finally, here are some questions about framework issues and policies in general:

▶ At what point do you make your policies clear to the client?

▶ Do you require your client to agree to these conditions, or do you make them a negotiable condition of proceeding?

▶ Do you make this agreement verbally, on paper, or both?

▶ Do you make this agreement in the form of a contract or in another way?

What should a therapist do if the client does not follow a framework policy? First, framework policies must be upheld in some way. If a policy is not going to be upheld, dropping or revising it should be considered. The therapist who ignores the disregarding of a policy is sending a message that the specific policy is not important and that all the other policies the therapist has may not be important either. This weakens and may eventually undermine the therapeutic framework, harms the therapeutic relationship, damages mutual trust, and subtly makes the client less secure. For example, if the therapist lets the client slide on paying for sessions, this can lead to mistrust because the client learns that he or she cannot fully depend on what the therapist says, even when the loosening of the frame seems to be an advantage for the client.

Furthermore, framework policies that are poorly formed or not upheld can become fodder for resistance and a battleground for negative transference. This allows the therapeutic process to become chaotic and embroiled in emotional issues.

For example, the massage therapist may extend a favor to a client and—despite a policy requiring payment at the close of each session—may allow a payment to be missed or even waived. The therapist may expect the client to feel grateful for this favor, but instead the client may interpret the action to mean that the payment policy is unimportant to the therapist. The client may be so unaware of the policy's importance that he or she may even pay (another therapist) for another type of massage to sample it or may purchase an expensive item and come in and tell the therapist about it before paying the balance due. This can create resentment in the therapist, followed by guilt when trying to enforce the policy later. An argument can ensue if the client demands an explanation for the therapist's eventual demand to be paid, or the client may act out by not showing up for the next session or canceling it at the last moment. Not clearly establishing and upholding a policy on payment results in emotional conflict and argument that weakens the therapeutic alliance between the therapist and client.

Ensuring the client's consent to the therapeutic frame is vital. To do this, review the frame carefully with each new client at the outset. After going over your policies, ask the client something like, "Do you have any questions about my policies?" This allows some time to ensure as best you can that the client understands the policies. Then, receiving the client's explicit agreement to your policies is important. A simple way to do this is to directly ask the client something like, "Do you agree to these policies?" If a problem related to upholding the policies arises later, you can then return to the fact that the client agreed to it, rather than something you have just imposed. By doing this, you will have prepared the ground for appropriately upholding your frame policies if and when you need to. Some therapists, taking the idea of acknowledgment and consent one step further, ask the client to sign a document detailing their agreement.

If the problem is a misunderstanding, referring the client to the initial discussion of policies usually helps. However, if the problem arises from the client's difficulty with entitlement issues or boundaries or the client's character structure, explaining that the client has agreed to the rules may not have as much impact because the underlying issue is something that is more emotional and irrational in nature. In such a situation, the fact that the client agreed to the rules will not prevent the client from trying to do whatever to get what he or she wants, even if it means irrationally maintaining that the prior agreement is irrelevant. In this case, *you must hold firm*. This may be difficult because such a situation often involves manipulation that may "hook" you emotionally. Remembering that the frame serves a positive purpose for both therapist and client may be helpful, especially in difficult moments. This is illustrated in the following scenarios. The first scenario illustrates the type of situation in which a hidden motive underlies a client's not following a policy.

Scenario One: Monty

Monty, a client, forgets to bring his checkbook. The exchange takes place at the close of the session. We assume that Monty is not simply being deceitful to get massages without paying.

Monty: I forgot my checkbook.

Therapist: Would you like to drop a check in the mail or bring it next week, Monty?

Monty: Okay, sure.

Next session.

Monty: I forgot my checkbook.

Therapist: I hear you forgot it, but paying me on the day of service is really important as we agreed when we started. Would you please drop a check for these past two sessions in the mail today?

Monty: To tell you the truth, I wasn't really happy with the last massage. My leg didn't stop hurting and it felt sore.

Scenario One: Monty

Therapist: I need to talk about a couple things. First, I understand that your leg didn't stop hurting and that you may have expected the massage to make the pain go away completely. However, your leg needs more than one or two massages before it will feel noticeably different. Your body needs the time and additional massage. Second, my policy about paying at each session is still in effect. It doesn't change based on the results of each session.

Monty: I need to think about what you said.

Therapist: Good. I'm hearing that you may not have understood before now that massage is a process rather than something that fixes a problem right away . . . however, I still need to uphold my payment policy. Can I expect to receive your check in the mail before the next session?

Monty: Okay. What about my next session?

Therapist: We can set up a time now, or you can give me a call after you've thought about it and then we'll look into setting up another session.

Here is another scenario that is a common problem for massage therapists and illustrates how clear the frame needs to be. The massage therapist in the scenario customarily leaves the last 5 minutes of the appointment for the client to get dressed, briefly discuss the session, if needed, make future appointments, and leave.

Scenario Two: Shawna

The client, Shawna, is still lying on the table with 5 minutes left in the hour.

Therapist: I need to let you know that it is time to end.

Shawna: But it's not the end of the hour yet. It's only 3:54.

Therapist: As I explained when I went over my policies with you, the hour includes 5 minutes at the end so you can get dressed and we can end. That allows me to begin each client's session on the hour. I know from my experience that this works best for everyone. For example, then I can be ready for you when you come in for your session.

Shawna: Okay, but I wish I knew that before.

Therapist: I can understand how you feel. That's why I always discuss my policies during the first session.

Shawna: Okay, you did do that.

If this is a misunderstanding, this explanation will probably be sufficient. If it is an entitlement issue, i.e., if the client feels a full hour is something she deserves or has an inherent right to receive, then she may resist and possibly manipulate. The therapist still needs to stand ground, *even if it means risking losing the client. If the therapist does not stand ground, it is almost certain that problems will continue to surface*, as illustrated in the next scenario of this case study.

In the following scenario, the client, Mario, who has an entitlement issue (someone who feels he is entitled to or deserves extra attention or special treatment), is disputing that the hour includes some time to finish up after the massage is over. In contrast to the previous scenario with Shawna, Mario is more resistant.

Scenario Three: Mario

Mario: Hey, you stopped before the hour was up. Look, if I pay for an hour, I expect a full hour.

Therapist: Mario, I made my policy clear at the beginning of our first session, which is the massage portion of the session ends 5 minutes before the hour is up. The time it takes you to dress and get ready to leave is part of the hour.

Mario: Well, I've been to other therapists who gave me a real hour.

Therapist: I understand that someone else might have a different policy, but this is my policy. I have found from experience that it works fairly because it makes it possible for me to be ready and on time for each client.

Mario: Well, maybe I'll just go back to one of them.

Therapist: That's your option. I don't want you to leave, but it's your choice if you don't want to follow the policies we agreed on.

Mario: But the other therapists are out of state where I used to live!

Therapist: I would be glad to give you the names of other massage therapists in this area.

Mario: Do they give real full hours?

Therapist: I don't know. Each massage therapist has their own policies. You'll need to discuss it with them.

At this point the client may say:

Mario: I'd like those names.

Or, alternatively the client may say:

Mario: But I think you do good work and you're convenient for me to get to.

Therapist: I would be glad to continue to work with you, but I need you to agree to my policies, including the one about the hour. My policies allow me to conduct my practice in such a way that I can continue to offer my best service to my clients.

Mario: Okay, I can go along with it.

Therapist: Good, would you like to set up your next appointment now?

There *is* some risk that the client may stop coming if you uphold a policy. It is important that you accept this possibility and understand that the frame is part of the process, just as much as the techniques and the massage table you use are. Just as you cannot work without them, you cannot work effectively without a frame. A final consideration is whether you would want or be able to effectively work with a person who is not willing to agree to your frame. In this situation, the client not coming back may be an acceptable outcome.

Eventually, the final frame issue that arises is ending therapy. This may be the most anxiety-provoking phase of therapy to deal with. The massage therapist may feel very uncomfortable talking to a client about this when it comes up, feeling that he or she is being unprofessional, pushy, or invasive—trying to "sell themselves" or "overcome the client's objections." Termination of a relationship also can bring up feelings about rejection, or separation, which a person may want to avoid at all costs. The number of factors that affect how and when someone should leave further complicates the situation. The challenge for the massage therapist in dealing with the ending of therapy is determining: (1) whether questioning the client's decision to end is appropriate; (2) if it is appropriate, then, to what extent the therapist can question the client's decision to end; and, (3) whether the client's reasons for ending are warranted or a form of resistance to the work.

In the frame of psychotherapy, it is generally considered appropriate, even necessary, to examine carefully the reasons a client gives for leaving before the client actually leaves, because anxiety and other factors arising during therapy may cause a client to want to quit. In other words, the client's wish to leave may be a form of acting out or resistance and needs to be dealt with accordingly. In some cases, the desire to quit is a way for the client to bring up certain issues, such as negative feelings. Sometimes, a client's wanting to quit brings out issues that lead to a spurt of progress because these were issues that were causing the process to be stuck. *In contrast, the massage therapist does not have a contractual permission to delve into some of these emotional areas. Doing so may even be outside the scope of practice.*

Given the limitations a massage therapist may have in dealing with a client leaving, strategies that differ from those traditional in psychotherapy need to be used. Three factors that come into play are the context of the work, the motivation of the client, and the commitment of the client. The context of the therapy may dictate how massage therapy ends. Massage therapy, in some cases, is contracted on a session-by-session basis and has open-ended goals. Unless there is a very specific treatment plan, there may be no agreement to a certain number of sessions, specified goal, or end point. Furthermore, massage is often done with experiential goals, rather than progressive ones. For example, the client may want to feel relaxed at the end of a session, so that the goal is the same for each session, rather than seeking to work toward a result over a span of several sessions or time. In this context, the ending could come anytime and probably is based primarily on the client's subjective perspective.

However, in some cases, massage therapy does have specific goals that the client and therapist have agreed upon. They may have estimated or specified the number of sessions needed to reach that goal. In this context, the ending is likely to be discussed at specific points in time during the course of therapy. If the massage therapist does primarily long-term work with clients, he or she may need to state at the beginning that occasionally the client might want to leave before the work has been fully effective or completed. In that case, the therapist may want to ask the client to agree to come for one or two more sessions after a notification to end so that there is a cushion of time to consider the decision and to have closure if the therapy does end.

People also have very different motivations for coming for massage therapy. It may be to feel better, manage stress, maintain health, heal a muscle strain, have more energy, or explore personal development and growth. The client's motivation clearly relates to his or her goals, and the goals influence the client's expectation of how many massage sessions to be coming for and how willing the client is to work through difficult or challenging aspects of the process.

Depending on their motivation, clients also have differing degrees of commitment. As massage therapists, we need to keep in mind that not everyone is as committed to massage therapy as a process as we are. For some people, massage therapy may be only a phase in their lives, something new to try, or viewed as a nonessential luxury. People interested in sampling the smorgasbord of change and growth often move on, no matter how good the work is. For them, there is always something new, better, or more enlightening around the next corner. In any event, noticing any gap between a client's motivation and commitment can be helpful. If a client's motivation is personal growth, but his or her commitment is to come once a month for 6 months, the incompatibility of the commitment to the motivation is really a problem that is better to deal with at the beginning, rather than at the end.

In evaluating whether or not to discuss the client's reasons for ending, the therapist needs to ask him- or herself the following questions:

▶ What was the client's original motive for coming for massage therapy?

▶ Has this motive changed during the course of our work?

▶ What is the client's commitment to the process? If you do not know, then what does the client's motivation imply about what the commitment could be?

▶ Is the client's motivation consistent with the commitment? For example, if a client is coming for massage therapy once a month to feel good, the commitment may be minor. On the other hand, if a client is a 57-year-old who is coming for maintaining health, then the commitment is probably ongoing.

▶ Is there a specific agreed upon goal? Has that goal been met? If so, is there another goal that needs to be negotiated?

▶ Was a specific number of sessions estimated or discussed?

▶ Are there any other relevant contextual questions that need to be considered?

The preceding questions are intended to help you bring up what needs to be considered in reaching a decision. We would like to provide specific directions on how to decide whether or not to question a client's reasons for leaving, but in truth we cannot because ultimately the therapist's judgment is required. Essentially, the breadth, depth, and gravity of these issues, which vary for each client, determine what is appropriate. If, for example, the therapist is doing sports massage as a maintenance regimen, it is difficult to confront reasons such as, "I don't have time," "I can't afford it," or "I think I'll try something else and see if that works better or faster." However, if the massage therapist is doing sports massage as part of a rehabilitation program, this frame may allow the therapist to have more leeway in addressing the issue of ending. The fact that rehabilitation might not yet be complete, and the client may not yet have reached full functionality, gives the therapist more cause.

A much more difficult situation is one in which emotional release has taken place or a client has chosen to share psychologically sensitive personal material in relation to the massage work. It is possible that a client may want to leave because he or she feels threatened, either consciously or unconsciously, by what is coming to the surface or otherwise into awareness. In this situation, the massage therapist has to walk a fine line. The therapist may say to the client that his or her impression is that the emotional material coming up in massage may be influencing the client's decision to leave. The therapist may ask the client whether he or she has a psychotherapist or another form of appropriate support to help or work through the material. For example, the massage therapist may say something like, "In my experience, when someone has had a strong emotional experience in massage, has been revealing lots of psychological material, or is experiencing thoughts and feelings breaking through into awareness, he may feel scared, overwhelmed, or awkward and suddenly want to leave, probably believing that leaving will allow things to calm down. What is really important is that you have continued support to help you work through this material. Are you seeing a psychotherapist? Another reason I am asking is, as a massage therapist, I am not qualified to help you delve into and analyze the underlying emotional issues that may be happening for you. You can do this with your/a psychotherapist, though. Based on what you discover, you may or may not want to continue massage therapy." Note that this statement presents important information in a neutral manner to the client without trying to get them to stay, which could be a self-serving motive.

An announcement that a client wants to leave can bring up feelings of rejection, self-doubt, low self-esteem, resentment, sadness, or neediness for the massage therapist, sometimes even when the departure is expected and appropriate. How a massage therapist feels about and then deals with a client's termination may be related to how he or she deals with people leaving in general, outside of therapy. If a client ending therapy has a serious emotional impact on the therapist, the therapist should discuss it with a supervisor, psychotherapist, mentor, or trusted peer.

Depending on the nature of the therapist's practice, a client's departure also can have a negative impact on the therapist's livelihood. We encourage massage therapists to think through how to deal with the financial fluctuations resulting from clients coming and going. If the therapist does not have financial affairs in order, then the therapist may be susceptible to influencing the client not to leave in order to serve his or her need for monetary security.

Therapeutic frames and boundaries are not always bent or broken by the client. *Sometimes the therapist violates his or her own boundaries and frame.* Following are some of the warning signs a massage therapist is slipping on boundary and frame issues.

▶ Believing an exception is justified because it will help the client's progress—an "emotional rescue"; it almost always backfires
▶ Allowing relationship entanglements to develop, particularly "sticky" dual relationships
▶ Developing a sense that a particular client is "special," which justifies making exceptions
▶ Not collecting fees in a timely manner, for example, doing so "in exchange" for favors provided by the client
▶ Giving physical expressions of affection without permission or in an inappropriate manner, such as hugs that are a bit too tight or linger a bit too long
▶ Dressing or behaving in a way calculated to be attractive to a particular client
▶ Making flirtatious comments, for example, about a client's dress or physical features
▶ Interjecting sexually oriented words, phrases, or comments into conversation with a client
▶ Sloppy draping, uncovering more than should be
▶ Working closer than normal to areas of the body ethically restricted from being touched
▶ Being lax with a client's privacy, such as leaving a door slightly open while the client is undressing or placing a mirror in the dressing area where the reflection can be seen from elsewhere
▶ Locking doors that usually are not locked during other clients' sessions to provide (consciously or unconsciously) possible concealment, rather than privacy
▶ Minimizing or not caring about the effect of a lax boundary or frame, which may be an indication of burnout, stress, or distraction by a personal problem or crisis

The therapist should consider such violations or slips as calling attention to an issue or problem that the therapist needs to think about and work on. These often reveal that the underlying problems are (1) countertransference issues, that is, the therapist is not getting needs met personally or professionally in some way, or (2) the boundaries and frame are poorly designed, unclear, confusing, or not upheld properly.

Dealing with frame and boundary issues can be thorny, and ensuring that our own motivations are not coloring our judgment of our behavior as therapists is challenging. Professional isolation is our enemy when it comes to such issues. When unsure about these matters, supervision or consultation with trusted colleagues is of great importance and is an important step in ensuring that our actions are in each client's best interest and not self-serving for us or in some other way exploitative or harmful (see Chapter 3 for a discussion on seeking supervision). The line between the two is not always clear.

Here are a couple examples of differentiating between serving the client and being self-serving. Time issues are a common frame component, such as ending a session on time. Compare and contrast, for instance, allowing a session to run over the allotted time for a client who is clearly in an emergency situation and needs immediate assistance versus spending increasing amounts of session time with a client who is particularly attractive to you and even scheduling sessions at the end of the day so that you will not be disturbed by other clients arriving for their sessions.

Self-disclosure is another common frame issue, namely, that the therapist refrains from discussing personal information about the therapist with the client, thus keeping the focus on the client. Compare and contrast sharing with a client who has suffered a great loss about a personal tragedy you overcame with assistance despite feeling at first you could not recover from it versus sharing with an attractive client about the difficulties you are having in your marriage and how unsympathetic your spouse is to the many stresses you are under. Here is a brief aside about self-disclosure: disclosure by the therapist has transference as well as countertransference ramifications. A certain amount of self-disclosure reduces fantasizing about the therapist by the client, whereas overdisclosure feeds into it. A sound balance in disclosure—not too much, not too little—is ideal.

To help guide you in decision-making when confronted with ethical dilemmas involving boundaries and frame issues, you can ask yourself questions such as these:

▶ Will taking this action help my client?
▶ Will taking this action exploit or harm my client? Are there any other adverse consequences that might result? Could anyone else be harmed?
▶ Is this course of action consistent with our therapeutic agreement or contract and frame and with the client's expectations of me and of massage therapy?
▶ Am I being dishonest or deceptive toward my client or anyone else by acting in this way?
▶ Am I treating this client differently from others, either negatively or positively?
▶ Have I adequately addressed my self-care or could my failing to do so impair my judgment and decision-making?
▶ Whose needs are being met?
▶ What would my colleagues think if they knew about this?
▶ Does this action meet the standards of the profession?
▶ Will this action create an inappropriate dependence on the massage therapy, or on me, or will it help promote an appropriate level of dependence or independence for my client?
▶ Am I imposing my values upon my client?

In the next chapter we will explore the basis of the psychology of the body—the connection between mind and body.

REFERENCES

Gray, A. (1994). *An introduction to the therapeutic frame.* London: Routledge.

Hunter, M. & Struve, J. (1997). *The ethical use of touch in psychotherapy.* Thousand Oaks, CA: Sage Publications.

Katherine, A. (1993). *Boundaries: Where you end and I begin.* New York: Parkside Publishing.

Lazarus, A. & Zur, O. (2002). *Dual relationships and psychotherapy.* New York: Springer.

May, J. (2002). *Explorations in ethics for body psychotherapists.* St. Louis: Self-published.

Smith, D. & Fitzpatrick, M. (1995). Boundary issues: An integrative review of theory and research. *Professional Psychology: Research and Practice, 25* (5), 499–506.

Smith, E., Clance, P.R. & Imes, S., eds. (2001). *Touch in psychotherapy.* New York: Guilford Press.

Taylor, K. (1995). *The ethics of caring.* Santa Cruz, CA: Hanford Mead Publishers.

Wolberg, L. (1995). *The technique of psychotherapy.* New York: Jason Aronson.

The Bodymind Connection

Chapter 5

Akey principle of the psychology of the body is that *the mind and body are interconnected: whatever goes on in the mind is reflected in the body and whatever goes on in the body is reflected in the mind*. Therefore, touch affects not only the conscious mind, but also the *unconscious* mind. We often conceptualize the unconscious as some kind of vague bubble located in some unspecified place in the ether. However, if we think about it carefully, the unconscious also must be located in the *body*, not only the mind.

In other words, we generally understand that the conscious mind is connected to and part of the nervous system, and the nervous system exists in the entire body, not only in the head. Building on this concept, since the unconscious mind is using essentially the same physical pathways, then the unconscious mind is also located in the body. Furthermore, as we accept the idea that the mind and body are interconnected and the mind and body reflect each other and as we also accept that the mind has conscious and unconscious components, then we can conclude that the unconscious mind is also connected to the body. In this chapter, we explore the bodymind connection: what it is, how it develops, and why it is important for massage therapists to acknowledge, understand, and respect.

AN EXPERIENTIAL EXPLORATION OF THE BODYMIND CONNECTION

Later in this chapter, we provide an extensive description of the bodymind connection. Reading about it will help you to understand it intellectually, but it won't help you to

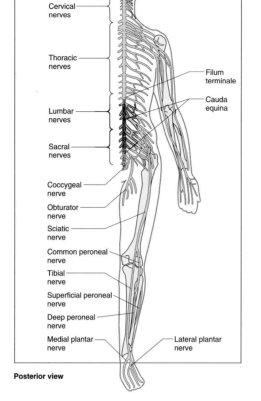

Anterior view

Posterior view

Figure 5.1

The nervous system net. *The nervous system forms a web that interconnects the entire body. It is not merely centered in the head by itself.* (From Willis MC: *Medical Terminology: The Language of Health Care.* Baltimore, Williams & Wilkins, 1996.)

acknowledge the workings of the bodymind connection in your own being and in your day-to-day life. Thus, we provide some exercises that should help you to experience the bodymind connection directly, in a way that follows common sense. We encourage you to perform each of these exercises with careful and thoughtful introspection as you proceed through the section. After all, the key to the search for ways to help others is knowing yourself first and best. *These exercises are in italics to let them stand out from the rest of the text in the following paragraphs.*

We all carry some tension. Some of it is necessary to maintain posture and carry out other physical functions. However, most people have more tension than is necessary to simply carry out physical functions. *Take a moment to focus on your shoulders. Are they tense at all? Do the same with your neck. Is your neck tense at all? Do the same with your forehead. Is your forehead tense at all?* In this experiment, nearly everyone finds some tension in some part of the body that has nothing to do with performing or sustaining any required physical activity.

Now let's try something a bit different. *Raise your arm overhead. Now raise your arm again, but this time focus on the amount of effort this action requires. See if you become aware of any overuse: are you using more effort or energy than is needed to accomplish this simple action?* This experiment shows that we tend to override the body's natural way of movement, which requires only the amount of effort it takes to complete the desired action, and substitute a tenser way of movement. This substituted pattern is our *characteristic* pattern. We return to the idea of a characteristic pattern when we discuss armoring and character in later chapters, but it is fundamental to our understanding of the bodymind connection.

Now a critical question: Why do we substitute a characteristic pattern that actually is less efficient than a natural pattern? It is not our muscles' fault. The nervous system controls the voluntary muscles; in other words, muscular activity or tension is translated from nervous activity or tension. *Let's try another experiment. Raise your arm overhead again. This time, be as aware as you can of the overuse. Now try raising your arm overhead again, but this time relax your muscles and raise your arm so it takes the least amount of effort.* This experiment shows how eliminating excess tension through conscious awareness is possible. This same idea could be extended to daily activities and movement. Interestingly, this is what many therapies do essentially, especially somatic education methods, such as Alexander Technique, the Feldenkrais Method, Trager Mentastics, Rolf Movement Therapy, Aston Patterning, and Body Mind Centering.

Let's try another type of experiment to demonstrate the bodymind connection while drawing on a common experience. *Imagine yourself driving in congested traffic, such as during rush hour. Give yourself a moment to get into the feeling of it. How tightly are you gripping the steering wheel? Now take a moment to focus on tension in your shoulders . . . then your jaw. Note any tension you feel.* You will likely notice that you use your muscles in ways that are not needed simply for driving, making a much greater effort than necessary. This triggering of muscular tension may happen whether or not you are conscious of it. Indeed, people are often not conscious of it.

What about the connection between the *unconscious mind* and the body? This calls for a somewhat different sort of experiment. *Give yourself some time to fully sense these. Think back to some time in the past, which could be the very recent past or farther back in time. How did you react when you were angry? Then do the same with other feelings: frightened . . . humiliated . . . frustrated . . . nervous . . . or pressured?* You may notice that your heightened emotions cause an unconscious increase in tension (although because of our instructions, you may be conscious of them). Usually, people report that their tension increases in the shoulders, face, upper torso, and/or jaw, and it results in shallower breathing. You also may have noticed your responses have something to do with emotions.

Let's take our experiment one step farther. Sometimes we have an unconscious fear of expressing our emotions in a natural way. *Again, give yourself enough time to fully sense these. Let your mind wander back in time again to past emotional events. This time, go back to events that took place when you were a child. Notice how your parents or other adults who took care of you handled your natural expressions of emotions, such as anger, sadness, fear, and joy. Taking one of these emotions at a time, how did you respond with your body to their responses or actions?* We know from doing this experiment with many participants in workshops that emotional responses deemed inappropriate were often suppressed with a slap, cold stare, threat, or a discouraging or critical verbal response. In essence, such responses amount to the withdrawal or threatened withdrawal of love, whereas responses deemed as acceptable are rewarded. If you responded as did many others who have done this experiment, then you also unconsciously used your body as a shield of protection by tensing your muscles, altering your breathing, masking your facial expression, or changing your posture to a more closed, controlled, defensive attitude. This shift likely changed your outer emotional expression and inner feeling. *Now take a moment to shake out and release any residual tension from the exercises, take some full breaths, and relax a bit before going on.*

The patterns of tension and emotional reactions to life situations are determined early in life. The catch is that although such reactions may be intended to provide some measure of protection, they are not the best for coping with stress later in life. For example, burdened shoulders can lead to chronic soreness, along with an inability to say no. A collapsed chest may conserve energy and protect the heart emotionally, but may lead to feeling depressed and having low energy.

We are conditioned from infancy to think of certain feelings as bad and dangerous because they get us into trouble with the persons we are dependent on and to whom we want to be and feel close. Box 5.1 lists some of the phrases parents use to let children know what not to feel. Such feelings come to be seen as the enemies of good relations, and we end up internally afraid of or threatened by such feelings . . . *our own feelings.* These are the feelings that end up getting rejected and defended against.

What do we do when we feel emotions, but do not want them perceived? We engage in subtle—or not so subtle—tensing of the muscles that would express these

Box 5.1

EVERYDAY STATEMENTS THAT TELL CHILDREN FEELINGS ARE BAD AND DANGEROUS

The following are some "classic" statements parents and other care-givers often make to children. Although they may be well intentioned, such statements can convey the message that the child's feelings are somehow unacceptable to the caregiver.

▶ Don't let me hear you say you hate your baby brother/sister!
▶ If you can't say something nice, don't say it at all!
▶ You shouldn't feel discouraged about it!
▶ Don't feel bad; things will get better!
▶ There's nothing to be afraid of!
▶ Keep a stiff upper lip!
▶ Hold your temper young lady/man!
▶ You'd better swallow your pride!
▶ That doesn't *really* hurt, does it?
▶ Stop crying or I'll give you something to cry about!
▶ You should be ashamed!
▶ I don't care what you think/feel/want/know/believe!

Feel free to add your own past messages that you heard when you were a child to the list.

Emotion versus Feeling

The words **emotion** and **feeling** are often used interchangeably in the English language. However, when these words are used in the context of the bodymind, we like to make a distinction between them that is not necessarily apparent when looking in a dictionary. A feeling involves awareness or consciousness, which is an internal event. An emotion involves the expression of a feeling, which is an external event. We make this distinction because it is possible to be emotional without being feeling, that is to say, a person can express anger, sadness, fear, or joy without consciously experiencing—feeling—these emotions. Sometimes, an emotional person is not a very feeling person. Conversely, a person can be feeling without being emotional. A person can be angry or sad without showing it outwardly.

When we use emotion and feeling in this book, we are usually making this distinction between them. For example, in the text, we used the sentence, "Blocked emotions and feelings are held, stored in the body as muscular tension." We purposely used both words—not to be repetitive, but to indicate that both emotions *and* feelings can be blocked. We say this not to be doctrinaire, but to point out and use the nuances of these two words.

emotions. In other words, *muscle tension is used in the conscious suppression of emotion* (Gross and Levenson). While we are still very young, we learn that it works—we succeed in suppressing the emotions, neither feeling, expressing, nor showing them. In this sense, *we are all deceivers*. If we are afraid to cry, we learn muscular actions that block the expression of crying, such as diaphragmatic tension, and muscular actions that conceal the expression, such as tensing muscles around the mouth, throat, and eyes. If we are afraid to strike out, we may inhibit muscles that produce a hitting movement, such as the pectoralis major, deltoid, and tricep, and tense opposing muscles such as the rhomboids to resist any forward arm swinging movement. In this way, tension is used to help us cope by stopping and hiding responses that could get us into trouble or otherwise lead to unwanted consequences.

Furthermore, once we learn such patterns, we use them characteristically, that is, each time the target emotion is triggered. Eventually, these patterned responses typically become unconscious, so they take place without our knowing it. In other words, *muscle tension also is used in the chronic (unconscious) repression of emotion* (Weinberger).

Thus, *a conscious, learned response progresses to an unconscious, involuntary habitual pattern*. The resulting emotional repression, postural changes, and muscular tension turn into pain, and possibly stress, which can cause someone to turn up for massage or to seek psychotherapy!

In summary, each response to stress involves an increase in muscular tension. Blocked **emotions** and **feelings** are held, stored in the body as muscular tension. When the muscles are tense in this way, the natural energy flow is blocked too. This is the basis of the slang term, "uptight." A person who unconsciously blocks a great deal of emotion and feeling gets uptight.

CHARACTERIZING THE BODYMIND CONNECTION

The idea that the body and the mind are interconnected is the fundamental principle of body-oriented psychology. This literally entails that the activity of the mind is reflected in the body and the activity of the body is reflected in the mind. In the past, Western religion, philosophy, and science have tended to split the body and mind, seeing the mind as dominant over the body and relegating the body to an inferior—even servile—position. This **mind-body split**—meaning to see the body and mind as separate entities—characterizes the mind and body as antagonists, usually with the mind attempting to control a crude, instinctive entity that, if unrestrained, could endanger the individual. A common saying expressing this condition is "mind over matter."

One result of this attitude in most Western cultures, including in the United States, is that many people are unaware of what their bodies are expressing. The following case study is an example.

Clint

We were leading a workshop on reading the body, in which we look at the correlation between the physical and emotional structures of the bodymind. During the part of the workshop in which we discuss what we call "body splits"—discrepancies in the emotional expression of two different areas of the body—we were observing Clint, who had volunteered.

Clint was outwardly a very mild-mannered, quiet-spoken man. When we, along with the group, observed Clint (he was wearing only swim trunks to aid observation), Clint's front side looked soft and his facial expression very meek. The overall group response to the front half of his body could be summed up as, "We see you as a friendly, big Teddy Bear."

Then we asked Clint to turn around, so we could look at his back half. The feeling in the room changed. Clint's back was very muscular and tense, and his back appeared to be bristling. Looking at Clint's back half, the overall group response was, "We see you as angry." At this point, Clint turned around, and with a grin, said, "I'm not angry, I hardly ever get angry." We asked Clint to turn around so he had his back to us again and we could not see his face (and be deflected by his friendly facial expression). The group repeated several times, "We see you as angry." This time, still with his back turned to the group, Clint bellowed, "Angry, I'M NOT ANGRY!"

After a brief moment of silence, the group, Clint included, spontaneously broke into laughter—the sort of laughter that happens when everyone comes to a realization. Besides demonstrating how a body split shows contrary expressions in two areas of the body, the point about "putting your feelings behind you" so you are not aware of a feeling had been made.

The mind-body split may also be reflected in attitudes toward sexuality and bodily functions. The mind is seen as struggling to gain control over bodily impulses and functions that are seen negatively as impure, threatening, and arising from the body, not the mind. This often manifests as what can be called the "fear of the organic," which is expressed as discomfort with things that are liquid and soft—gooey, mushy, sticky. A fear of loss of control, that the body will take over and lead one to degeneration and decay, is underneath this discomfort with the organic aspects of life. To the mind that is in such a state, the life of the body is like being buried in a compost heap of feelings.

In the twenty-first century, the historical concept of the mind-body split has been fading. Even scientists in "traditional" fields such as medicine and biology have come gradually to acknowledge and investigate the bodymind connection. See as examples *Molecules of Emotion* by neuroscientist Candace Pert, neurologist Antonio Damasio's *Descartes' Error: Emotion, Reason, and the Human* and *The Feeling of What Happens: Body and Emotion in the Making of Consciousness*, and psychiatrist Alan Schore's *Affect, Regulation, and the Origin of the Self*, which are only a

Body Psychotherapy

Simply put, **body psychotherapy** integrates the recognition and utilization of the body into the theory and practice of psychotherapy. Body psychotherapy takes into account the complexity of the intersections and interactions between the body and the mind. This is reflected in a developmental model, theory of personality, hypotheses as to the origins of psychological disturbances, as well as a variety of evaluative and therapeutic techniques used within the framework of the therapeutic relationship. There are many different approaches or schools of thought that make up the field of body psychotherapy. The names of some of these are: Bioenergetics, Bodynamic Analysis, Core Energetics, Hakomi Integrative Somatics, Organismic Body Psychotherapy, Radix, Reichian (Orgonomy), and Rubenfeld Synergy.

The scientific knowledge base of body psychotherapy has developed over the last 75 years, derived from the results of research in biology, anthropology, proxemics, ethology, neurophysiology, developmental psychology, neonatology, perinatal studies, and many more disciplines.

A wide variety of techniques are used within body psychotherapy. Some of these involve touch, movement, and breathing. Therefore, a link exists with some manual therapies, somatic disciplines, and complementary medical disciplines. However, although these may also involve elements such as touch and movement, they do not include the psychotherapeutic aspect, so they also remain distinct from body psychotherapy.

The work of a body psychotherapist could be described as such: The body psychotherapist supports the client's internal self-regulative processes and accurate perception of external reality, based on a belief that an essential *embodiment* of mental, emotional, social, and spiritual life exists within the client.

Through his or her work, the body psychotherapist makes it possible for alienated aspects of the client to become conscious, acknowledged, and integrated parts of the self. According to the European Association for Body Psychotherapy, the body psychotherapist should have the following qualities and abilities:

1. An intuitive awareness and a reflective understanding of healthy human development
2. The knowledge of different patterns of unresolved conflicts originating from childhood, recognizing the resultant specific chronic splits in mind and body
3. The ability to maintain a consistent frame of reference and a differentiated sensitivity to the interrelatedness of:
   a. Signs in the organism indicating vegetative flow, muscular hypertension and hypotension, energetic blockage, energetic integration, pulsation, and progressive stages of natural self regulative functioning
   b. Phenomena of psychodynamic processes of transference, countertransference, projection, defensive regression, creative regression, various kinds of resistance, and other defenses*

(*Adapted from the official description of body psychotherapy of the European Association for Body Psychotherapy)

few among many scientific studies of the bodymind. Perhaps one of the most succinct statements on the scientific knowledge of the bodymind is by Bessel van der Kolk, a psychiatrist and researcher at Boston University,

> Brain, body, and mind are inextricably linked, and it is only for heuristic reasons that we can still speak of them as if they constitute separate entities. Alterations in any one of these three will intimately affect the other two. For example, emotions and perceptions are both psychological functions and parcel of the neural machinery for biological regulation. Their core consists of homeostatic controls—drives and instincts. Mental processes are products of the brain and body, which continuously interact with each other through nerve impulses and through chemicals carried by the bloodstream: neurohormones and other neuromodulators (p. 216).

Of course, the idea that the body and mind are connected has been for decades the fundamental principle of body-oriented psychology and **body psychotherapy**. Now that we have completed our experiential exploration into the bodymind connection, let's explore the phenomena behind it.

Phenomena Constituting the Bodymind Connection

All of us have ample everyday experiences of the mind and body being connected, as demonstrated by the exercises in the preceding section. We have only to observe that our bodies are responding to our thoughts fairly constantly. For example, think again of driving in heavy traffic. As you have observed, although the physical act of driving is not very demanding, you often grip the steering wheel with enormous physical tension and force that greatly surpasses what is needed to steer the car. On top of that, your shoulders probably have much more muscular tension than is needed to hold and turn the wheel. Your jaw may also be tense, even though you do not need your jaw at all to drive (though you may use it to yell at other drivers!). *The source of the tension is your emotions*, responding to how you feel about the experience, not to physical demand.

This example illustrates three phenomena of the bodymind connection. The first is that your body is continually reacting to whatever you are thinking. If you think of things that provoke anger, you may notice a variety of physical reactions: tightening of your hands up into fists, tensing of your arms and shoulders, thrusting of your jaw, inflating of your chest, stiffening of your neck, and/or tightening of your mouth. These may range from being very obvious and gross to subtle and fine, even to the point of being hardly noticeable at all. Or, they may have become so habitual that they remain invisible, part of the background, until a conscious effort is made to observe them. In summary, what is going on in the mind is going on in the body; that is, the body is *expressing* what is going on in the mind (Figure 5.2).

This characteristic of the bodymind connection was illustrated by Nina Bull's classic studies at Columbia University. Subjects in a light hypnotic trance were given the suggestion that they would experience the feeling indicated by one of six words (given one at a time)—fear, anger, disgust, depression, joy, and triumph. The researcher also suggested that the subject would show the feeling as an emotion in outward behavior. Researchers recorded the subjects' actions and then asked the subjects to describe their experience. They concluded that unpleasant feelings always involve not only psychological, but *bodily* conflict and frustration. In other words, Bull found that with all three such feelings studied (fear, anger, and disgust) primary muscular movement is suppressed or blocked by secondary movement restraining the impulse to act. In depression, a more complex pattern of blocked movements was reported. For the pleasant feelings of joy and triumph, the subjects' bodily response was very different. Conflict and frustration were not present, and there were no blocking movements. In other words, the patterns of pleasant emotional responses showed expansion, while the unpleasant patterns showed contraction (Bull).

The second phenomenon constituting the bodymind connection is that our *entire* mind is reflected in the body. Not only our *conscious* thoughts, but also our *unconscious* anxieties, insecurities, desires, and other feelings, beliefs, thoughts, and values are reflected in our bodies (Figure 5.3). The simplest way of observing the body reflecting the unconscious mind is to watch the unconscious habits of people you know well. For example, does your boss clear his throat when he is talking to clients or customers? Does a classmate continually twist her hair when she responds to a question? Do you know someone who picks at himself with his fingers when he is nervous, or tightens her face when she is not saying something she is thinking?

These gestures can range from being relatively inconsequential to very complex and loaded with meaning about the person's character and personality. This is because the activity in the unconscious ranges from material that we either cannot or do not need to be aware of, to material of which we *do not want* to be aware. This is where things get interesting and involves a fundamental idea in body-oriented psychology! *Thoughts and feelings we do not want to be aware of are still manifested in the body. They do not simply go away.* For example, most of us have seen someone who has a tense jaw, tense shoulders, and a raised voice, but does not have any awareness that he or she is experiencing anger. In fact, if the anger is pointed out, the person may deny it or even be taken aback by the observation (as Clint did in the case study).

This characteristic was demonstrated by a study conducted by Malmo and Shagass. Studying subjects during psychotherapy sessions, the researchers measured and recorded muscle tension in the subjects' legs and arms and correlated the measurements with certain themes that came up during the sessions. They found that when the discussions turned to sexuality, muscular tension rose significantly in the subjects' legs. When anger was the subject, muscle tension increased in the subjects' arms. Furthermore, the more the subjects denied they were feeling anything related to the subject, such as sexuality or anger, the more their muscular tension increased. The subjects' defensive responses showed that unconscious, as well as conscious, mental activity manifested in a bodily response (Malmo and Shagass).

Figure 5.2
The bodymind connection. In response to seeing the thuggish bully Spike, the person thinks, "there goes that bully Spike," and has an emotional reaction of fear. The fear engenders a protective and fearful response in the body that involves a tightening of the entire body, raising the shoulders, and adopting an anticipative defensive position of slightly raising fists.

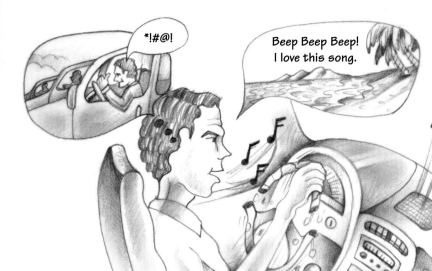

Figure 5.3
The unconscious aspect of the bodymind connection. *If we accept that the mind and body are interconnected and that an unconscious mind exists, then unconscious as well as conscious thoughts are reflected in the body. For example, someone driving in heavy traffic may have simultaneous conscious and unconscious thoughts. The conscious thought may be about something mundane like the tune on the radio, whereas the unconscious thought may express the frustrations of driving. The driver is whistling away while tensely gripping the steering wheel into dust, expressing the unconscious frustration.*

The third phenomenon constituting the bodymind connection is that what is going on in the body is also reflected in the mind. Expressions by and sensations in the body will become reflected in thoughts. Try the following experiment to illustrate this phenomenon. *Form your hands into fists, then tighten your fists as much as you can. If you also tighten your forearms, that is okay. Hold the tension for 10 minutes if you can, a bit longer if you wish. After the time period is up, reflect back on your thoughts during the exercise. Many people, when they do this experiment, report that they start having angry or aggressive thoughts.*

This experiment demonstrates the "two-way" nature of the connection between the mind and body. Thoughts can stimulate body responses, and body actions and sensations can stimulate thoughts. For example, stress due to worrying about something may cause your forehead or shoulders to get tense, *and* a tense forehead or shoulders may make you feel stressed, or reinforce a stress pattern. In this way, the bodymind connection is a continuous loop, rather than a causal relationship. One can intervene in the loop at any point—for instance, with massage therapy—and create change (Figure 5.4).

A team of psychologists at Clark University studied the emotional effect of the body on the mind. They instructed people to put their facial muscles into the configurations typical of several emotions, such as fear, anger, disgust, and sadness. After a brief period, the different facial expressions produced the moods they portrayed. The researchers also showed that these responses consistently correlated with a *specific* facial expression, so that they were not random correlations. While simulating the facial expression of anger, for example, subjects said they felt anger, but not any other feelings, such as disgust, sadness, or fear (Duclos et al).

Another one of Nina Bull's studies came to similar conclusions. Also using light hypnotic induction, it involved asking subjects to "lock" their bodies into a pattern described by the researcher. They devised patterns corresponding to the six emotional states of fear, anger, disgust, depression, joy, and triumph. However, these instructions did not include any description of the emotions that these patterns represented. Participants recorded feeling the emotions that the locked patterns represented. For example, participants tightening the abdominal muscles while rotating the body reported feeling "disgusted." In addition, subjects blocked in a specific pattern representing one emotion found that they could not experience any other emotion, especially pleasant ones. Bull concluded that when our bodies are in a specific chronic emotional blocking pattern that (1) we are predisposed to feeling that emotion and (2) we can experience only that emotion until we clear that pattern.

William James, the first great American psychologist, was one of the first to observe this two-way nature of the bodymind connection. In 1892, he said, "Common sense says we are insulted by a rival, are angry and strike . . . the more rational statement is that we feel sorry because we cry, angry because we strike, afraid because we tremble . . . stopping the expression of emotion often makes it worse. The funniest event becomes quite excruciating when we are forbidden by the situation to laugh, and anger pent in by fear turns into ten-fold hate. Expressing either emotion freely, however, gives relief."

Factors Affecting the Shape of the Body

Several factors influence the actual shape of our bodies and how our bodies respond to touch. Learning to interpret the shape of the client's body can enable the massage therapist to determine which therapeutic approach or strategy is best suited to that individual client (which we discuss in subsequent chapters). The five factors that affect the shaping and appearance of the body are: psychological history, genetics, nutrition, physical history, and culture.

IS SAMMY RUNNING BECAUSE HE'S SCARED . . .

OR IS HE SCARED BECAUSE HE'S RUNNING

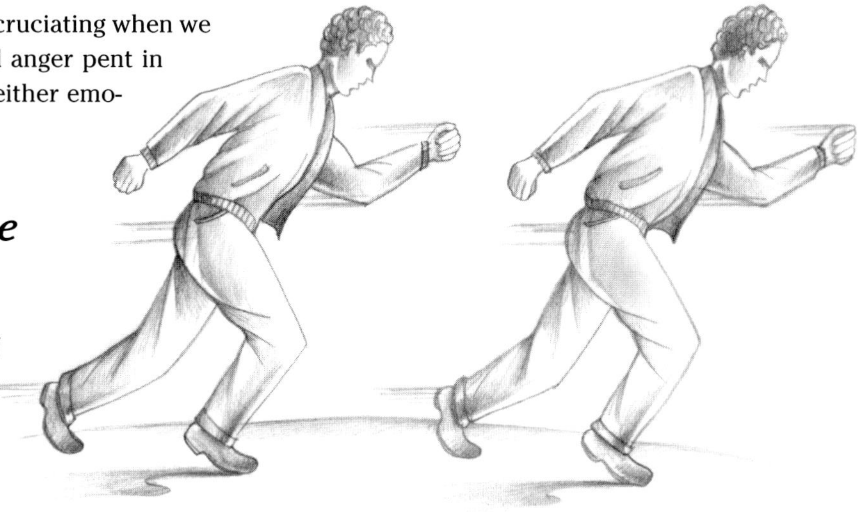

Figure 5.4
The James-Lange theory . . . Is Sammy running because he's scared . . . or is he scared because he's running?

Psychological History

Our bodies have a psychological historical context. Our *psychological history*— that is, the sum of our past psychological experiences, our interpretations of those psychological experiences, and the feelings they provoked, whether conscious or unconscious, remembered or unremembered—influence the shaping of our bodies. Many clinicians and researchers agree that there is a relationship between specific body patterns and psychological traits. For example, in one study, psychotherapists and clinical researchers were asked via a survey whether they could correlate specific body characteristics with personality traits. Significant agreement was found that they could do so. For example, 93% correlated a person's feet being solidly on the ground with feeling secure, 91% correlated raised shoulders with fear, 91% correlated a downward turned mouth with depression, 88% correlated a perpetual ("pasted on") smile with negative attitudes, 87% correlated a tight jaw with anger, and so on. The *lowest* figure was 66% and correlated tight arms with anger, which still showed a considerable level of agreement (King).

Our psychological history is the factor at the very heart of this book, so we accordingly devote the most content to it throughout. As we mentioned in Chapter 1 and will explore in later chapters, patterns in thoughts and feelings that we deem threatening or otherwise unacceptable in the present are similar to those that were somehow regarded as unacceptable in the past. These patterns surface not only cognitively and emotionally, but also in patterns of muscular tension in the body, which we call *armoring*.

However, the psychological history is not the only factor that shapes the body, and we do not intend to give the impression that it is. We do not want to be reductionistic. When we see or touch the body, besides the psychological history, we are also observing the effects of genetics, nutrition, physical history, and culture in shaping the body. Each of these four topics could be the subject of book-length discussion. However, because these topics are not the primary focus of this book, our discussion of each is accordingly briefer.

Genetics

Genetics alone determines many of our physical features, such as facial features, hair color, tall or short stature, and tendency to be angular, rounded, or bulky in body composition. Genetics also in part dictates to what diseases or conditions we may be predisposed. Some of these conditions can lead to a chain of events that affects the shaping of the body. For example, a person who lacks good binocular vision and depth perception will have difficulty developing good eye-hand coordination, which is essential to do well in many sports. The child who cannot participate in sports may not have an opportunity to fully develop his or her body. Another example is the high and tightly constricted chest that is a classic holding pattern of someone with asthma. The holding pattern is a reaction to the asthmatic condition and possibly the anxiety about having an asthma attack. Not only does genetics shape our bodies, but our *response* to our genetic conditions shapes our bodies as well.

Nutrition

It is well known that nutrition can affect the body in various ways, especially while a child is growing. Undernourishment or overnourishment in early childhood can result in marked developmental effects. As a more dramatic example, a prolonged shortage of food can cause symptoms that include extreme emaciation. The loss of insulating body fat makes undernourished people highly vulnerable to death or damage resulting from a drop in core body temperature when the air falls below 60° to 65° F. Young children who survive usually develop adult short stature (along with some degree of permanent brain damage).

A lack of specific kinds of nutrients can result in changes in body structure, along with various life-threatening health problems. For instance, when babies and very young children have a diet extremely low in protein, they are likely to develop kwashiorkor. Typical symptoms are edema due to water retention, especially in the abdomen, stick-like legs and arms with little fat or muscle mass, and loss of hair and skin pigmentation in patches. Children with kwashiorkor also are likely to have retarded growth.

Specific vitamin deficiencies can result in serious health problems for children, which lead to bodily changes. For example, inadequate amounts of vitamin D can cause a bone disease known as rickets, which can affect postural appearance because the bones can deform.

Dietary changes can also have a positive effect. This has been the case in Japan as nutrition improved while prosperity progressed during the post-World War II era. In each generation since 1945, children have been significantly taller. In 1986, 14- to 15-year-old Japanese boys averaged 7 inches taller than did comparably aged boys in 1959.

Some physical effects of nutritional stresses are generally reversible, whether they occur in childhood or adulthood. For instance, people suffering from mild, long-term undernourishment typically lose excess body fat and are very slender. Later, if their diet increases to a consistent level of excess calories, they are very likely to retain more body fat, eventually becoming obese.

Physical History

The shape of the body is also reflected in each client's history of physical activity, that is, developmental factors, activities in which a person typically engages over time, and specific physical events, such as traumatic accidents. Developmental factors refer to how our bodies are shaped by interactions with our environment while we are children. The body of a person who was very physically active as a child differs from a person with similar original physical composition who was sedentary as a child (although these differences could lessen if their physical activities as an adult are very similar). What makes developmental physical adjustments to our bodies possible is the fact that as humans we have a high degree of physiological plasticity. Our interactions with our environment while we are growing can physically mold us. Having said this, we must also recognize the interplay between physical history and genetics. Our adult bodies are the result of genetically inherited traits that were shaped to a certain degree in each of us by our environment as we grew up. The degree of importance of each factor can be difficult to evaluate, as reflected in the ongoing nature-versus-nurture debate that remains firmly unresolved.

The effect of physical activities as adults, such as occupational activities and physical habits, also demonstrates the moldability of the body. Different kinds of activities or sports, for example, build different groups of muscles. A person who swims a lot will probably develop very muscular shoulders, whereas a carpenter or plumber may develop muscular forearms.

On the other hand, some activities contribute to muscle breakdown and typical injuries. Intensive, frequent computer use may lead to carpal tunnel syndrome, whereas a career as a ballet dancer may lead to plantar fasciitis. Massage therapists also are likely to encounter clients with chronic neck tension who cradle the phone between their neck and shoulders at work, clients with shoulder and back problems who habitually lug heavy shoulder bags, or clients whose sleeping positions cause them a variety of physical problems. In turn, these activities—those that result in injury and those that do not—subsequently affect the shape and appearance of the body. For example, if someone has an elevated left shoulder, it may be because that person fell out of a tree when a child, rather than signifying some psychological significance.

Culture

Each **culture** carries rules of behavior, stated and unstated. Regarding the body, culture directly influences its shape and appearance. In addition, body language, expression, personal space, energetic patterns, gender behavior, and other aspects can indirectly affect the shape or appearance of the body.

Cultural influences *directly* affect the shape or appearance of the body or parts of the body in many ways. For instance, wearing leather shoes that enclose the feet can make them become narrower. Similarly, the practice of women wearing shoes with pointed toes and high heels, which are often too small in size, commonly results in a variety of painful deformities and biomechanical defects. This Western cultural practice is driven by the belief that small feet and a contoured leg line are attractive for women. However, this cultural practice can exact a price. The American Academy of Orthopedic Surgeons has reported that 9 of 10 women in the United States wear shoes that are too small for their feet, and 7 of 10 subsequently develop foot deformities, such as bunions or hammertoes. As another example, men and women in the United States, motivated by a culture that values a youthful and athletic appearance, use fitness regimens that build large, highly toned muscles in certain areas of the body or subject themselves to surgical procedures to attain desired alterations of their bodies.

A more extreme example of cultural practices that directly affect the shape of the body, at least from our Western cultural viewpoint, is the now-banned Chinese custom of tightly wrapping or binding the feet of young girls with cloth to hinder

Culture

Culture is the "sum of beliefs, practices, habits, likes, dislikes, norms, customs, rituals, and so forth that we have learned from our families" (Spector). The word culture stems from the Latin *colere*, translatable as to build on, to cultivate, to foster. People's actions, as well as the structure and appearance of their bodies, are consciously and unconsciously subject to cultural influence.

Various components constitute a culture (Maletzke):

▶ National character and basic personality
▶ Perception
▶ Time concept
▶ Space concept
▶ Thinking
▶ Language
▶ Nonverbal communication
▶ Values
▶ Behavior: norms, rules, manners
▶ Social groupings and relationships

Culture is determined not only by ethnicity or nationality, but also by factors such as geography, age, religion, gender, sexual orientation, and socioeconomic status.

normal growth. While foot binding caused permanent crippling and painful deformities of the foot bones, it also produced tiny feet that were considered to be very attractive and extravagant in the dominant Han culture of China. Parents crippled their daughters with good intentions, for extremely small feet would make them more attractive marriage partners for rich men of high social status.

Body language can differ from culture to culture, so misunderstandings and miscommunications are particularly possible. An example of a major misinterpretation happened when the former Soviet leader Nikita Khrushchev visited the United States at the height of the Cold War. He greeted the press with a clasping of his hands, shaking them over each shoulder. This expression is understood to be a sign of friendly greetings in Russia. In the United States, however, this is a gesture of the winner in a battle or contest; consequently, the U.S. media reported his gesture as an aggressive signal that the U.S.S.R. would prevail over the United States.

Examples of misunderstood body language are numerous. Many are based on proverbial sayings that cannot be translated literally. For example, the French phrase "*ça t'a passé sous le nez*," which in English translates literally as "that has passed under your nose," also is a vernacularism meaning "you missed your opportunity." The gesture for it is passing a hand under the nose, which makes no sense to members of a non–French-speaking culture. Put in another perspective, its American counterpart could be "you blew it," accompanied by a gesture of blowing air between pursed lips, while shaking the head slightly sideways. This might be incomprehensible to a person from a French-speaking culture.

The total amount of body language expressions used also varies according to culture. Asian cultures, for example, are less inclined to use any at all, whereas southern Europeans are far more likely to use them.

Touching behavior varies in different cultures. According to anthropologists, the most widespread touching ritual is the handshake. Handshakes differ in degree, length, and strength, depending usually on the level of intimacy. A moderate handshake in Spain could include the use of a double grip, which might cause confusion for a German, and would utterly confound a Polynesian. A strong handshake is stronger in Spain than in northern Europe and might be interpreted as overfriendly by northern Europeans, whereas the strong handshake of the northern European might be interpreted as perfunctory by the Spaniard. Similarly confusing would be a confrontation of a non-contact culture, such as a northern European one, with a contact culture, in which frequent touching is a sign of friendship or politeness.

Eye contact is another body-oriented cultural variable. In most Western cultures, direct eye contact signifies listening and attention, whereas failure to make eye contact is interpreted as a sign of dishonesty or weakness. However, direct eye contact is seen unfavorably by various Asian cultures. The duration of the eye contact is also a cultural variable, since it might become perceived as aggression when sustained for too long or as an uninterested attitude when perceived as too short. Other cultures may consider sustained eye contact as disrespectful or a sign of hostility, impoliteness, or lack of respect for authority. An example of how eye contact behavior can influence body appearance is that of avoiding eye contact, which can reinforce a posture that favors keeping the head downward. In U.S. American culture, this body position might be interpreted as submissiveness, but in a culture that favors avoiding eye contact, this could be seen as respectful or humility.

Culture also influences *how people structure the space* around them. Generally, low-context cultures have a tendency to prefer greater distances between persons than high-context cultures, although Southeast Asian cultures, which are high context and prefer a large distance, are the exception (in a low-context culture, what is said is what is meant; conversely, in a high-context culture, subtle cues are used, often nonverbal, so what is said must be placed in the context of all other cues to understand what is meant). For example, shaking hands is something that can be uncomfortable for Chinese (high context), whereas even a tap on the shoulder, often practiced by U.S. Americans (low context), can be interpreted as threatening in northern European countries (lower context).

We also know that *how people dress* affects their bodily appearance. Modes of dress are also interpreted differently among cultures. In most Western societies, suits and formal attire reflect professionalism, are required often for business activities, and represent a civilized manner. The perception of such dress, however, is also different regarding various styles. For example, a British person might judge the Italian style of dressing to be flamboyant, ridiculously fancy, or *nouveaux riche*. This could be completely different in other cultures. In Arab societies, a *ghutra* (a white, fine cotton headcloth) and *thobe* (a long, generally white, robe) might be preferred.

Culture also supports *energetic patterns*. Cultures that favor individualism and success-seeking behavior reward individuals who have a high energetic charge. This kind of culture reinforces body phenomena such as holding one's head high, keeping one's chin up, and having a hard, prominent chest. These bodily behaviors require maintaining a relatively high energy level. Other cultures are more collective and support group-oriented behavior that would disapprove of an individual striving for personal prominence or being nonconforming. Such cultures often have a saying, "The head that sticks up, gets chopped off." In this case, the head up, chin up, chest forward body is less likely to be found. In effect, culture normalizes body behaviors, making those behaviors seem invisible, meaning people take them for granted to the extent that they are not consciously noticed as long as they conform to the norm.

Cultures also usually have powerful parameters for *gender behavior*. These dictate not only dress, but how a person walks and talks and in which kinds of activities each gender can participate. Sometimes these parameters change. Thirty years ago, a girl who participated in sports might have been stigmatized in some way. Therefore, the condition of the musculature in girls and women at that time was considerably different from that in the present day. Now girls and women are encouraged to play sports and to take care of their bodies by working out. This naturally affects bodily appearance.

Cultures can also have *subsets of characteristics*. For example, a national culture often

---

Box 5.2

ASSESSING CULTURAL BELIEFS ABOUT HEALTH AND ILLNESS

Every culture includes specific beliefs and practices related to health and illness. These beliefs and practices dramatically shape one's perception of health and illness. The following eight areas can help you assess cultural variations in both your clients and yourself, which will help you understand your clients better and to communicate with them, especially those from different cultures than your own. Using this list, try identifying your cultural identities, beliefs and practices in each of these eight areas. Then, try doing the same for one of your clients, perhaps one that you know well.

1. Origins of the client's culture (identify the culture)
2. Value orientations, including view of the world, ethics, and norms and standards of behavior, as well as attitudes about time, work, money, education, beauty, strength, physical contact and touch, dress, and change
3. Interpersonal relationships, including family patterns, demeanor, and roles and relationships
4. Communication patterns and forms
5. Religion, spirituality, and magic or shamanism
6. Social systems, including economic values, political systems, and educational patterns
7. Diet and food habits
8. Health and illness belief systems, including behaviors, decision making, and use of healthcare providers*

(*This list is adapted from Boyle and Andrews)

also has urban-rural cultural differences. Walking in an urban area is a considerably different experience from walking in a rural one. In a city, one might be more rushed, vigilant, and habitually tense. A rural environment has other factors with which to contend. Peoples' bodies adapt to each environment accordingly.

The phenomenon of culture shock applies not only to being in a different national culture, but also to moving between cultural subsets. The sheer newness of the environment, as well as changes in levels of stimulation, danger, and expectations can cause stress that manifests in the body.

Finally, the therapist's perceptions can be affected by cultural factors, especially when encountering clients from another culture. In such cases, the therapist may need to shift from his or her own cultural lens. The ability to do this becomes especially important if the therapist wishes to communicate effectively and understand the client.

Ashley and Luciana

Ashley was excited to hear a foreign accent on her telephone answering machine requesting a massage appointment. Luciana said she had gotten Ashley's name from an association's locator list on the internet and that she had massage before when she lived in Italy. Ashley had never worked with anyone from another country before.

When Ashley came into her waiting room, she saw a bright-eyed and energetic woman who immediately stuck out her hand and said, "I'm Luciana. Happy to meet you."

As they sat down, Luciana immediately began chatting. Ashley noticed that Luciana's face was very close to hers as they talked. The closeness made Ashley uncomfortable and she wondered what was going on. She liked Luciana, though, and the massage went very well. Luciana came for more sessions, and each time Luciana got very close physically to Ashley as they talked.

Ashley became very disconcerted and went to her supervisor. "I don't understand," said Ashley. "I'm sure it's not a sexual thing or anything like that, but she gets too close to me. Maybe she doesn't have good boundaries."

"Or maybe she has *different* boundaries," said her supervisor. "She comes from Italy, right? I've been there. People there have a very different sense of personal space while they speak, and they don't use as much space as we do. It can be pretty unnerving when someone gets so close to you while they're talking, but you get used to it."

"Oh," said Ashley. "I wouldn't have thought of that."

"Yes," said her supervisor, "When you deal with people from different places and cultures, you have to put what you see and feel through a new filter, or at least adjust your own. Some things carry across cultures and some things don't."

In particular, the massage therapist also needs to understand the effects of his or her own cultural background and how it influences his or her perceptions of the body and health, as well as how these same cultural considerations would apply to clients. Box 5-2 will help you be aware how culture shapes perceptions of health and illness.

As our exploration of the bodymind has shown, when we touch the body, we touch the mind. In massage, this can result in the phenomenon known as emotional release, the subject of the next chapter.

REFERENCES

Boyle, J., & Andrews, M. (1989). *Transcultural concepts in nursing care.* Glenview, IL: Scott, Foresman/Little, Brown College Division.

Bull, N. (1962). *The body and its mind.* New York: Las Americas Publishing.

Duclos, S. et al. (1989). Emotion—Specific effects of facial expressions and postures on emotional experience. *Journal of Personality and Social Psychology, 57*(1) 100–108.

Gross, J.J. & Levenson, R.W. (1997). Hiding feelings: The acute effects of inhibiting positive and negative emotions. *Journal of Abnormal Psychology, 106,* 95–103.

Hall, E.T. (1967). *The silent language.* New York: Fawcett.

James, W. (1892). *Psychology.* New York: Henry Holt & Company.

Juhan, D. (1987). *Job's body.* Barrytown, NY: Station Hill Press.

King, C.A. (1972). *An investigation of selected associations between personality traits and human muscular skeletal structure.* Doctoral dissertation, University of Miami, Coral Gables, FL.

Maletzke, G. (1996). *Intercultural communication.* Opladen, Germany: Westdeutscher Verlag.

Malmo, R.B. & Shagass, C. (1949). Physiologic studies of reaction to stress in anxiety. *Psychosomatic Medicine, 11,* 9.

Marrone, R. (1990). *Body of Knowledge.* New York: State University of New York Press.

Marsh, P. (1988). *Eye to eye.* Topsfield, MA: Salem House.

Ridley, M. (2000). *Genome.* New York: Harper Collins.

Schore, A. (1994). *Affect, regulation, and the origin of the self.* Hillsdale, NJ: Lawrence Erlbaum Associates.

Spector, R.E. (1991). *Cultural diversity in health and illness.* Norwalk, CT: Appleton & Lange.

Van der Kolk, B.A., McFarlane, A.C., & Weisaeth, L. (1996). *Traumatic stress: The effects of overwhelming experience on mind, body, and society.* New York: Guilford Press.

Weinberger, D.A. (1990). The construct validity of the repressive coping style. In: Singer, J.L., (Ed.) *Repression and dissociation* (pp.337–386). Chicago: University of Chicago Press.

Williams, R. (1981). *Contact, human communication, and its history.* New York: Thames and Hudson.

6

Chapter

Emotional Release

At this point in this book, a more detailed examination of emotional release is in order. Nearly all massage therapists who have practiced for any length of time have encountered emotional release. For example, a client may suddenly become sad, perhaps even cry, during a session, or an apparently relaxed client may suddenly stiffen in fear. Or, more subtle manifestations, such as bodily tremors or vibrations, may suddenly appear. Or, a client may become sharply critical or difficult without warning, seemingly out of nowhere. Some emotional releases may be very expressive and demonstrative, including sobbing or yelling. Others may be more subtle, manifesting simply as holding the breath or a fist tightening up.

What takes place in an emotional release is generated from the internal state of the client. It can be related to recent events, but more often it is related to the past. What summons the emotion into consciousness is the massage; that is, *the triggering event is the massage itself.* This can surprise the client as well as the therapist, because the client may have his or her conscious mind focused on something else. For example, the client may be thinking about what to do after the massage, when moments later suddenly he or she experiences feelings about the loss of a loved one. Or, during the course of the massage the client may experience a gradual building of emotion that finally manifests as an outward expression.

Emotional release can be entirely spontaneous, occurring without willful initiation by either the client or massage therapist. In contrast to a psychotherapist who may use techniques *designed* and *intended* to evoke an emotional response, the massage therapist never *deliberately* attempts to provoke emotional release. Because emotional release is frequently encountered in massage therapy, you should have a thorough understanding of why it occurs, how it manifests, and how to work with it. These topics are the subjects of this chapter.

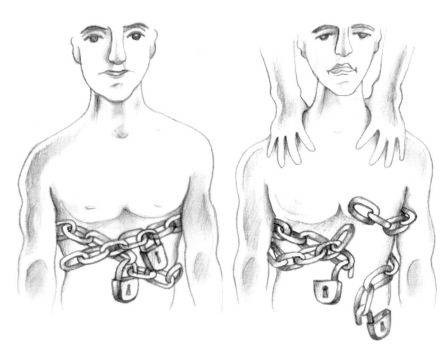

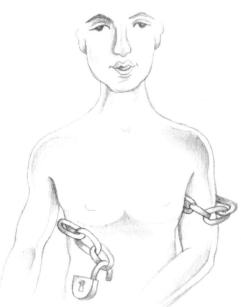

WHY EMOTIONAL RELEASE HAPPENS IN MASSAGE

Figure 6.1
Intervention. *The intervention of massage can change the status quo. If tight chest muscles are assisting the unconscious to block emotional expression (left), massage can intervene by loosening the tension and allowing the emotional expression to be released (center), leading to relief and a feeling of greater openness (right).*

As we stated in Chapter 1, massage is an intervention. This means *massage is capable of disturbing or altering a pattern of experience, as well as a pattern of defense or protection.* Specifically, massage intervenes in the patterns of the body—muscular and otherwise—that organize or hold each person's psychological experiences, including those of both the conscious and unconscious mind (see Chapter 5). When such a pattern is disturbed, it creates a space for new experiences to occur. Since the unconscious mind is actively involved in controlling experience and emotional flow, thereby maintaining the status quo, alteration of a person's bodymind patterns can threaten or loosen unconscious control of feelings and memories. If this control weakens, then what is stored or blocked in the unconscious can surface to consciousness and may be expressed emotionally in the form of what we know as emotional release. Altering these patterns can be like moving a stone that is blocking the middle of a stream, whether the client has any idea that stone is there or not (Figure 6-1).

Something as simple as a supportive touch to someone who has not previously had such touch can jolt a pattern of emotional deprivation and compensation. For example, what manifests as a compensatory attitude of "I don't need anything" can provoke tears with the touch of the therapist. In addition, touching the skin can have subtle energetic effects. For example, someone who is described as "being wired" and has a very nervous quality becomes more calm and centered through touch itself. The following case study is an example of supportive touch and emotional release.

Gloria and Lorraine

Lorraine had been going weekly to Gloria for massage for eight sessions. At the initial session, Lorraine told Gloria that she wanted massage therapy for general relaxation. Lorraine had a very difficult job as an office manager at a law

Gloria and Lorraine

firm that caused her to experience a high level of stress, particularly in the past year when one of the partners left the firm on bad terms. Lorraine was aware that the people she worked with sometimes counted on her for more than she was capable of providing. However, she would try her hardest to come through for them anyway.

At the beginning of the ninth session, Gloria began by sliding her hands underneath Lorraine's scapulae and keeping them there without moving her hands for 5 minutes. Gloria saw Lorraine's face begin to change color and becoming more reddish and also noticed Lorraine very slightly biting a sliver of her lower lip. She then noticed Lorraine attempt unsuccessfully to fight back tears. Saying, "This has never happened before, I'm so sorry," Lorraine alternately fought back her tears, erupting finally a few moments later into full crying.

"It's okay to cry," said Gloria in response to Lorraine's apology. Gloria kept her hands under Lorraine's scapulae, waiting for the crying to subside, not saying anything further. This sequence of fighting tears and then crying repeated for several minutes.

"What was that?" asked Lorraine, as she finished crying.

"I don't know exactly what you were feeling, but I do know that sometimes relaxing deeply makes room for feelings to come up," Gloria replied.

"When you put your hands under my back, I began to feel how tired I was . . . *bone-tired*," sighed Lorraine, "It just sunk into me how I've been doing so much without any help, holding the office together. I've been running around like crazy for practically a year, and I haven't done anything to take care of myself. I guess I've been waiting for other people to notice that I needed something too."

"I'm really glad you got in touch with that . . . and by the way, you did do one thing to take care of yourself, you came in for massage," Gloria said. A moment later she continued, "Are you ready to go on with the massage, or do you need a few more moments?"

"Just let me lie here for one minute."

"Good, just let me know when you're ready," Gloria replied, waiting quietly for Lorraine to let her know.

Other aspects of massage can also increase the likelihood of emotional release. For instance, the massage therapy room may feel like a safe space for the client. After all, the therapist hopefully has made a purposeful effort to be supportive, nonjudgmental, caring, and trustworthy while providing the power of touch in an ethical manner. Such an environment and relationship can allow a client to let go on an emotional level.

HOW EMOTIONAL RELEASE MANIFESTS

Emotional release manifests many ways in the body. It can take several years of experience, possibly helped by instruction from a supervisor or teacher, to learn to become aware of all possible manifestations, but our intent here is to acquaint you with at least some of them. In any one individual, not all these manifestations may be present simultaneously. Sometimes, there is only one.

Some manifestations of emotional release are obvious. The most evident are clear emotional expressions, such as tears, raising of the voice, nonverbal sounds, and large movements. These may reveal that the client has become obviously sad, angry, fearful, disgusted, or joyous. Sometimes the client knows what the emotion is connected to, and sometimes he or she does not.

Other manifestations during massage can be more subtle. A change in breathing sometimes signals that an emotional release is about to occur. Or, there may be changes in color: an area may become flushed or pale. The client's body temperature may change: for example, the hands, feet, and face may become cold or hot. Muscle tightening may occur in other parts of the body as the emotions are beginning to flow, as if the holding will stop or slow the flow. Typical areas that tense to hold or block emotions are the jaw and mouth, hands, and belly. Fluttering of the eyelids generally indicates that an energetic shift is taking place that may eventually surface in another form of emotional release. The client can start doing squirming-like movements on the table, as if to escape or contain the coming emotion. Similarly, the client may attempt to ward off the feelings by twiddling thumbs, tapping fingers, pulling hair, or making various other hand and finger movements. Conversely, some part of the body may start moving or twitching, as if to express an emotion. Usually, these movements are not under conscious control. The client may also begin talking, but the content is often unrelated to what is happening in the case of subtle signs.

CHARACTERISTICS OF CLIENTS LIKELY TO EXPERIENCE EMOTIONAL RELEASE

Any client can potentially have an emotional release, but certain clients have a greater propensity for emotional release than others. It may be stating the obvious, but the reason the client gives to you for coming for massage therapy can give an indication. A client whose presenting problem is primarily physical is less likely to have an emotional release, at least at the outset. However, if the physical problem is strongly limiting the client's important life activities, then the effect of the physical problem may have emotional consequences that could surface in an emotional release.

Zack

Zack, a massage client, had chronic shoulder pain that had progressed to the point of limiting his ability to write and operate a computer keyboard. Since Zack was an attorney, this increasingly hampered his work. As the tension was released in his shoulder area and the condition began to improve, Zack described intense feelings of frustration and anger surrounding his inability to work normally. However, a short time afterward, other feelings surfaced during a session related to how his shoulder injury ended what had been a very active athletic life. Zack had enjoyed playing softball for many years, and the shoulder injury curtailed his ability to play. This led to feeling grief, loss, and sadness about the end of his playing days.

People who suffer from chronic pain are also somewhat more likely to experience emotional release. When the massage therapy begins to disrupt the underlying physical pattern(s) behind the pain, then emotional patterns related to the chronic physical pattern may surface.

Rose

Rose was a client with chronic osteoarthritis who came for massage therapy to get pain relief. Rose was holding an enormous amount of tension around many of her joints to guard against the pain. As massage began to help Rose release the muscular tension around the joints, she began to cry, first with relief from the pain, and then with the awareness that she had been holding herself together just as her mother had done. When Rose realized this, she said, "It feels good to let go. I guess I don't have to hold myself together all the time as I saw my mom do."

In this particular case, Rose did not come for massage therapy with any expectation of emotional release or psychological insight. However, as the massage released the tension around Rose's joints, not only was her pain relieved, the stressful feeling of holding herself together also was relieved. The reality that she held herself together came back into her awareness, which in turn allowed her to make a conscious realization that her mother had done the same thing. The realization allowed Rose to consider and choose another way of dealing with her discomfort than her mother's way.

Invalidation

Invalidation is the direct or subtle verbal and nonverbal negation or "putting down" of a person's thoughts, feelings, experiences, or character by another person. Verbally, one person says essentially to the other that his or her feelings are inappropriate or incorrect. For example, a child says, "I'm sad," but the parent responds, "No, you're not." Or, a child says "I'm scared," but the parent responds, "There's nothing to be afraid of." Or, one person says, "I had a really rough time," and the other person responds, "What are you talking about, it wasn't so bad." Some nonverbal examples of invalidation are rolling the eyes and sighing conspicuously. An invalidating response sends a message that the person should not feel what he or she feels, is wrong to feel what that way, or even that someone else knows better than the person how he or she feels.

Invalidation hurts. Such comments, intentionally or unintentionally, often lower the self-esteem of the affected person. Invalidating comments or gestures can lead people to cover up what they feel and whom they are when they believe or anticipate that they will be put down. Over time, invalidation leads a person—especially children—to confusion about the reality of his or her perceptions of the world and self.

Invalidating responses by a therapist are practically always made with good intentions, for example, to calm fears or to be optimistic, but just as often have a negative impact. For example, a client may say, "I feel better, but I'm really worried I'm going to start hurting again before long. I just don't know if this will last." An invalidating response would be, "There's nothing to worry about, you'll be fine," or "It'll last, you'll see, don't worry." Besides the negative effects described above, the therapist's invalidating response closes off the possibility of further discussing the client's thoughts or feelings.

Possible responses that are not invalidating are: "How worried are you about it?" and "What are your concerns about how you're going to feel?" This open-ended response *acknowledges the client's feeling and leaves the door open for the client to say more if he or she wishes*, while in contrast an invalidating response may cause the client to shut down.

Chronic pain presents its own set of emotional implications, which can become as complicated as those that are developed from early childhood problems. Chronic pain sufferers develop psychological patterns to cope with the physical pain, just as people must similarly develop ways to cope with long-term emotional pain. Consequently, when massage begins to intervene by affecting tension, the client can experience any number of changes that can lead to an emotional release. For example, simply restoring a person's level of vitality can bring with it a sense of intense relief and release. However, because people who suffer from chronic pain tend to diminish their level of feeling and awareness as a way of numbing out their pain, when physical feeling returns, they then begin to feel their emotions more fully. They can burst out in a flood of emotion as they "thaw out." Sometimes chronic pain sufferers are surprised to discover that a large amount of the pain they are feeling in their body is the result of defensive guarding against the injury and its emotional effects rather than the injury itself. Another result of improved vitality to be aware of is that it can also be accompanied by fear concerning whether the improvements will last. Usually, it is best to acknowledge the client's feelings, but to avoid well-meaning, but **invalidating** responses (see definition) that there is nothing to worry about.

Another phenomenon contributing to the likelihood of emotional release in clients with chronic pain is the fact they often develop a pattern of "normalizing" their pain, meaning that they adjust to it to the point where their pain becomes a normal part of everyday life. Such normalization causes them to accept the status quo without complaint or reaction. However, when the client begins to go through a change process, the chronic pain becomes less normalized, and emotional reactions can well up. Releasing the emotions related to the chronic pain then becomes an important part of the healing process, resulting in a higher level of healthy functioning. Releasing emotions may also open up unconscious attitudes that the client has held toward the injury or disease. For example, even though a client may rationally know that the injury came through no fault of his or her own, he/she may unconsciously perceive it as a form of punishment or something deserved. If an emotional release helps to relieve the sense of guilt, then the client may become free to live without the chronic pain.

Clients who receive massage therapy to reduce stress and whose presenting problems are nonspecific also have an increased probability to have an emotional release. Stress is clearly a common problem. However, many people either do not know what causes their stress, or they have some idea of the causes, but deny the impact. As they receive massage, they begin to make connections between the tension and its sources, both past and present. The client may then begin to experience feelings regarding the sources of the tension, and these may be expressed in emotional release. If the stress has an emotional origin, then the probability of emotional release is further increased. However, if the client is well defended psychologically, then the probability may be decreased.

Clients in psychotherapy are usually used to exploring their emotions and thus may become more likely to experience emotional release. Such clients may have even come to massage because they read or heard that it may enhance psychological awareness. These clients may therefore be somewhat predisposed to . . . even wanting to . . . experience emotional release. If a client is in psychotherapy, finding out what type it is may be useful. Certain types of psychotherapy emphasize expression of emotions more than others (Box 6.1). If a client is coming for massage therapy because of a recommendation or referral from a psychotherapist, it can be helpful to obtain permission from the client to speak with the psychotherapist. Knowing why the psychotherapist has recommended or referred for massage therapy and what benefits the psychotherapist believes the client will receive from massage therapy can be useful. More information regarding referrals from a psychotherapist is presented in Chapter 11.

Box 6.1

EXPRESSIVE PSYCHOTHERAPIES

The following are many of the therapies that emphasize emotional expression. This list is provided to help you identify whether a form of psychotherapy that a client may be doing is an expressive psychotherapy. Additional information is available through the website and/or email address provided here.

Bioenergetic Analysis: Originally arising from a collaboration by two of Wilhelm Reich's students, Alexander Lowen and John Pierrakos Bioenergetic Analysis was primarily developed by Lowen. Bioenergetic analysis sees tension patterns in the body as diagnostic aspects of psychological structure and works with these patterns through touch and mobilization to bring about strong emotional release. The concept of grounding within the body is a major tenet of Bioenergetics, which helps anchor and integrate emotional release and psychological change in the individual. Website: www.bioenergetic-therapy.com

Biosynthesis: Founder David Boadella encountered many of the primary body psychotherapy developers such as Reich's student Ola Raknes, Gerde Boyeson, Lowen, and Stanley Keleman in the 1950s and 1960s. Boadella later moved away from catharsis-oriented forms of therapy. Drawing on the work of clinicians Francis Mott and Frank Lake in prenatal and perinatal psychology, Boadella incorporated all these threads into Biosynthesis. This form of therapy works with emotional expression, movement potential and integrative insights through techniques called centering, grounding, and facing. Website: www.biosynthesis.org

Bodynamic Analysis: Based on the research of Danish childhood educator Lisbeth Marcher into the somatic aspect of psychological development, Bodynamics focuses on the "key interaction between each muscle in the body and that muscle's corresponding psychological function" through specific mapping of the body. Bodynamics emphasizes developing psychological and somatic resources that may have been skipped in an individual's childhood development. Email: info@bodynamicusa.com

Bonding Psychotherapy: Based on the work of Dan Casriels, Bonding Psychotherapy works with the neurobiological and psychosocial need for attachment. Bonding Psychotherapy takes place only within a group setting and focuses on emotional release and corrective attachment experiences through the body. Website: www.Bondingpsychotherapy.com

Core Energetics: Psychiatrist John Pierrakos with the contribution of his wife, Eva Broch, expanded his previous work in Bioenergetics into a more spiritually focused form of body psychotherapy. Core Energetics works with body and soul to bring about strong emotional release of negative feelings so that the natural and positive core self can emerge into the awareness of the individual. Websites: www.core-energeticsintl.org or www.coreenergeticinstitute.com

Box 6.1 *(Continued)*

Dance Therapy: Evolved from the work of Rudolph Laban, Marion Chace, May Whitehouse, and others, dance therapy and movement therapy use psychomotor expression as the primary form of intervention, leading the participant to explore both personal psychological and universal themes. Dance Therapy is the "psychotherapeutic use of movement as a process that furthers the emotional, cognitive, social, and physical integration of the individual." Website: www.adta.org

Drama Therapy: Using techniques from drama and the theater, drama therapy allows the individual to unfold his/her personal story with goals of dealing with problems, deepening awareness, allowing catharsis, learning to express feelings appropriately and in context, and improving understanding of roles and interpersonal skills. Email: info@nadt.org

Gestalt Therapy: Gestalt Therapy developed from the work of Frederick (Fritz) and Laura Perls, weaving together strands from Kurt Goldstein (neurology and Gestalt psychology), Karen Horney (psychoanalysis), Wilhelm Reich (psychoanalysis and body psychotherapy), Max Wertheimer (Gestalt psychology), and Martin Heidegger (existential philosophy). Gestalt Therapy emphasizes psychological and somatic processes as they occur in the here-and-now. Healing takes place within the framework of continuous awareness and the bringing together alienated parts of self as they are experienced both psychologically and physically. Website: www.aagt.org

Hakomi: Hakomi body-centered psychotherapy was originated by Ron Kurtz, synthesizing strands of technique and theory from Reich, Psychomotor, Bioenergetics, Feldenkrais, Rolfing, Ericksonian hypnosis, and Neuro-Linguistic Programming. Its emphasis is on "mindfulness," which allows the individual to become aware of core patterns of emotional, cognitive, and somatic response to experiments that are designed evoke such patterns. Website: www.hakomiinstitute.com

Integrative Body Psychotherapy (IBP): Developed by Jack Lee Rosenberg, Integrative Body Psychotherapy addresses the somatic core sense of self as the foundation of healthy experience. IBP specifically tracks interruptions to this somatic sense of self, stemming from psychological and emotional patterns arising in childhood. It integrates verbal and cognitive work with breathing, movement, and awareness regarding boundaries and presence. Website: www.ibponline.com

Medical Orgonomy: Medical Orgonomy was formed by some of Wilhelm Reich's students, such as Ellsworth Baker, and its practitioners consider it a direct extension of Reich's work. Medical orgonomists, who are all physicians, work directly with breathing and muscle tension in the body to bring about emotional release, particularly of anxiety and anger. Website: www.orgonomy.org

Organismic Psychotherapy: Developed by Malcolm Brown and Katherine Ennis Brown, Organismic Psychotherapy's theoretical base is derived from Gestalt phenomenology (Kurt Goldstein),

Another type of person comes to massage therapy with a nonspecific complaint or goal. This client may have a vague sense that something is wrong that has something to do with the body or bodily experience, but typically has no idea what the underlying problem actually is. This type of client is drawn to massage therapy because he or she intuitively senses that massage may help. This intuition is often correct because the client is sensing a need to reconnect with his or her body. In such cases, the disconnection with the body serves as a defense; therefore, reconnecting with the body through massage can then lead to the blocked emotional content surfacing. The underlying causes of the disconnection with the body may also become apparent.

DEALING WITH EMOTIONAL RELEASE

Before we offer any guidelines for dealing with emotional release, we want to point out that we are strictly and deliberately avoiding suggestions for responses that fall within the realm of psychotherapy. There are several extremely helpful and effective steps that a massage therapist can take that do not violate a scope of practice or ethical boundary.

Dealing with emotional release presents a paradox, as it is both very complex and very simple. Years of study, training, and experience are required to be able to work with someone to *resolve* the release and the issues involved, but at the same time, basic qualities and abilities can *help the client move forward* toward resolution. You do not have to have a Ph.D. in psychology to be helpful, but you do need common sense, empathy, and integrity.

Increasing Self-Awareness

Just as there is no single standard massage that works for everyone, there is no single way or exact formula to deal with emotional release. Each situation is different. However, we can certainly recommend that in preparing yourself to deal with emotional release, you begin by increasing your self-awareness. Specifically, we suggest you answer the following questions:

What kinds of emotions do I feel comfortable with?

What kinds of emotions cause me to feel uncomfortable or threatened?

What level of intensity of emotional expression can I tolerate?

What are my beliefs about emotions themselves?

Knowing how you feel about emotional release and specific emotions is important. You need to know and understand how you respond in the presence of sometimes dramatic expressions of emotion. Box 6.2 provides a self-assessment exercise to help you explore how you respond to various emotions that may arise during an emotional release. After you are aware of your responses and after you read about withdrawal in the next section, you will be more attuned to which emotional responses of your clients you need to be especially careful with in how you respond. We encourage you to do what you can to become more comfortable with these particular emotions. Insight into what causes your discomfort is one step that will help.

Avoiding Judgment, Withdrawal, and Psychotherapeutic Intervention

Since emotional release usually is not under the client's conscious control, it is imperative that you avoid judging the client who is experiencing it. Being judgmental can be one of the most damaging responses that a massage therapist can make during or about an emotional release. With considerable inhibitory power, it can cause the client to abruptly stop the emotional release by tightening their body, blocking their breathing, and cutting off the energetic flow of the emotion. Prematurely shutting

Box 6.1 (Continued)

humanistic psychology (Abraham Maslow and Carl Rogers), Jungian Analytical psychology, and the work of Wilhelm Reich. It emphasizes that change takes place throughout the entire organism and works with mobilization of the body and nurturing touch to bring about both active and expressive emotional discharge and deep, quiet internal emotional release. Email: x204guitar@aol.com or Website: www.bodypsychotherapy.org

Pesso Boyden Psychomotor System: Coming from a background in dance, Albert Pesso and Diane Boyden formed a highly structured group psychotherapy using movement, role playing, and other elements to help individuals experience what needs remain unmet from childhood and, using body and verbal techniques to symbolically satisfy the needs for support, nurturance, protection, limits, and belonging. Email: PBSP@aol.com

Primal Therapy: Founded by Arthur Janov, author of *Primal Scream*, Primal Therapy emphasizes emotional release and catharsis relating to early painful childhood experiences. Primal Therapy believes that deeply feeling this pain releases neurotic patterns and allows new, healthy patterns to establish themselves. Website: www.primals.org

Psychodrama: Jacob Moreno created Psychodrama as an early form of group therapy. An action oriented psychotherapy, psychodrama employs guided dramatic forms to examine personal problems, bring about emotional expression, psychological insight, and amplifies learning on cognitive, emotional, and behavioral levels. Website: www.asgpp.org

Radix: Charles Kelley, a student of Wilhelm Reich, originally founded Radix Work in Feeling and Purpose as a system of education rather than therapy, while later Radix practitioners also see it as a psychotherapy. Radix built upon Reich's work in armoring and character structure and sees the unblocking of emotion through working with the body as a way of opening to life energy and well-being. Website: www.radix.org

Rubenfeld Synergy: Ilana Rubenfeld synthesized the work of F. M. Alexander (Alexander Technique), Moishe Feldenkrais (Awareness Through Movement and Functional Integration) and Fritz Perls (Gestalt Therapy) into a type of work that flows between touch, gentle movement, and verbal dialogue between therapist and client. Emotional release may be present when there is a shift in bodymind consciousness. Website: www.rubenfeldsynergy.com

Sensorimotor Psychotherapy: Extended from the original Hakomi therapy, Pat Ogden, together with Ron Kurtz and Bill Bowen, integrated information and techniques from somatic practice. It strongly distinguishes between treatment of developmental issues and the treatment of trauma. Interfacing with the work of Bessel van der Kolk, Peter Levine, and others, it has created a specific set of theories and techniques for the treatment of trauma. Website: www.sensorimotorpsychotherapy.org

down the emotional release can lead to a sort of "emotional indigestion," which causes the client to feel fragmented and anxious, as if something is brewing just under the surface. In some instances, the uncompleted process also can lead a person to believe there is something "dangerous" lurking inside. Another effect is that it can recapitulate the original scenario in which the client learned to repress the emotion in the first place, which reinforces the defensive pattern. Part of the original scenario can include the client feeling that he or she did something wrong or is disliked. Judging can stimulate one or a combination of the following feelings within the client: anxiety, fear, shame, humiliation, guilt, dissociation, anger, despair, emotional paralysis (freezing up), depression, confusion, or being rejected.

Although judgment is inappropriate, having limits on what the client does while in your workspace is appropriate and recommended, as we discussed in Chapter 4. For example, a client may become very angry during an emotional release. Although he or she may not be able to control the *feelings* of anger, the client can control the *actions* that stem from the anger and indeed may need your guidance in doing so.

Another extremely detrimental response to a client in the midst of emotional release is withdrawal. We learn early in our lives that withdrawal can be an expression of disapproval and even a form of punishment. Parents and other caregivers commonly withdraw their attention, affection, and approval from children to demonstrate their disapproval of the child's actions, thoughts, or feelings. Thus, withdrawal by the client's massage therapist may reenact the original situation that caused the client to repress the feelings that he or she is presently displaying. Such a response, whether or not it reenacts the past, may be devastating, even shaming, to the client, leading him or her to believe that not only the expressions of the emotions, but *the emotions themselves are "bad."*

The client who perceives the therapist withdrawing from emotional expression may also feel abandoned and alone. This too can cause the client to shut down the release process, essentially leaving a part of the emotional process "undigested." As we saw with judgment, this emotional indigestion can have a rebound effect later on, which can manifest as anxiety or depression.

Typically, less experienced massage therapists withdraw because they fear that the client will become lost in an emotional tailspin, crying or ranting endlessly, and possibly directing the emotion at the therapist. Only rarely does such a scenario occur. However, it is the *fear of emotional release*, sometimes compounded by *the therapist's fear that he or she will not know what is right to say or do*, which undermines the therapist's confidence and interferes with the ability to deal with the client's release appropriately. The client is also affected when the therapist withdraws because of fear. The client is often left feeling that his or her emotional condition has overwhelmed the therapist, thereby inhibiting the client from further emotional expression. In

---

Box 6.2

EXPLORING HOW YOU RESPOND TO CLIENTS' EMOTIONS AND BEHAVIORS

The following are some emotions and emotion-based behaviors that may cause you to feel uncomfortable. Imagine a client exhibiting each emotion or behavior, and notice how you react. Try to observe your emotional, cognitive, and physical responses. Do any of these emotions or behaviors make you feel as though you want to withdraw? If so, notice *how* you withdraw. Then see if you can imagine how your withdrawal might affect a client expressing the emotion. Finally, ask yourself what makes you feel and respond in this way.

- Weepiness
- Sobbing
- Irritation
- Screaming rage
- Great excitement
- Deep depression
- Fist-pounding anger
- Flirtatiousness
- Terror
- Hysteria
- Withdrawal
- Inquiries into your personal life
- Nervousness
- Chattiness or talkativeness
- Mistrust and suspiciousness
- Joy
- Wild laughter and silliness
- Childishness
- Pain

addition, the client may infer from the therapist's reaction that his or her emotional condition is too much for the therapist—perhaps for *any* therapist—to handle. Another reason why a massage therapist may withdraw is feeling uncomfortable with the kind of feelings being expressed by the client, such as the feelings we asked you to explore in Box 6-2. In this case, withdrawal can be a way of saying, "I don't want to deal with this, and/or I don't want to deal with you."

Riccardo

This case study is a little different because it is a second-hand account of a massage therapy session. One of our clients, Riccardo, is a psychotherapist. He shared the following story about the massage experience of one of his clients.

Riccardo said, "I have a psychotherapy client who recently went for her first massage. During the massage, she began to cry spontaneously. The massage therapist seemed to become overwhelmed very quickly and withdrew emotionally. She [the client] felt very alone and abandoned, as if she had done something wrong. Attempting to please the therapist and reassure the therapist that she was okay, she stopped crying. The sad thing is that she said that she does not want to try massage therapy again, since she is concerned that she might have another emotional release and overwhelm the massage therapist. This is an unfortunate turn of events because I believe massage therapy can be an excellent adjunct to psychotherapy, and she would have benefited from using the massage to feel more in touch with her body."

A confident therapist conveys to the client that the emotional release is not boundless or dangerous, that it will complete itself, *and* that the therapist is not overwhelmed, frightened, or repelled by it. This "contains" the process for the client, allowing him or her to "disintegrate" safely, effectively, and creatively and then reintegrate with a new perspective. The therapist conveys this truth nonverbally, simply through the calm presence that stems from his or her confidence. Our use of the word disintegrate may seem a bit unsettling, but we use it in the sense that most people in our society are too well held together and need to let go. Safely "falling apart" can be a benefit to emotional health, even more so when we reintegrate after a release and put ourselves back together in a more open, effective way.

Another element in communicating confidence is feeling comfortable with both emotional expressions in general and specific emotions. This is a reason why we asked you to explore how you respond to specific emotions in Box 6.2. The more comfortable you can learn to be with such emotions, the more present you can be for your clients.

The third response for the massage therapist to avoid is a psychotherapeutic intervention. By *psychotherapeutic intervention*, we mean asking psychological questions, probing, making interpretations, offering solutions, and giving advice. Many massage therapists have participated in workshops in which emotional release has occurred during class or a demonstration by the instructor. Based on their experiences at such workshops, attendees may be inspired to duplicate what they have seen, thinking that it is good or powerful to provoke emotional release. However, such activity crosses over into the realm of psychotherapy. There is a great difference between an emotional release arising spontaneously from the client and the deliberate stimulation of release by the therapist.

Most massage therapists who stray into using psychotherapeutic interventions in response to emotional release do so with the best intentions. Based on discussions about emotional release with many massage therapists, we believe most therapists act out of a strong sense of responsibility to the client, which in turn drives the therapist to aggressively respond. This often results in the massage therapist feeling that he or she must use powerful, directive techniques and thereby overdo it.

Psychotherapeutic intervention may be especially tempting when working with clients who suffer from chronic pain conditions, such as recurring migraine headaches, fibromyalgia, arthritis, lupus, and so on (however, remember that chronic pain may have an *undiagnosed* physical cause), but it must be strictly avoided. During initial sessions, a client with chronic pain may talk about the physical patterns she is aware of that are related to the problem. As the work progresses and the client's awareness expands, she may begin to have spontaneous insights into the emotional factors surrounding the problem. This is appropriate and beneficial. However, if the therapist aggressively pursues the underlying causes for the chronic physical patterns without the client already fully accepting the idea that emotional factors are contributing, then the client's response could either be inhibited or defensive. The client may well terminate the therapy.

Instead of using psychotherapeutic intervention, we urge you to focus on maintaining a proper therapeutic environment. This is achieved by providing support, promoting the client's grounding, and integrating the experience. We turn to these subjects next.

Providing Support

The most vital part of providing support to a client experiencing an emotional release is to BE PRESENT. What being present means is the ability to communicate non-verbally to the client that you, as the therapist, are there, listening, watching, being accepting, concerned, centered, and focused on the client. No matter how intensely emotional things become for the client, the message you send is that you will remain focused and able to handle whatever comes up. This requires that you be comfortable within yourself with the expression of emotion. You must also deeply understand that emotional releases, as dramatic as they can be, are not harmful, but rather, are part of a natural process of releasing blocked emotions that are intricately involved with chronic tension patterns. With experience, you will come to recognize that emotional releases have a distinctive beginning, middle, and end. Trust that this process has its own flow and primarily requires you to simply be present in a supportive manner, rather than play the role of someone who must "run the show" or solve the problem.

Reflective listening is an important technique for providing support to the client experiencing emotional release. Carl Rogers, a psychologist who was a major force in the development of humanistic psychology in the 1960s, found that having a sense of feeling understood and being seen by another person was indispensable and significant to his clients' growth. He used a technique known as *reflective listening* to impart this vital sense of feeling understood and being seen. Reflective listening not only became a basic part of psychotherapy in general, it also influenced other helping professions, organizational psychology, political discourse, some spiritual pursuits, and education.

Rogers' seemingly very simple technique focused on the act of one person accurately reflecting what another person said and felt. In essence, the listener becomes a mirror for the speaker. In mirroring another, the listener does not interpret the speaker. The listener feeds back to the speaker what the listener feels is the essence of the speaker's thoughts and feelings.   Reflective listening includes the following qualities:

▶ Presence
▶ Acceptance
▶ Support
▶ Empathy
▶ Understanding
▶ Accuracy

Reflective listening leaves out the following from the conversation:

▶ Analysis
▶ Interpretation
▶ Judgment
▶ Comparison
▶ Advising
▶ Placating
▶ Confronting

Reflective listening does not involve simply parroting what the other person says. The listener (the therapist) may, however, paraphrase what the other person says with an aim to truly understand the speaker (the client). The listener must have and convey an *authentic* interest in the speaker and what the speaker is saying.

You can begin a reflection with the following phrases:

What I hear you saying is . . .

My sense of what you're saying is . . .

My understanding is . . .

Do you mean . . .

The speaker often gives a verbal or nonverbal confirmation when the reflective listening is effective. The speaker may say, "That's right" or nod and may even repeat a bit of what was said in the previous sentence and then go on, often in more detail and depth. If the speaker signals that the listener is not accurate, the listener can simply make a new statement that takes into account the speaker's correction. For example, the listener can say, "Oh, you meant . . ." The speaker will signal that the listener has understood correctly by moving on in the conversation. If the listener's reflections are not effective, the conversation will feel as if it is not progressing. In this case, the listener can inquire whether the speaker feels something has been misunderstood or not heard. Sometimes, this gets the conversation "back on track."

You can best practice reflective listening with three people: a speaker, a listener, and an observer. The speaker can put out a thought or a feeling, and the listener can reflect that feeling or thought. The speaker can reflect back subjectively to the listener whether the listener accurately reflected the speaker, while the observer can provide an objective observation when needed. As the exercise goes on, the roles can change.

Besides simply being there for the client or listening reflectively, another form of support can be maintaining some form of contact, such as holding the client's hand or feet and keeping the other hand in contact with the client (e.g., on the belly,

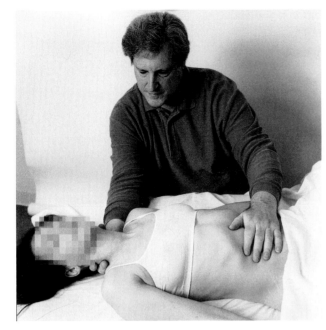

Figure 6.2
*Technique useful during emotional release: placing **a hand under the neck and on the belly** of the client. The hands are giving "still-handed" touch, meaning that the hands are not moving or applying pressure other than from the weight of the hands. (Standard draping procedures were not used in this photo so that the placement of the therapist's hands would be visible.)*

under the neck, or on the upper back (Figures 6.2 and 6.3). If the client is looking around anxiously, also establishing or maintaining eye contact can be important.

Any directions you give or actions you make also need to be supportive. An appropriate direction, for example, would be to encourage deeper or slower breathing. The important thing is that by your actions you are nonverbally assuring the client that it's okay, or "I'm with you." It may also be helpful to respond briefly to comments the client is making. For example, if the client is mentioning someone or somewhere ambiguously, you might ask the client to mention a specific name or place. If you notice an area of tension or emotional blocking developing, touch that area or ask the client to move or focus on that part of the body.

Promoting the Client's Grounding

Emotional release often disorganizes and disrupts the person's grounding. When it occurs toward the end of the session, noticing the time and helping the client "wind down" the release before the session time elapses are important. Being "thrown out" too quickly into the world after an emotional release can be a shocking and disorienting experience, possibly prompting subsequent anxiety or depression. Furthermore, the client may be so unfocused that he or she may have difficulty operating a car or otherwise getting home. One client we know about left a massage therapy session too quickly and sat in her car for 2 hours, unable to drive home.

As the emotional release is ending, or if it is close to the end of the session, bring the client back into the "here and now" (time) and "into the room" (space). Ground the client by focusing on the hands, feet, and eyes, which are the points of contact with the environment. For example, you can hold the client's hands or feet and make eye contact until you sense the client feels the contact (Figure 6.4). If you do not feel that the client is making contact, encourage the client to focus on feeling the contact created by your touch. Have the client stand for a few minutes with knees slightly bent while looking around the room. Make sure that the client is actually focused on what he or she is looking at, because he or she might be looking without actually seeing. A suggestion could be made to notice concrete details of objects in the room, such as color and size. While the client is standing, suggest that the client feel his/her feet making contact with the ground, or if sitting or lying, feel the body making contact with the chair or table. After the client stands for a few moments, suggest that he or she is ready to walk around the room. If needed, you can do some more touching to ground the client. Finally, while doing any of these grounding techniques, it is also very important to suggest that the client keep breathing and keep experiencing the breathing.

Integrating the Experience

Finally, the manner in which you as the therapist say goodbye and end the session is important. Being excessively businesslike *or* overly emotional can create an uncomfortable departure or closure for the client. The client needs to feel that you are present, that you were able to handle the emotional release, and that you believe something constructive took place. Convey to the client that the emotional release was not destructive or disruptive to the relationship, the therapy process, or either of you. Also, confirm that you will continue to be present for the client and that the process will continue. This helps the client feel positively about the release, affirming that what happened is a genuine part of the client's life and process.

The client also may have had no idea that an emotional release was a possibility during a massage session. In either case, talking about the release is imperative to assist the client in integrating the experience. If there is not enough time at the end of the session to talk about it, then the therapist can suggest that they both discuss what happened at the beginning of the next session. Such a discussion can be brief, the purpose being to assure the client that emotional release is a spontaneous and valid part of the therapeutic process. The emotions that surfaced during the emotional release may have been among those deemed unacceptable or intolerable aspects of the client's psyche, so their revelation can stir up reactions ranging from slightly to extremely threatening and upsetting. This helps the client integrate what happened. If the client does not want to talk about it, then the therapist needs to state that talking about it probably is important and that the therapist is available to talk about it at another time if the client changes his or her mind.

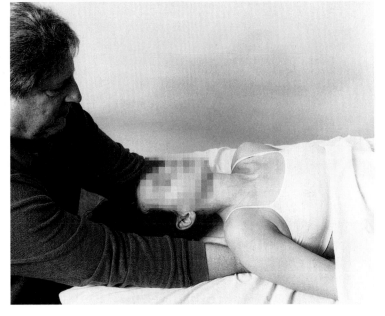

Figure 6.3
*Technique useful during emotional release: **Hands under the scapulae** of the client. The hands are giving "still-handed touch," meaning that the hands are not moving or applying pressure other than from the weight of the hands. (Standard draping procedures were not used in this photo so that the placement of the therapist's hands would be visible.)*

What should such a discussion about emotional release include? First, an invitation by the therapist to the client to talk about what might have felt uncomfortable and what might have felt beneficial about the emotional release. The therapist also needs to invite the client to share any insecurity related to the therapist's reactions to the emotional release. This is an opportunity for the therapist to assure the client that no judgments have been made about the client or the experience.

Sometimes, a person who has never experienced emotional release may fear that he or she is going crazy or that the release is a symptom of a serious problem. Another possibility is that the client may have no idea why the release occurred. In such situations, the client may need to have the experience "normalized;" that is, the therapist points out that an emotional response to the work is not abnormal.

In some cases, the client may believe that the therapist "caused" the emotional release. In such cases, the therapist explains that the release resulted from spontaneous reactions taking place within the bodymind of the client and was not produced by the therapist.

Most important, the follow-up discussion is *not* an analysis by the therapist of the client and what happened during the session. This can be one of those moments when the massage therapist needs to refrain from using psychotherapeutic interventions. Occasionally, something may surface in an emotional release that the client needs to work on with a psychotherapist. In such a case, the client may need the help of the massage therapist in finding someone to help integrate the experience. Making referrals to mental health professionals is discussed in Chapter 11.

Integrating the experience also means letting go of expectations for further release. If the client felt some sort of gain coming from the emotional release, such as more emotional freedom, deepening insight, physical well-being, greater

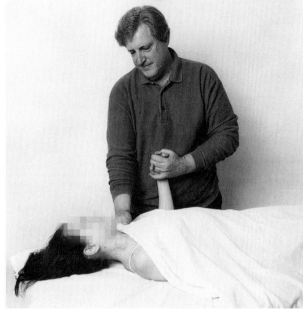

Figure 6.4
Grounding technique: Therapist looks into client's eyes while holding hand. Contact with the hands and eyes facilitates grounding; that is, it helps bring the client into the "here and now" of the present moment.

energy, or clearer thinking, he or she will be motivated to continue working with and exploring the territory opened up by the emotional release. However, this does not mean that future sessions will involve emotional release. For one thing, replicating a previous session is not possible. Letting the client know that emotional release is not a matter of technique, but rather of emotional readiness on the part of the client is important. This readiness is not just in the conscious mind! The unconscious considerably influences whether or not an emotional release will occur; therefore, *no matter what the massage therapist or the client consciously wants, an emotional release in nearly all cases will happen only when the unconscious is ready*. This last point also is important for therapists who may fear that an emotional release may be harmful. Unless the therapist is inappropriately forcing the issue, an emotional release is unlikely to occur unless the client is ready for it. It is as if most people have unconscious "brakes" that protect their psyches.

Finally, during the discussion, clients should be asked if they have any other questions. Pose this question in an open-ended manner, meaning that the question should be nonspecific enough to allow the client to put things in his or her own words. Some clients do not bring up certain material if they answer only specific questions from the therapist (Box 6.3).

Box 6.3

DEALING WITH EMOTIONAL RELEASE

Tips for dealing with emotional release.

▶ **Be present!**
▶ **You do not need to "do" anything.**
▶ **Feelings are not harmful.**
▶ **Keep breathing, remain centered and grounded (yourself).**
▶ **Encourage the client to keep breathing.**
▶ **Facilitate grounding (by the client).**
▶ **Allow time for quiet, if needed.**
▶ **Allow time for talk, and to ask questions, if needed.**
▶ **Use reflective listening when appropriate.**
▶ **Be supportive, nonjudgmental, and accepting.**
▶ **Maintain a safe space for the client.**
▶ **Respect what has happened, remember this may be a very important event in the client's life.**
▶ **Refrain from giving advice.**
▶ **Own your feelings, i.e., honestly acknowledge and take responsibility for how you are feeling (to yourself).**
▶ **Refrain from withdrawal, judgment, and using psychotherapeutic methods.**
▶ **In the long term, increase self-awareness and work to become more comfortable with the feelings with which you are not comfortable.**

EFFECTS OF EMOTIONAL RELEASE ON THE MASSAGE PROCESS

If a client has an emotional release, what implications does this have for subsequent sessions? Will the client continue having emotional releases? Will the client speak about it in the next session? Does having one emotional release "take care of" the problem? Will the client come back? Does the massage therapist need to refer the client to a psychotherapist or counselor?

Expansion and Contraction

Emotional release brings a sometimes euphoric, emotional, somatic, and cognitive expansion. For a little while, the client may feel free, emotionally expansive, and able to see new options in life. On the other hand, we have seen clients again and again in our practices in whom this expansion is followed by a contraction that leaves the client feeling bewildered, disappointed, or angry. The defense system that was put in place in childhood is tenacious. The defense system embedded in the client's unconscious may experience openness as a threat to the organism and attempt to close or shut down the expansiveness. The client can experience this as a slow erosion of good feeling, a return of negative internal chatter, or a sudden tightening of the body accompanied by anxiety. Letting the client know that such a contraction might occur helps the client cope with contraction without being surprised.

Kenisha

While Graham was working with Kenisha's belly, Kenisha began to cry. Graham stopped any movement he was making and let his hand rest on her abdomen in a warm and supportive way. Kenisha's crying became deeper and deeper until she was finally wailing. Kenisha's cries began to diminish spontaneously. Graham's hand had never left her abdomen.

"Could you hand me a tissue," Kenisha asked as she wiped her nose. "Wow! I never knew how much I missed my father. It's like he left and I've been waiting for him to come back. I've been waiting for 12 years. I've put my life on hold and didn't realize it. A big space has opened in me. Now maybe I can let myself go back to school. I don't have to wait any more."

"That's great," said Graham, keeping his hand on her abdomen. "Sounds as if you've had a big opening. It's important to know that this place of openness and awareness lives in you all the time and you just need to know how to find it again. You may close up a little in a few days, but if that happens you still know it's there."

The next week Kenisha came back for her regular massage. "You were right," she said to Graham. "That great open feeling didn't last, but I remembered what you said. Even though not feeling as good was a little disappointing, I remembered that you said that place was within me. That comforted me. I'm going to keep working to find it and learn how to keep the open feeling longer."

Resistance

Some people have a high level of psychological curiosity and an inner motivation to engage psychological issues. An emotional release stimulates and motivates them to continue working further. Not much concern is needed in this case. But for some clients, emotional release results in resistance, not only to the emotional release, but also to the massage therapy itself. In Chapter 3, we discussed resistance in detail as one of the psychological defenses of the client. Here, we focus on resistance as a response to emotional release.

Resistance can manifest overtly or covertly. The most blatant form of resistance is simply not showing up for the next session, maybe even never coming back. Although this is unfortunate, the massage therapist usually cannot do much about it. If this happens to you, do not automatically assume it means you did something wrong. Instead, it usually indicates that the client was just not ready to go further. This does not contradict what we stated earlier about emotional release not taking place when there is a lack of emotional readiness. The client who terminates therapy may well have been ready to have an emotional release, but may not be ready to let the process go *further*. In other words, the client's defenses were triggered by the emotional release and caused the client to avoid any further vulnerability.

Another form of resistance by the client is avoiding discussion of anything related to the emotional release and the previous session. He or she will get right back into the routine as if nothing happened. A client also may try to gain assurance from the therapist that it will not happen again. This, of course, the therapist cannot promise, especially when the emotional release came about spontaneously. It would be more effective, in this case, for the therapist to encourage the client, if the client wishes, to talk about how he or she felt about the emotional release and why he or she would like to be assured it will not happen again. Doing this may help the client be more in touch with his/her feelings and integrate the experience.

Resistance may also occur in the client's body. The client may be exceptionally tense in a session after an emotional release, particularly if he or she does not know what instigated it. The client's guard may be up, consciously or unconsciously. If you notice this, inquire whether the client has any feelings—such as anxiety or fear—about another emotional release or is attempting to prevent an emotional release by remaining tense. This can create an opening for the client to discuss feelings about the emotional release or for you to encourage the client to relinquish the tension, so that he or she can be more relaxed and receptive during the massage.

If a client has an emotional release and either does not make another appointment or misses the next appointment, we recommend phoning the client. The purpose of the call should be to find out how the client is and whether the client needs help to deal with his or her experience from either the massage therapist or a mental health professional. Some clients react with anger to an emotional release, because they are frightened or embarrassed by it. This anger may be expressed toward the therapist and can take the form of blame, accusations of incompetence, or manipulation. It is important that the massage therapist not become defensive, but listen to the client in a reflective manner, as we previously discussed. If the client's anger subsides enough to take in what the therapist is saying and discuss the release openly, the opportunity may arise to give the client some general information about emotional release and typical responses to it. This may allow the client to gain a wider perspective and may help him or her integrate what happened. If the client is completely unreceptive to talking to you, then gracefully end the call without forcing the matter.

Fear

A client may experience either a generalized sense of fear or specific fears after an emotional release. Such fear may arise several hours or even days after the session and may surface in dreams, even nightmares. It can be an intensification of a familiar fear known to the client, or it can attach itself to a new object in the client's psyche. A delayed experience of fear could occur if fear was underlying the emotions that came up during the emotional release. Similarly, the client may experience free-floating anxiety, which is anxiousness that is not related to or attached to anything specific.

Fear as a reaction to an emotional opening up occurs because the new or freed feelings threaten the client's defenses. This threat can manifest as fear of impending doom, fear of doing something wrong or destructive, or fear of being found out for doing something wrong. Fear can also be in response to or anticipation of the sheer intensity of the release. Before the release, emotions can build up in intensity owing to the blocking effects of the client's defenses. By not allowing a regular flow of feeling, a sort of "emotional pressure" builds. An analogy would be that water breaking through a breached dam has much more energy and force than water flowing freely in a running stream.

Another fear that commonly surfaces is that of being judged as weak, sick, monstrous, or otherwise unacceptable. If the client can tell the therapist that he/she fears that you are judging him/her, then you as the therapist can help. If you suspect that a client feels you are judging him or her, but cannot verbalize this, then ask the client directly if he or she is concerned about what you are thinking. Bear in mind that the client may fear you are judging him or her because he is judging himself. This defense is *projection*, as discussed in Chapter 3. Again, the idea is not to perform a psychotherapeutic intervention, but to help the client clarify a misperception so as not to get stuck.

One fear clients commonly have about the effects of emotional release is a fear of losing control, "going crazy," or becoming overly emotional at an inopportune moment. In these instances, the therapist can explain to the client what causes the emotional release process and why the release is not harmful. Helping the client understand that the emotions surfaced because of the safety and containment of the therapeutic setting and the loosening of blocks, not because the client was "losing it," is also important.

Jana

As Carolyn applied light pressure to Jana's chest, she noticed that Jana was beginning to hold her breath. Instead of Jana's chest relaxing as Carolyn intended, Jana's chest became very hard and inflated. Carolyn also noticed that Jana's jaw was becoming very set. Jana was clamping her lips together and a little tear was trickling out of her left eye. Carolyn lightened her pressure, but kept her hand on Jana's chest. "How are you doing?" Carolyn asked Jana.

Jana spoke through her teeth, "I don't know. I'm really scared, upset. I feel like I'm going to lose control."

Carolyn had experienced this with other clients, so she felt fairly calm. "Losing control means different things to each person. Can you tell me what it feels like to you?"

Jana's breath was still held and she still spoke through her teeth. "I feel like I'll explode. I feel like I'll cry forever. I feel like they'll put me away."

"You know," said Carolyn, "Feelings will sometimes come up in a massage, feelings we've put away for a long time. It's as if we stuff them behind a wall. The wall acts like a dam, and the feelings build up a lot of pressure so it feels as if when they break through and we let them out, they'll destroy everything. But in my experience, this is a safe place to let these feelings come through if they need to. They won't destroy anything, and they won't last forever. You really will be okay if you get angry here or if you cry. See if you can work with me to let you body relax and see what happens."

"I'm pretty scared. How do I know that you know what you're doing?"

"Well, as I said, this is a natural occurrence in massage. I've worked with people before who have had feelings on the massage table."

"Well, okay," said Jana begrudgingly, "I guess I'll try."

"Okay," said Carolyn as she cupped Jana's jaw and supported it, "I'm just going to support you and we'll see what happens." Jana's jaw began to relax in Carolyn's hand and her lower lip began to tremble. Jana began to cry—a little at first and then more heavily. The tears were angry in the beginning and then softened into grief. Jana's crying lasted a few minutes, then it subsided. Carolyn took Jana's hand and looked into her eyes. "What's happening now?" she asked.

Jana

"I feel a lot better. I'm surprised. I didn't die," exulted Jana.

"And you didn't go crazy," said Carolyn, with a smile.

"No," said Jana, with great relief and satisfaction, "I didn't. I actually feel better."

"Do you want to talk about what you experienced?" asked Carolyn.

"No," replied Jana.

"You don't have to tell me the details now or even ever, but I really would like to talk together about the process you went through. We could do it at the end of our session today or the beginning of the next one. That's an important part of continuing to have this be a safe place for you."

"Okay," Jana agreed.

"Now, let's finish the massage," said Carolyn.

If Jana had not been able to stop the flood of emotions after the session, Carolyn's most appropriate action would have been to refer her to a psychotherapist. One reason is that psychotherapy, with its particular set of treatment methods, provides greater psychological containment, and therefore security. Another reason is that—as we have repeatedly stated—probing into the root causes of a client's fears crosses over the boundary line between massage therapy and psychotherapy. In this case, Carolyn helped her client get past her fear, but without pushing her to respond in a particular way.

Many people who have had opening emotional experiences in massage welcome the suggestion that they engage in psychotherapy and go on to make great strides in their personal growth, thanks to the impetus provided by their experience with massage therapy. However, some people may feel insulted or judged by the suggestion that they might benefit from psychotherapy. In such cases, emphasizing that you do not consider the client to be crazy, deficient, weak, or whatever the client fears may be true about himself is important. State unequivocally that, as a massage therapist, helping the client work through what opened up is outside of your area of expertise and that you are therefore making the referral in the best interest of the client. You can also assure the client that the massage therapy can continue and you will not abandon the client.

Euphoria

Euphoria is another feeling that may follow emotional release. Although it is one of its more pleasant byproducts, it is not the most dependable. *Unless the euphoria is grounded, the client is likely to crash into disappointment or depression, experiencing the contraction we discussed earlier. Encouraging the client to enjoy the euphoria, but also letting him or her know it is not the final result of the work, is important.* If the client has a history of depression, the euphoria may cause the client to look for the same result again. In such cases, explain to the client that euphoria is not the antidote to feeling down or depressed. A client with depression may also try to expand the euphoria. Although this rarely happens, if unstable behavior develops and the client seems "too high" and frenetic, a referral may be needed (see the section on mania in Chapter 10). With all euphoric clients, promoting grounding is important.

Other Responses

In addition to the effects just discussed, clients may react to an emotional release with a variety of *psychological defenses*. These include resistance, which we touched on briefly above, projection, denial, transference, and many more. These defenses may also occur in clients who have not actually experienced a release, but who sense that the massage is unearthing emotions that they feel unable to handle.

One such defense that we have so far only touched on is **dissociation** (see the definition). Dissociation may occur as a result of emotional release. One might recognize dissociation by the person having a "spaced-out" quality or seeming to be out of contact and unable to focus (Figure 6.5). Dissociation indicates that the emotional release or its content has been overwhelming or overpowering. It is unusual for dissociation to occur in a person who does not usually use dissociation as part of his or her defenses. Some other manifestations of dissociation can be denial that something significant has taken place, or "changing the subject" and unemotionally talking about something other than what is related to what happened. Generally, a client dissociates so as not to experience feelings. If a client appears dissociated, then use grounding techniques.

Emotional release sometimes opens up areas of a person's life that the person believes are too painful to deal with. The client believes if he feels this pain, then he will be caught in a swamp, abyss, or bottomless hole out of which he will be unable to climb. In this case, depression might result from emotional release because of the impact of experiencing that part of his life. This form of depression is different from clinical depression, which may have biochemical origins. It can actually be a reasonable reaction to something that was truly saddening. We discuss depression in more detail in Chapter 10.

At the beginning of this chapter, we stated that emotional release results from disturbing or altering a pattern of defense or experience. Such patterns of defense combine both the psychological and physical dimensions of the bodymind in forming *armoring*, which is the subject of the next chapter.

REFERENCES

Allison, N. (1999). *The illustrated encyclopedia of body-mind disciplines.* New York: Rosen Publishing.
Diagnostic and Statistical Manual of Mental Disorders. (1994). Washington, DC: DSM-IV.
Knaster, M. (1996). *Discovering the body's wisdom.* New York: Bantam Books.
Levy, F. (1988). *Dance/movement therapy: A healing art.* Fairfax, VA: AAHPHERD.
Rogers, C. (1965). *Client centered therapy.* Boston: Houghton Mifflin.
Van I., Marianus, H. & Schuengel, C. (1996). *The measurement of dissociation in normal and clinical populations: Meta-analytic validation of the Dissociative Experiences Scale (DES).* Leiden, The Netherlands: Algemene Pedagogiek.

Figure 6.5
Dissociation. *A person dissociates by not being "in" his body and retreating into a disembodied world of thoughts and fantasies, but not feelings.*

Dissociation

Dissociation is a bodymind phenomenon that occurs when an individual compartmentalizes bodily sensations, perceptions, memories, affects, and distinct psychological states and detaches them (dis-associates them) singly or in combination from each other, from present experience, or from conscious knowledge. Dissociation ranges from the ordinary (spacing out, highway hypnosis, "running on automatic," daydreaming, reveries) to the religious (shamanism, voodoo, some forms of meditation) to a response to traumatic or stressful situations (short- or long-term amnesia, fragmentation of personality, disembodiment). Most abnormal dissociation is a result of trauma or stress. Dissociation manifests on the bodily level in the form of disembodiment as a defense against feeling overwhelming pain or fear (to not be in one's body is to not feel).

When dissociation impairs a person's functioning, it is considered a *dissociative disorder*. The *DSM* (a psychological diagnostic manual) generally defines a dissociative disorder as "a disturbance or alteration in the normally integrative functions of identity, memory, or consciousness. The disturbance or alteration may be sudden or gradual, and transient or chronic."

A certain amount of dissociation is considered normal. Nearly everyone experiences dissociation, albeit on a minor level, at least occasionally in life. For example, we daydream, fantasize we are another person, or imagine we are somewhere else. Some mental health professionals consider dissociation to be a healthy defense mechanism under certain circumstances, provided that the dissociation itself does not cause impairment of functioning.

Armoring

7

C h a p t e r

Armoring can be defined as chronic patterns of involuntary tension in the body that dampen or block emotional expression, alter perception of both the outer world and the inner psychological world, diminish or eliminate kinesthetic awareness and other sensations, and restrict range of motion and movement. Simply put, armor is a defense against **affect** that is manifested in the entire body (see the definition). Armoring is a useful concept because it portrays how the psychological *and* physical elements of people *dynamically interact* to form resistance to thoughts, perceptions, and feelings.

Affect
Affect is the expression of feeling, emotion, or mood.

NATURE OF ARMORING

Our definition of armoring reveals that it has three key characteristics: chronic, involuntary, and defensive. Let us examine each of these qualities more closely.

Chronic Nature of Armoring

The chronic nature of the armor patterning—the way armoring reasserts itself despite temporary relaxation—gives armoring a quality that is different from simple muscular contractions, spasms, and tension. This chronic patterning is a manifestation of the *resistant* nature of the armoring and the psychological defenses that armoring reflects. The patterning takes many different forms (to be discussed later in this chapter and in Chapters 8 and 9).

Involuntary Nature of Armoring

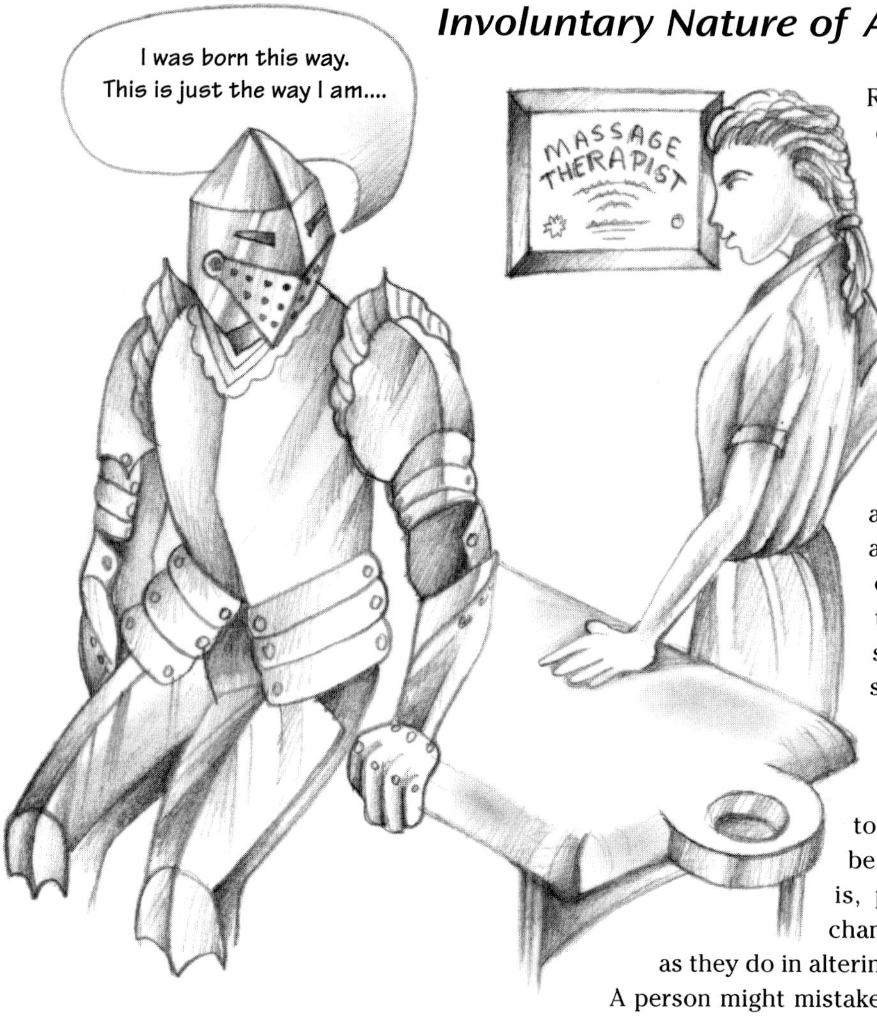

Figure 7.1
Identification with armoring.
People usually think their armoring is an inherent part of their personality without realizing that the armor is a defense.

Research has affirmed that somatic defenses, like many physiological changes associated with emotion, happen automatically and outside awareness (Damasio, LeDoux). The *involuntary* nature of the armoring demonstrates the conflict and disconnection between the conscious and unconscious motivations occurring within the same person. As we discussed in earlier chapters, while the client's conscious mind may want to let go of and gain relief from the tension caused by a pattern, the unconscious part of the client's mind might find such relaxation threatening and resist letting go of the tension. If the client is caught between a conscious desire to let go and an unconscious need to resist letting go, then the involuntary tension of the armoring can be frustrating to the client . . . and perhaps also to the therapist. A similar frustration may be felt in the psychological dimension; that is, people can have as much difficulty in changing certain thought patterns or behavior as they do in altering chronic muscular tension patterns.

A person might mistake this automatic quality of armoring for a personal trait. For example, two very common claims people make about the armored aspects of themselves are, "That's just the way I am," or "I've always been like that." These statements reflect the unconscious quality of the armoring and the extent to which people identify with their armored traits. They believe the armored traits are inborn, natural parts of themselves, rather than defenses *against* inborn, natural parts of themselves (Figure 7.1)

Defensive Nature of Armoring

As our definition stated, armoring defends against many aspects of human existence, and primary among these are our awareness and expression of our feelings. The impact of armoring on awareness may be so profound that the person becomes unable to feel parts of the body. Armoring may even cause a person to experience the body as numb or anesthetized, or him- or herself as figuratively invisible or even nonexistent (i.e., "If I do not feel my body, then I will not be noticeable and I will be safe").

Jackie

Jackie was a client of ours who suffered from low self-esteem. As a child, she received very little positive feedback from her busy, successful parents. She felt as if she was barely noticed around the house. When she did make bids for

Jackie

attention, her mother tended to criticize her and her father tended to ignore her. Trying to be noticed brought her much emotional pain, so she learned to do without. Jackie developed a pattern of withdrawing into her room, where she spent hours by herself.

As an adult, Jackie struggled in her career and in relationships with men. She came to realize that she felt distinct discomfort whenever she stood out or was noticed. Thus, she developed a manner that helped her to escape notice, as if she were invisible. She was stiff and inexpressive, with a frozen, doll-like quality that did not invite others to interact with her. She actually had developed a manner of not being noticeable, as if she were invisible. If she did get noticed, her reaction would be to somehow undermine or undo whatever it was that brought her the attention. For example, she would blow big sales that would have won her special recognition from her firm, suddenly become tongue-tied when meeting an attractive man, avoid wearing brightly colored clothes, and sit in the back row at adult education classes and meetings. Once she began to recognize her invisibility and self-denial, she gave herself the nickname "The Invisible Spartan," since she had learned to stealthily soldier through any situation with the scarcest sustenance.

The effects of armoring can make people feel mechanical to the point where they perceive their bodies more as machines than organic beings. For example, when Jackie suffered a pulled muscle in her shoulder, she said, "This part won't work, how can I get it fixed?" Clients similar to Jackie also describe themselves with terms such as glassy, wooden, frozen, steel-like, shapeless, or distorted. Note the inorganic or lifeless quality of such descriptors. Armoring's effect on awareness also distorts body image and often underlies the problems accompanying poor body imaging.

Scientific studies have also affirmed that somatic and visceral feedback plays a critical role in the experience and repression of emotion. Body armor inhibits both bodily activation in emotion, and somatic and visceral feedback that accentuates, intensifies, and ultimately makes emotional experience conscious (Damasio, LeDoux). Kinesthetic awareness, which depends on bodily activation and visceral-somatic feedback, is one of the building blocks of self-perception. We depend on kinesthetic awareness, that is, sensing what is going on in our bodies and guts, in many ways *to know how we feel*. If armoring reduces kinesthetic awareness, this results in a reduced awareness of critical internal issues of existence, security, belonging, and self-acceptance as well. Damasio, LeDoux, and Gerson all have shown that emotional experience is accentuated, intensified, and ultimately made conscious through bodily activation of emotion and somatic and visceral feedback. Therefore, by inhibiting both bodily activation and visceral and somatic feedback, armoring affects the experience and repression of emotions. *Kinesthetic and psychological awareness are linked.*

Armoring not only restricts movement physically, but also figuratively. If you are unable to move parts of your body in certain ways, you may also lose or never develop the ability to imagine or visualize that movement and any expression related to that movement. For example, armoring in the area of the posterior shoulder girdle, such as the rhomboid muscles, inhibits movement that involves reaching forward. Expressions such as hitting or reaching out are also inhibited. Sometimes, the movement is so inhibited and the kinesthetic awareness so diminished that reaching out would never even come to mind. Not being able to reach out can create a mind-set in which reaching out for support is not possible. In this way, armoring

Box 7.1

EXPERIMENTING WITH PHYSICAL AND PSYCHOLOGICAL RANGE OF MOTION

These three exercises can help you explore the relationship between physical and psychological restrictions. We have used artistic license in coining the term "psychological range of motion" to reflect this correlation.

1. Rigid and Flexible

▶ We can see both rigidity and flexibility in the body as states of being. Try making yourself rigid in an exaggerated way. Try walking around and doing familiar movements for a little while. Notice any subtle changes in your thinking and feeling.

▶ Now let go of the exaggerated rigidity and become as flexible in your body as you can. Become flexible in an exaggerated way. Try walking around and doing familiar movements for a little while. Notice any subtle changes in your thinking and feeling.

▶ Write down all the attributes you can think of when you consider rigid thinking.

▶ Write down all the attributes you can think of regarding flexible thinking.

2. The Head and Neck

▶ Try stiffening your neck so that you can only look straight ahead. You cannot turn your head to the left or right. Walk around for a little while and notice how this concretely affects your perception, thinking, and feeling. What can you see and what can't you see? How much of an adjustment do you have to make with your body to perceive what is at your sides? As you are moving through space, what ends up happening to your direction and speed?

▶ Try holding your neck so that you are looking down and staring at the ground. Walk around for a little while in this way, and notice how this affects your perceptions and mood. What can you see and what can't you see? What are you missing by keeping your head in this position? What kinds of adjustments do you have to make to see anything but the ground?

3. Arms and Shoulders

▶ Try reaching out. Is this a familiar movement? Does it feel restricted? Do you reach out all the way? What are your hands doing? Are they open to taking something? Are they limp? Are they tense? Do you let yourself reach out to people? Do you reach out for good things in life? Do you reach to achieve?

▶ Try reaching up. Is this a familiar movement? Does it feel restricted? Again, feel your hands? What are they doing? Do you let yourself reach for higher things in life-goals, knowledge, spiritual actualization? Is this range of motion comfortable for you?

▶ Try reaching back. Is this a familiar movement? Does it feel restricted? Do you let yourself reach into your memory and your past to discover resources, insight, or feelings? Does it feel all right to reach back, or is it too painful?

limits individual potential. Many varieties of thought, feeling, and emotional expression, in effect, are eliminated from that person's emotional repertoire. To explore this phenomenon for yourself, see the exercises in Box 7.1.

Armoring also defends by dampening or blocking emotional expression energetically. If we look at the body as having three layers (discussed in more detail in the final section of this chapter)—ectoderm (skin and nervous tissue), mesoderm (muscle, bone, and other connective tissues), endoderm (digestive tract, respiratory tissues, and most other internal organs)—armoring also affects the body energetically. According to body psychotherapist Malcolm Brown, originator of Organismic Psychotherapy, armoring has the effect of "shrinking" **vegetative energy** (see the definition on page 135) on the endodermal or "core" level. This shrinking of the vegetative energy reduces a person's capacity to feel his or her needs. Diminution of the vegetative energy also decreases the quality of aliveness and capacity for self-direction. Without enough energetic flow, feeling is not sustained or may not even be perceivable. In turn, without feeling, expression is limited.

We often speak of people being "open" or "closed" to describe their relationship to *outer* reality, including other people, emotions, perceptions, and ideas. Armoring may create either a very dense boundary or an overly porous one between oneself and the world outside oneself. It also may affect what we perceive. For example, persons who, because of their armoring, habitually walk with heads down tend to perceive mostly what is at their feet and directly in front of them. Their perception has become selective and limited. Or, the armoring pattern within a person allows him or her to perceive *some* of the emotions of other people, but not other emotions. A person may see a heightened sense of anger in others, but not be able to perceive love or gentleness coming from the same persons. Conversely, some people only see the pleasant qualities in others and reject obvious hostility or other negative emotions with which they may be uncomfortable. In this sense, they "wear rose-colored glasses."

Armoring's effect on the perception of *inner* reality comes from blocking the feeling, sensing, or identification of both physical and emotional inner conditions and needs. The greater significance of this is *not being able to feel or sense that our body interferes with our ability to know what we want in life.* Fritz Perls, in his book *Ego, Hunger, and Aggression*, used hunger to explain the relationship between feeling and self-direction. Perls observed that if one cannot feel (meaning sense) one's stomach, cannot feel hunger or being filled up, or cannot feel what one wants or needs to eat, then confusion will exist about what the person wants out of him- or herself, others, and life overall. The logical flow of this idea is that if we cannot feel our bodies or bodily sensations, then we cannot feel what we want or need; and if we cannot feel what we want or need and thereby do not know what we want or need, then we will have difficulty determining what our direction in life should be. In this sense, *through interfering with inner feeling, armoring interferes with self-direction.*

Vegetative Energy
The autonomic nervous system is described in older texts as a vegetative system. The term "vegetative" therefore describes a biophysical, fundamental level of functioning and existence. Writers such as psychiatrist Wilhelm Reich and neurologist Kurt Goldstein have used the term vegetative energy to describe life energy or an energetic life force that infuses an individual with vitality, which is a difficult quality to capture in words. Some contemporary writers, such as Damasio, use the terms somatic and visceral in reference to this core energetic flow.

HOW ARMORING DEVELOPS

In some movies with a psychological theme, the lead character is commonly portrayed as having lost the memory of a single powerfully traumatic event that happened in childhood and was the main cause of a psychological problem that has ruined or twisted the character's adult life. These movies reflect the popular view that associates psychological troubles with such singular traumatic events. They portray the notion that finding the "smoking gun" or "snake under the rock" solves the psychological mystery when the traumatic event that caused it all is finally uncovered. Although this certainly can happen, it is *not* the most common pattern of origin for armoring. In real life, it is more likely that painful events repeated many times cause psychological damage that is not necessarily catastrophic in scale or highly dramatic, but is cumulative. To help you understand the origins of armoring, we provide here a simplified story of a child and his mother in a difficult emotional situation. This story has been synthesized from those of many clients.

The child is named Johnny and he is 4 years old. He is with his mother, and his father has just left the family. Johnny's mother is not only emotionally crushed and overwhelmed, but she also has no idea how she and Johnny will survive economically. She is depressed and anxious and does not know what to do. As with all children, Johnny needs to make contact with his mother frequently in small ways—a look, a touch, a hug. His mother, however, is too distraught and tense to be able to respond to Johnny's approaches. Indeed, they irritate and anger her, and she treats Johnny's attempts at connection as distractions (Figure 7.2).

In our scenario, Johnny approaches his mother to tell her something. Perhaps he tugs on her skirt to get her attention. Johnny's mother turns and looks at Johnny with angry and rejecting eyes. Johnny is shocked and scared. He may never have seen his mother directing such anger at him. He may not even recognize the person he is encountering at this moment as the mother he knows. One thing is certain. His mother's angry look scares Johnny, and the physical manifestation of his reaction is that Johnny's shoulders rise almost to his ears, his breathing diminishes, and he backs away slightly. The rising of Johnny's shoulders, his diminished breathing, and his backing away are **organismic** responses to a threatening situation (see the definition).

Johnny's mother's irritation might temporarily diminish and Johnny's fear along with it. However, the situation that Johnny and his mother are in does not change. Johnny's mother remains overwhelmed, confused, angry, and depressed. Thus, when Johnny goes to his mother for comfort, he often finds that she gives him an

Organismic
Natural, instinctual responses arising from the organism, resulting from the holistic interaction between the mind, body, and soul are termed organismic. One of the first to introduce the idea of organismic functioning was Kurt Goldstein, the neurologist and Gestaltist, who wrote about the holistic functioning of the nervous system in his book *The Organism*, in which he challenged the reductionistic thinking of his day. One of the persons to expand upon Goldstein's teachings is the psychologist, Malcolm Brown, who developed Organismic Body Psychotherapy and wrote *The Healing Touch*.

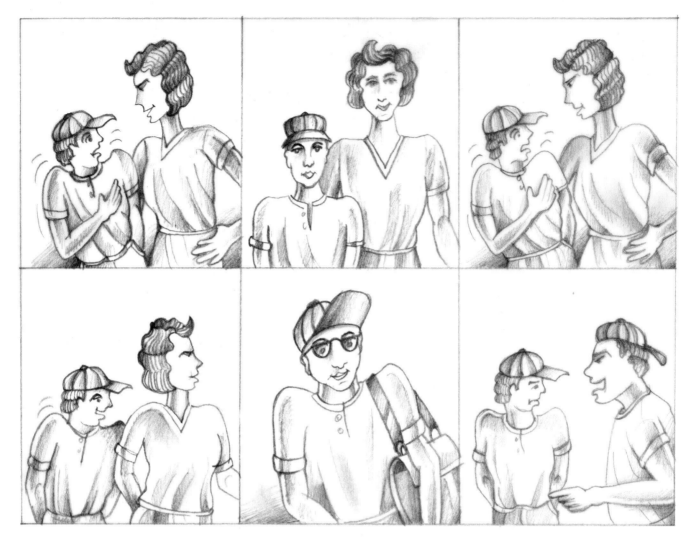

Figure 7.2
Johnny's storyboard: How Johnny became armored. *An illustration of how armor develops. At first, Johnny's emotional response to his mother's anger subsides after she calms down. However, after happening repeatedly, Johnny's anxiety and fear (depicted as raised shoulders) remain locked in his body. His social environment, symbolized by the bully picking on him, reinforces his image of himself as timid and weak and the world as a hostile place. His armor hardens more in response.*

angry response, especially with her eyes. Each time he feels afraid, his shoulders rise and he backs away. As with most daily life, even in bad situations, there are respites from the tension and Johnny's fear can subside temporarily, and with it, his shoulders lower to a normal level. He again assumes a normal physical stature.

If we notice the animals that are pets in our homes, such as cats and dogs, we can observe mammalian responses to danger. We can see that there is a strong and observable body response to danger, but when the danger passes, so does the bodily response. For example, a passing dog may arouse a sleeping cat to a state of alert. The cat springs up, arches its back, and bares its teeth as its fur stands up. However, as soon as the dog has left, the organismic response to threat quickly subsides, and the cat may return to sleeping almost immediately.

Humans, however, remember and learn in a different way. Humans usually have more difficulty returning to a state of relaxation so quickly or easily, especially when the triggering situation is recurrent. When the situation Johnny and his mother are in does not change, and thus the emotional atmosphere remains the same, Johnny begins to anticipate the look his mother will give him when he approaches her. He may not know consciously that this is what he is doing. If someone asked him, he might not be able to say that he is scared. Even before he approaches his mother though, he feels bad and his shoulders rise. Johnny is anxious now. His body looks scared. Johnny's situation reflects the fact that *anxiety is associated with an increase in muscle tension* (Borkovec and Lyonfield).

Johnny is caught in a "Catch-22." The figure he is attracted to and needs, his mother, is also a figure he is increasingly afraid of. His irresistible need drives him to approach her, but his overwhelming fear repels him. Approaching his mother feels bad, but as a 4-year-old he needs his mother. He is unable *not* to approach her. The bind causes anxiety to build within Johnny . . . and, in turn, the anxiety causes muscular tension to build within him. As their situation continues, Johnny's approach and his mother's response remain the same. It becomes a dance with which both are all too familiar. However, something more is happening now within Johnny. He *must* do something about the anxiety.

Humans cannot tolerate anxiety for prolonged periods. Instead, we tend to resolve it in one of two ways: we either experience or express the feeling, or we stop the feeling. Numbing is a common method of controlling the feeling, which quells the anxiety. Since Johnny feels he is unable to either experience or express his feeling, he begins to numb his body and his emotions.

Johnny's kinesthetic awareness is also affected. As the situation continues and his shoulders continually rise, he begins not to feel the pain of their tense positioning. In fact, he begins to carry his shoulders in an elevated position all the time without being aware of it. As Johnny begins to lose kinesthetic awareness, a simultaneous reduction in *psychological* awareness occurs. This reduction is extremely significant because Johnny is about to lose awareness of what he is really scared of—his mother.

Johnny *must* approach his mother. He depends on her for love, nurturing, and survival. He does not have the option of leaving the situation, one that also happens to be harmful for him. To know that the person he is absolutely dependent on is also a source of powerful fear is intolerable. Johnny consequently must begin to obscure his sense that his mother is the source of the fear. Ironically, to survive, Johnny must no longer identify the perceived source of danger (his mother). He will use the psychological defense of denial to protect himself from the threatening perception that his mother is a source of danger. As he does so, instead of his mother being scary to him, Johnny begins to identify himself as a scared person and consequently as a person incompetent to defend himself. This is a pivotal shift in psychological and bodily awareness, brought about by a *reduction* of the kinesthetic awareness that would tell him he is specifically scared, accompanied by an *increase* in nonspecific anxiety that tells him that he is a scared person. The longer he holds his shoulders up, the more he loses kinesthetic awareness, and, in turn, the more automatic holding his shoulders up becomes. The reciprocal relationship between the body and mind, as discussed in Chapter 5, can be seen in action here. The continual holding of the shoulders in a position of fear generates a continual feeling of fear (and vice versa). Johnny's body now is continually giving his mind the message that he is afraid, whether or not a source of fear in the immediate outer world exists.

We see a reflection of ourselves in others' eyes, and how they mirror us in turn strongly influences the formation of our self-image (for an insightful description of the formation of self-image, see Putney and Putney, *The Adjusted American: Normal Neuroses in the Individual and Society*). People around Johnny eventually read his body language. Children respond to his raised shoulders and generally fearful look by bullying and teasing him. This begins another feedback loop that reinforces the perceptions of himself that are already taking shape in Johnny's bodymind. From the bullying and teasing by kids around him, Johnny knows for sure that he is a scared and inadequate person and that the world is a dangerous place.

Johnny may be able to figure out ways to compensate for the anxiety he is feeling. One of these ways may be to split off from his body and go into his head. If he does so, he will not have to feel the constant fear coming from his bodymind. He may also enhance or emphasize his intellectual capabilities. We have all known "brains," "geeks," or "nerds" when we were children. They seemed to be "out of it." Some of them may have been in this type of situation.

Armoring generally happens when the child is in a dependent state and in a negative situation he can neither escape from nor change. Armoring is a way of adapting to chronic, painful conditions and becomes a critical coping mechanism.

It is this *survival*-oriented quality of armoring that makes it resistant to change. To be armored is to survive; therefore to de-armor paradoxically also makes a person feel vulnerable to what threatened the person in the past, *despite the person's desire to change.*

In this sense, the *armoring is the lifeboat to which a person clings for survival in the rough emotional seas of life.* To suddenly take away this personal lifeboat, even though it consigns one to drift in an ocean of misery, can be formidable. *This is the foundation of one of the great paradoxes of therapeutic change: to gain greater health, one must give up what at one time served to protect.* A caregiver who is dedicated to working with people to resolve their life conflicts, or to dissolve the armoring, is prone to "go after" that lifeboat. Appreciating the survival quality of the armoring allows the caregiver to honor the armoring and refrain from yanking it away. It also affords a greater appreciation of why armor is so persistent and resistant. This can be extended to massage therapy, because the effect of massage therapy on the bodymind also engages armoring.

Learning how not to go "trauma hunting" when working with armoring is also important. For example, giving the suggestion that someone has been sexually or physically abused without any conscious memory robs the person of discovering his or her own past through psychological work. It also inserts the agenda of the therapist into the therapy. Furthermore, this is not the cause of most armoring patterns. Rather than being like a snake under a rock, it is often the day-in, day-out repetition and reinforcement of emotional patterns that are harmful to the child.

However, people *do* suffer trauma. Massage therapy can be a highly effective way of complementing psychotherapy for people who have suffered such events. Going after the armor to smash it or attack it is a mistake however, especially with someone who already knows she has been traumatized. Such traumatized people must develop a sense of safety within the body, often very slowly. Whereas much armoring occurs from toxic emotional situations, trauma also includes harm to the body and soul. This makes approaching the body of someone who has experienced trauma particularly complicated. When this type of client feels safe enough, he or she may spontaneously begin to release emotions around the events that have traumatized him or her. Supporting such clients without pushing them into **catharsis** is important, because they may not be ready for it (see the definition). The supposed cure can be as harmful as the problem. Most psychophysical traumas involve what is currently known as *shock trauma* (Box 7.2).

Besides forming in reaction to negative aspects of childhood relationships, as illustrated in the example of Johnny, armoring can be formed in reaction to negative childhood events as well. Negative events can include going through parents getting divorced, moving and changing schools, losing a pet, failing or excelling in school, not having friends, and being harassed or teased by peers owing to any perceived difference from others. These may sound like typical childhood events that many people go through without lasting effects, but for some this is not the case. What usually distinguishes negative events that lead to armoring is the subjective intensity of the event, duration of the event, availability of support, internal resources, and whether the child can take an action that solves the problem at the time it happens. Children can make it through difficult events without leading to armoring if they can somehow resolve them or have adequate help from others in tolerating the negative situation in a creative way.

Catharsis

Catharsis is bringing fears and psychological conflicts to consciousness and giving them expression with the intention of alleviating them. From the Greek origin, *catharsis* literally means "to purge."

Another way that armoring may come into being is through the child identifying with one of his or her caregivers. This identification may be with the caregiver that the child either feels safest with *or* feels least loved by. As pointed out in Chapter 3, identification can be a normal part of development; however, armoring related to identification generally occurs when there is a psychological conflict between the caregivers. For example, a child may begin to identify with the parent who seems more powerful in the relationship between mother and father. The child may begin to hold his/her body in a posture that imitates the more powerful parent. The child's voice and mannerisms may become similar to those of the parent. As the child copies that parent, he or she may be simultaneously taking on the attitudes and feelings of that parent. For example, it is not unusual in massage for someone to remark, "Oh, I can feel my father in my back." When the child becomes too identified with one of the parents, it is more difficult for the child, and subsequently the adult, to find his or her own sense of identity.

Box 7.2

SHOCK TRAUMA

Dramatic and intense events can cause *shock trauma*, a response to an event that is perceived by the organism as life threatening. Examples of events that can lead to shock trauma reaction are premature birth and other similar birthing problems, physical and sexual abuse, severe accidents, exposure to violent and traumatic events, severe personal illnesses and hospitalizations, and sudden illness and death of loved ones. Our responses to life-threatening events are to fight, flee, or freeze. Shock trauma locks the bodymind into one or any combination of these responses. Although the somatic response to shock trauma almost always involves some sort of dissociation between body and mind, it is not the same response as armoring that develops in reaction to negative aspects of relationships in childhood. Symptoms of shock trauma range from flashbacks of the traumatic event, fragmentary body memories, intense and uncontrollable fear or anger reactions to ordinary nonthreatening events, to loss of body sensation. In body psychotherapy and psychotherapy in general, shock trauma is treated differently than other childhood problems, such as negative aspects of childhood relationships.

Since identity is felt through the body as well as the intellect, one can begin to develop a better sense of self through massage by eliminating patterns of adaptation that have been adopted from the parents. Massage can do this by facilitating the client becoming aware of the pattern, releasing the body pattern associated with the identification, and experiencing what it feels like to be without the pattern, thus allowing new possibilities and choices.

The type of armoring that develops also depends on *when* harmful events happen in the child's life. What may be scary and threatening at 2 years old may be less troublesome at 7 years. We all go through critical developmental stages in our lives. We all experience total dependence and vulnerability when we are born and during the first weeks of life. We all experience being dependent for food, love, and other forms of care. We all experience weaning away from our dependence and developing autonomy. We all experience the struggle to control our feelings, yet remain a feeling person. We all develop our sexuality. If we do not journey through and complete each of these "way stations" in life, our emotional development is curtailed and we end up with deficiencies in certain areas of our emotional abilities. If we encounter difficulties at any of these points of development, then the emotional themes of that point influence the formation of armoring. Also, any previous damage affects our abilities to complete the next developmental task. Although we all grow up physically, we may have holes or deficits in our emotional development. Seeing that we can be for the most part whole, but have certain incomplete areas of ourselves that are enough to make us stumble, is important.

For example, if someone faced difficulty when being fed and taken care of, for example, from 6 months to 2 years old, then later in life that person may have difficulty in believing that he or she can get needs met. This can appear in many different ways. In relationships, this person may want more than anyone can give, or conversely, never expect to get anything. In the person's working life, he or she may not be able to connect efforts at work with being paid. The person may work too much and allow him/herself to be paid far less than he or she deserves or may expect inflated compensation just for showing up, feeling entitled to be taken care of. Most simply put, someone encountering obstacles in this stage of life will have difficulty in understanding how to get the world to work in both the realms of love and career (Box 7.3).

Almost like reading tree rings, at the body level we can see these stages by the types of armoring that occur, because each stage presents a different situation that leads to a different formation of armoring. Before looking at which stages associate with which type of armoring, we need to look at the components of armoring.

There is a tendency to associate armoring with tight, hardened tissue and with rigid, withdrawn behavior. However, armoring can manifest in many ways, and its components are complex.

COMPONENTS OF ARMORING: CHARGE, GROUNDING, AND BOUNDING

Three of the components of armoring we term charge, grounding, and bounding.

Box 7.3

DEVELOPMENTAL HIGHLIGHTS

We all pass through several critical way stations in our emotional development. There is some overlap between some stages. The following summary is adapted from the description of developmental stages in *Characterological Transformation* by Stephen Johnson.

▶ **womb to 6 months.** The key issues are existence (right to live), belonging, and security. The infant is completely dependent, and the infant's identity is merged with its caretaker(s) and environment.

▶ **6 months to 18/24 months.** Key issues are receiving nurturing and being physically and emotionally dependent while differentiation and individuation take place as a separate identity is formed. The baby perceives its caretaker(s) and environment as separate and is learning to positively manipulate its environment to get its needs met.

▶ **18/24 months to 4 years.** Key issues are continuing to differentiate and establish an independent identity, while at the same time the parents are attempting to instill appropriate social habits (e.g., toilet training). The toddler also gradually establishes greater autonomy.

▶ **3 years to 5 years.** A key issue is—if the relationship with the "mothering" caretaker is solid—that the child perceives his or her separateness and begins to reach out to the parent of the opposite sex. In a two-parent household, there *may* also be rivalry with the parent of the same sex. The foundation of how the child relates socially is laid down. The child has mastered delayed gratification and is gaining greater ability to control emotions.

Charge

Charge refers to the degree of aliveness in a person's body as a whole. A person who is well charged has a good quality of aliveness or vitality, but not too much or too little. Some massage therapists in some instances tend to refer to charge as energy. In this sense, the degree of energy someone is perceived to have relates to the charge that person has. Charge also can be seen in *parts* of the body, for example, in deadened legs. Different parts of the body can have different degrees of charge, although you may get a general sense of charge from the person's entire body. Charge can be a vague term to many people, so one way of observing charge is to ask yourself, "Is there much happening in this person's body or this part of the body?" (Figure 7.3).

Grounding

Grounding refers to the quality of presence a person has. Another way to put it is the ability to be in the present moment or how well one is attuned to reality. A person who is well grounded can be very present and appropriately realistic or can allow his or her imagina-

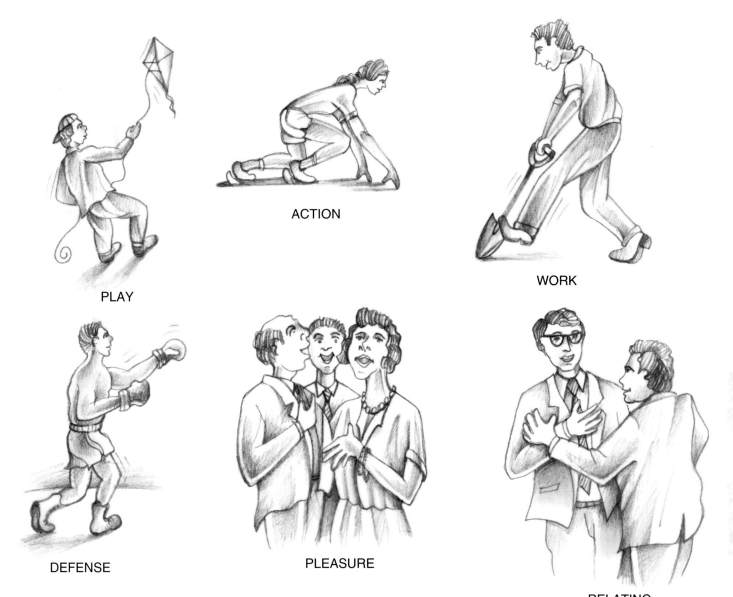

PLAY

ACTION

WORK

DEFENSE

PLEASURE

RELATING

tion to flow. One way of observing grounding is to ask yourself, "How much 'in the room' does this person seem?" or "Does this person seem to be in the 'here and now'?" On a deeper level, grounding reflects the degree of one's contact with reality. We are able to observe grounding in the parts of the body that make contact with the environment, such as the feet, legs, hands, arms, and eyes (Figure 7.4).

Figure 7.3
Charge. *Charge is vitality and aliveness. For example, charge fuels excitement and play, action, work, defending oneself, pleasure, and exchanging energy through relating.*

Bounding

Bounding refers to the ability to differentiate between what is oneself versus what is not oneself, or me versus "not-me." A person who is well bounded distinguishes accurately between his or her own feelings and the feelings of another person, yet can also gather what the other person could be feeling. On a deeper level, bounding reflects the solidity of one's identity. The parts of the body that bounding is related to in general are the skin and musculature (Figure 7.5).

Continua: Charged, Grounded, and Bounded

Charge, grounding, and bounding each occur within a continuum that ranges from excess to deficiency. In this sense, charge, grounding, and bounding each represent a polarity. The degree or amount of each can be too much, too little, or just right. If someone has an excess of one, this is termed *over*charged, *over*grounded, or *over*bounded. If someone has a deficiency of one, then the terms *under*charged, *under*grounded, or *under*bounded are used.

The charged, grounding, and bounding continua are not fixed, static states. A person's level or degree of charge, grounding, or bounding can change, depending on the circumstances of the moment. Being able to modify any of these so that the level is appropriate for the situation in the moment, and not too much or too little, is ideal. The psychologically healthy person operates in the middle range of each continuum and only in emergencies or extreme situations operates on the extremes of the polarity. For example, if a situation calls for understanding another person's perspective, that is, what it is like to be "in another person's skin," then being less bounded is appropriate. Consequently, the psychologically healthy person tends to be "well charged," "well grounded," or "well bounded." Armored persons tend to operate typically in the "over" or "under" ranges.

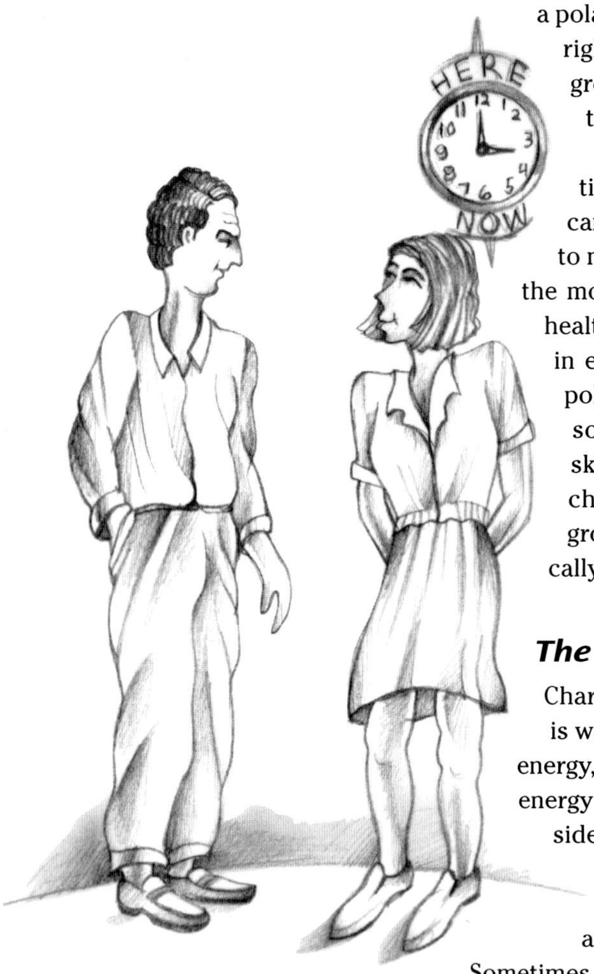

The Charged Continuum

Charge represents a person's degree of energetic aliveness. A person who is well charged can respond to situations with the appropriate amount of energy, spending neither all they have nor being unable to generate enough energy to function properly. Overcharge and also undercharge must be considered as being relative to what the well-charged position would be.

The overcharged person appears to be overenergized, which may manifest variously as being habitually frenetic, nervous, aggressive, energetic, perky, agitated, hot, racing, or overactive. Sometimes overcharged individuals seem to be in control of their energy, so we may not think of this as a problem. However, overcharge, whether the individual is in control or not, is a manifestation of an imbalance in the continuum. Depending on the client's body structure, which we discuss in Chapter 8, massage can affect overcharge through the use of still-handed touch, breaking up knots, or promoting the kind of relaxation that includes stilling the mind.

The undercharged person appears to be underenergized, which may manifest variously as being slow, collapsed, depressed, deadened, passive, low, indifferent, cool, or too mellow. If the undercharge is accompanied by flaccid muscles, then improving muscle tone and strength can help in combination with invigorating kinds of massage strokes. Holding a charge is more difficult without adequate muscle tone and strength.

As previously mentioned, people tend to see charge as energy, but energy is an amorphous term to many people. In classes that we teach, one method we use to help people sense energy in terms of charge, is to ask oneself, "Is there a lot happening or not much happening in this person's body?" If the answer is not much, this indicates an undercharge. If the answer is a lot or too much, the indication is an overcharge. We can observe overcharge in frequent and small movements, constant shifting, inability to sit still, or feeling extreme heat on the skin. We can observe undercharge in the lack

Figure 7.4
Grounding. *Grounding is about being in touch with reality through contact with the environment and the here and now (space and time). Our feet and legs, hands, and eyes make literal physical contact. "Having your feet on the ground" is a saying that reflects this basic wisdom.*

of aliveness, passivity of movement, lack of responsiveness, or a sense of stillness. Sometimes, we have students look at a person who has volunteered and together hum a tone that matches what they sense is that person's level of charge. When the class comes out with a high-pitched hum, this usually matches someone with a high charge, whereas a low hum indicates someone with a low charge. In our experience, the groups usually have been amazingly accurate when they do this exercise (Figure 7.6).

The Grounded Continuum

Grounding represents an individual's relationship between reality and fantasy. A well-grounded person has a healthy connection with reality and is also able to fantasize when appropriate to do so, meaning to use imagination unrestricted by time and place.

Overgrounded people are present, but *so* present that it interferes with their capacity for imagination. They have difficulty perceiving situations outside the literal "here and now" and tend to think and perceive literally and concretely. They also tend to be overfocused. Consequently, overgrounded people may have difficulty in taking a mental break and can get into a mental rut.

Undergrounded people are absent or "spaced out" and often a captive of their imaginations (therefore also of their projections). They have difficulty focusing on the "here and now" and tend to think and perceive abstractly or in fantasy. They also tend to have a diffuse manner of focusing. Dissociation and disconnectedness are more extreme forms of undergroundedness.

To help students get a sense of observing groundedness, we ask them to observe how "in the room," or present someone seems. When a person seems to be not present, this indicates undergroundedness. Conversely, if someone seems to be not able to figuratively "leave the room" and imagine what it is like somewhere else, this indicates overgroundedness. For example, if asked, "What do you think the weather is like in Jamaica right now?" the overgrounded person answers, "I can't" or "How should I know, I'm not there." The undergrounded person answers without difficulty. On the other hand, if asked, "Without looking, what is the pattern of the carpet in this room," the undergrounded person has difficulty, but the overgrounded person probably will not. The overgrounded person is stuck in the present reality. He or she cannot leave it, even for a moment. The undergrounded person cannot stay in the present reality.

Although overgrounded people seem to have better contact with reality, it is a forced contact. The overgrounded person is not well grounded, because the grounding is through his or her will, rather than the body. When one observes how an overgrounded person stands, the feet and legs seem to be pushing into the ground rather than being supported by it. In essence, the overgrounded per-

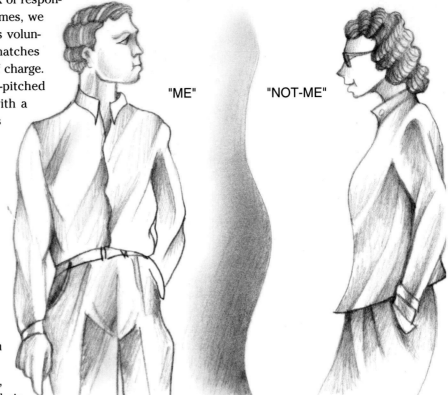

"ME"   "NOT-ME"

Figure 7.5
Bounding. *Bounding is related to the solidity of a person's boundary between him- or herself and the environment, which affects the ability to distinguish between what is "me and not-me." This distinction is essential for forming identity.*

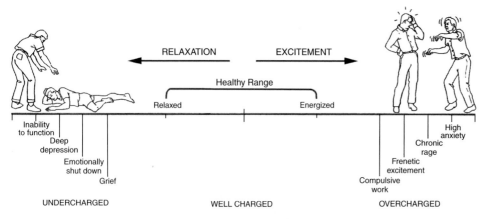

Figure 7.6
The charged continuum. *Charge ranges from undercharged (low energy states such as deep depression, inability to function, emotional shutdown, and grief) to well charged to overcharged (high energy states, such as high anxiety, chronic rage, compulsive work, or frenetic excitement). Sometimes, extreme undercharge can have an overcharge hidden underneath, or vice versa.*

Figure 7.7
The grounded continuum.
Grounding ranges from undergrounded (spaced out, dissociative, and in fantasy) to well grounded to overgrounded (absolutely literal, black-and-white, unimaginitive).

son is forcing him- or herself to be grounded. This can be related emotionally to a fear of flying off the ground or "losing control." This dependence on willpower deprives the overgrounded person of developing an experience of being supported by reality. In contrast, the undergrounded person may seem to be not quite on the ground.

Groundedness can be seen in the body by observing in particular the feet and legs, hands, eyes, and direction of energy because we make contact with the world with these areas of the body. When observing these parts of the body, note the degree and quality of contact made. In terms of direction, an overgrounded person's energy may seem to be directed into the ground, whereas an undergrounded person's may seem to be directed upward into the air. Consequently, massage that works with the feet, legs, hands, eyes, and direction of energy can affect grounding. With the overgrounded person, promoting relaxation, letting go, and a sense of lightness can be effective. With the undergrounded person, promoting increased sensation in these areas, a greater sense of contact, and sense of feeling support through these areas of the body can be effective (Figure 7.7).

The Bounded Continuum

Bounding concerns identity. Well-bounded people have a healthy sense of who they are and therefore who they are not. They can accurately identify their own issues and feelings and differentiate them from the issues and feelings of others, even when there is similarity. Healthy bounding allows for a healthy connection with another person, rather than merger, fusion, or lack of empathy.

Overbounded people have difficulty in identifying with anyone other than themselves. They have difficulty being in someone else's skin or walking in someone else's shoes. This may make them seem or be unempathetic, unsympathetic, or insensitive because they cannot imagine being in or having a feel for another person's situation. Consequently, overbounded people may be quite clear about whom they are and what they are thinking and feeling, but may have difficulty connecting with others.

Conversely, underbounded people often identify with everyone *but* themselves. They may seem very empathetic, but have no center and are unclear where the boundary between themselves and others is. They may project their own issues onto other people or take on others' problems as their own. They have a tendency to merge or fuse with others. Separation may be difficult for them. Underbounded people may also have difficulty with internal

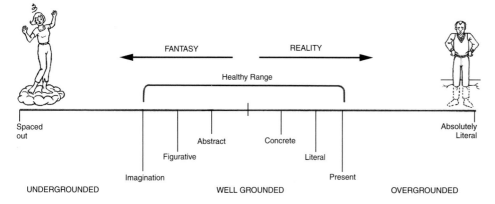

boundaries, because they may be flooded with emotions, may not sort out issues, and become easily overwhelmed. Consequently, underbounded people may be good at knowing what others are thinking or feeling, but may not always distinguish these perceptions from what thoughts and feelings are their own.

The skin is an important element of bounding. It forms the literal boundary between the individual and other people and the environment. An overbounded person figuratively (not literally) seems to have skin that has no pores and is impermeable. Overbounded skin is sealed tight. For an overbounded person, nearly all types of massage are helpful. Any response that leads the client to feel more open is a positive step. An underbounded person seems to have skin that is porous and absorbent (again, figuratively, not literally). Underbounded skin cannot be sealed. Working with the skin can facilitate bounding. For example, touching or pressing with the hands along the skin surfaces can affirm boundaries.

Similarly, the tone of the muscle tissue can also be related to bounding. Kinesthetic awareness and proprioception inform us about our muscle tone. In turn, muscle tone and proprioception affect how we stand and how we move in space. Our sense of muscle tone is intimately connected with our sense of identity. Poor muscle tone can be an indication of underbounding. Improving it may help an underbounded person. Consequently, improving muscle tone can give a person a better sense of bounding. Conversely, an overbounded person may have muscle tissue that has been held in a "dense" holding pattern. The pattern of the musculature numbs the tissue, so the person is less able to feel or sense what is outside himself or herself, thus contributing to overboundedness. Loosening the muscles and skin may help an overbounded person (Figure 7.8).

To help students learn to detect boundedness, we suggest they ask themselves, "Can this person walk in another person's shoes and, if they can, can they put on their own shoes?"

Figure 7.8
The bounded continuum. *Bounding ranges from underbounded (thin-skinned, hyperempathetic, merged, too sensitive, uncertain identity) to well bounded to overbounded (thick-skinned, callous, insensitive, isolated, inability to identify with others).*

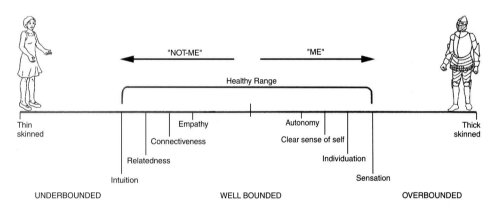

COMPONENTS OF ARMORING: TISSUE PATTERNS

Armoring generally manifests in the tissues in three forms that can be observed and palpated: knotty, sheath, and mesh. Some of these forms can be seen in combination in the same person and some do not frequently combine. Often, one type predominates.

Knotty Armoring

Knotty armoring is the type most common and familiar to massage therapists. It consists of hardened, contracted muscle tissue that is often described as ropy,

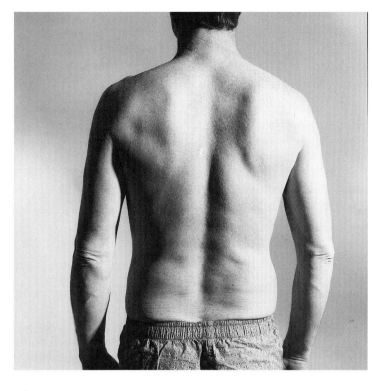

Figure 7.9
General knotty armor. *Knotty armor appears as general areas of muscular tightness in a system of knots to restrict movement or flexibility.*

Figure 7.10
"Held-back" knotty armor. *Systems of knots appear along the back of the body, either between the scapulae or in the hip and lower back areas, to restrict forward, aggressive, or expressive movement by the arms or legs. These movements include reaching out, taking in, pushing away, striking out, getting a grip, stepping forward, stepping up, and so on.*

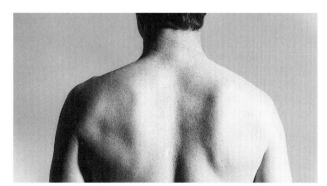

cable-like, wiry, lumpy, fibrous, or woody tissue that does not give or yield very much and often "snaps" or rolls over when pressed directly. What distinguishes the knotty pattern of armoring from simple muscle tension is the fact that the knots form a system, rather than being isolated focal points of tension. These systems of knots are designed to restrain movement—and therefore expression—or to rigidly hold up the person without succumbing to fatigue and collapse. Knotty armoring usually appears on the posterior of the body, but can sometimes affect the anterior side also (Figure 7.9) Two classic forms of knotty armoring are what we call the "held-back" and "held-up" patterns.

Held-Back Pattern

The *held-back* pattern is usually found in the upper back, especially between the scapulae (Figure 7.10). The pattern of knots restricts any forward expressive movement, including reaching out, reaching forward, pushing, hitting, or taking in. The significance of this restriction is that it interferes with actions related to connecting with the environment in a healthy manner, for example, connecting with others, taking in sustenance, and carrying out healthy aggression. These feelings and expressions are "held back" and not put forward and expressed. The knotted tension, typically located in the rhomboid or trapezius muscles, literally restricts the movement of the shoulder girdle in a way that the arms cannot be used in an optimal manner. This holding-back effect can be observed in the lack of follow-through in many arm and shoulder movements. For example, if someone with a held-back pattern is asked to do a hitting forward motion, the person's arms do not hit with full force. In effect, the person pulls the punch. Another example is if the person is asked to make a motion toward the mouth, as if feeding. The motion appears mechanical and lacking in some quality of aliveness, which might be perceived as desire, permission, or gusto. People with the held-back pattern, if they become aware of it, often report that they go through such motions without conviction.

The held-back pattern can also be found in the pelvis, as an anterior tilt, and in the posterior upper and lower leg. In these instances, in the pelvis it may signify held-back sexuality and healthy aggression on one's own behalf, whereas in the posterior leg it may signify holding back from moving forward. As in the upper back, in these parts of the body the holding-back pattern restricts forward expressive movement.

Armoring is not selective concerning bodily functions it protects or affects. Armoring in one place in the body can affect all other parts of the body in greater and lesser ways. For example, armoring in the rhomboids that occurs to prevent emotional pain caused by reaching out can also indirectly affect the diaphragm. This, in turn, can severely restrict breathing, which can manifest either as anxiety or depression. Indeed, armoring in the rhomboids can also affect the entire abdominal area.

Held-Up Pattern

The *held-up* pattern is usually found in the lumbar region of the back, especially in the paraspinal muscles (e.g., erector spinae). The knots are relatively large and involve the entire lower half of the erector spinae muscle group and are thick and bunchy. The pattern of knots appears to form rigid columns that hold up the back despite fatigue and restricts any tendency toward collapsing or falling. These columns replace the support provided by other areas of the body, such as the legs (Figure 7.11). The emotional significance of this restriction is that it does not allow the person to "let down." If one cannot let down, one cannot rest, give in to impulses, or surrender. The metaphor of falling is very important to understanding the held-up pattern. Most of our vulnerable qualities can be described with the falling metaphor, such as falling in love, falling ill, falling in defeat, falling down on the job, falling short, falling behind, and losing control. The held-up pattern associates falling with failing and feeling, both of which are forbidden. The held-up pattern is designed to be able to withstand pressure, carry weight (signifying responsibility), and achieve without showing any stress or strain ("don't let them see you sweat!").

Both systems of knots, held-back and held-up, are designed to favor *function over feeling*, achievement over emotion, and control over spontaneity.

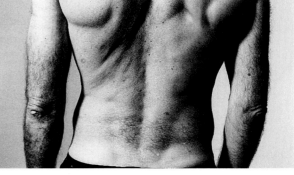

Figure 7.11
"Held-up" knotty armor. *Knots arranged in bunches within the erector spinae muscles that serve to stabilize the body against falling or collapse. These bunches appear to form columns or rods in the lower back. Falling serves as a bodily metaphor for resisting failing, feeling, being vulnerable, being defeated, losing control, falling in love or otherwise placing feeling over function.*

Sheath Armoring

Sheath armoring consists of large, slab-like or plate-like areas of thick, numbed tissue that often forms transverse bands. Since no single muscle other than the diaphragm crosses the body on the transverse plane, combinations of several muscles create these bands. The bands are usually found around the shoulder girdle area or the pelvic girdle, but when the formation becomes advanced, the sheath can envelop the entire back or even the entire body (Figure 7.12).

The quality of the tissue is firm and rubbery. When touched with pressure, the sheath armoring springs back. Another phenomenon that can be observed when digital pressure is applied to sheath armoring is that rather than compressing and springing back in a "pin-point" area, it does so in an area that is greater than the width of a finger or thumb. It absorbs the pressure, as opposed to resisting it as knotty armoring or rigid holding would. Sheath armoring obscures muscle definition, so very little surface anatomy can be seen usually on the person with sheath armoring. In the upper back, the sheath armoring appears to widen the space between the scapulae, rather than appearing as a contraction as in the held-back pattern of knotty armoring.

The sheath armoring has the emotional effect of *"holding in"* and deadening impulse. The sheath armoring does this by numbing, squeezing, pressing, smothering, or crushing the impulses. One cannot act on impulses if the impulses are continually being crushed before they come to awareness. Sheath armor does this so that the individual does not come into conflict with the will of others. Subordinating one's impulses to the will of others, while avoiding conflict, results in an inability to experience autonomy.

The sheath armor pattern is well suited to withstand pressure. It is as if nothing can get people with sheath armoring to release or give out their feelings. However,

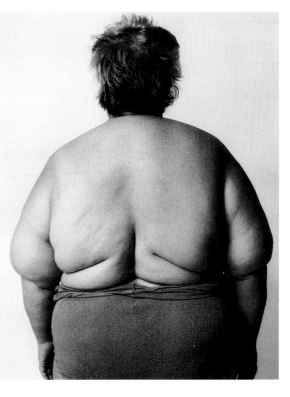

Figure 7.12
Sheath armor. *Sheath armor forms large plates of thickened tissue that obscure surface definition, giving it a smooth appearance. It engages several muscle groups in combination to make band-like rings around the body that squeeze or compress autonomous impulses.*

they still *feel* pressured. An apparently paradoxical situation is created in which people with sheath armoring subordinate their impulses to the will of others, yet can stubbornly withstand pressure and withhold their feelings no matter what. One may wonder how they can be so submissive to the will of others, yet getting them to do something can be so hard. However, it is the person's *will* that allows him or her to resist. If we see the relationship of sheath armoring to resistance, we can begin to see why the armoring is composed of dense tissue. It takes density to create a wall of resistance that can simultaneously block impulses and defy demands. Consequently, the person with sheath armoring can feel very "stuck," and those who try to get the sheath armored person to act or give in, such as therapists, can also end up feeling very stuck.

Mesh Armoring

Mesh is the third tissue pattern of armoring. This type is the most unusual and most difficult for the massage therapist to detect because the tension pattern does not reside seemingly in the musculature, although it is felt within the musculature. The person with mesh armoring tends to *appear* to be very emotional, but mesh armoring is actually an *energetic* defense *against feelings*. The important distinction that must be grasped to understand the dynamics of mesh armoring is that between emotions and feelings. Although the person with mesh armoring may experience him- or herself as feeling, the person is often emotional rather than "feeling." An internally experienced feeling state is expressed outwardly as emotion. The outward expression may not necessarily be connected to an internal feeling. Therefore, it is possible to be emotional *without* feeling. Normally, the emotional expression has some relation to experiencing the corresponding feeling from which it originates. However, in the person with mesh armoring, the emotion serves to *divert* both the person and the observer from awareness of the actual feeling. In this sense, the emotionality of the person with mesh armoring serves to block feeling.

Mesh armoring is a defense that uses a high charge of energy. This high charge resides in the musculature and at the skin level. It does not manifest as much in concrete muscular tension as does knotty and sheath armoring. The mesh-armored person may be extraordinarily limber, but still complain of an inability to relax. This combination of limberness and tension can be called the "onion-bag" or "string-bag" effect. When one puts a hand into a mesh onion or string bag, the bag stretches, but does not break. Similarly, the person with mesh armoring can stretch and stretch, but never break through the tension because the problem does not reside within the tissues. It is in the energetic field, which is why we did not provide a photo of mesh armor.

You can directly experience this high energy charge as an excessive amount of heat in certain parts of the body when you touch them. This charge can also be experienced through touch as a "buzzy" feeling, as if something were vibrating. Once the mesh-armored person becomes more attuned to the nature of the armoring, he or she may experience it as a form of static.

One of the features of mesh armoring, in addition to emotionality, is a hypersensitivity to body sensations. For example, the massage client may begin talking about the tension pattern in the left earlobe. For the massage therapist, this can be both seductive and confusing, since one of the goals of massage is to enhance body awareness. It is seductive in the fact that this exquisitely detailed body awareness on the part of the person with mesh armoring is actually a diversion from the more central problem that he or she cannot feel her body at a deep level beyond the musculature.

Armoring: The Disembodied, Collapsed, and Compressed Character Structures

Chapter 8

THE RELATIONSHIP BETWEEN ARMOR AND CHARACTER

The psychological equivalent to armoring manifests as *character*. Alexander Lowen says about the term character as it is used in the psychological sense, "The word character is related to 'characteristic' and implies that an individual behaves in a typical or predictable manner, whether good or bad" (*Bioenergetics*, p. 337). Wilhelm Reich described character as a chronic, automatically functioning mode of reaction, "[Character is] the sum total of typical attitudes, which an individual develops as a blocking against his emotional excitations, resulting in rigidity of the body, lack of emotional contact, and 'deadness'" (*Character Analysis*, p. 44). Lowen adds, "Character is also a psychic attitude which is buttressed by a system of denials, rationalizations, and projections and geared to an ego ideal that affirms its value" (*Bioenergetics*, p. 137). The term character is *not* being used in this book to mean moral strength, fortitude, reputation, an eccentric person, or a theatrical role.

Armor and character work together. Character emphasizes the *form* rather than the *content* of a person's psychological defenses. It is a person's typical way of *acting and responding*. Armoring is the *physical* structuring and manifestation of these characteristic *psychological* defenses; that is, armoring is the physical partner of psychological character defense. However, rather than being like a *static* suit of armor as worn by a medieval knight, armoring is an active and interactive *dynamic* defense system. As mentioned, armoring can be defined as chronic patterns of involuntary tension in the body that dampen or block emotional expression, alter perception of the outer world, alter perception of the inner psychological world, diminish or eliminate kinesthetic awareness, and restrict range of motion. Armor and character form an integrated defense system that simultaneously protects against the perceived forbidden internal impulses and the perceived threatening external stimuli of the outer world. As Reich puts it, "Armoring deflects and weakens blows of the outer world as well as the clamoring of inner needs" (*Character Analysis,* pp. 338–9).

Armoring and character develop because a perfect equilibrium rarely exists between the individual's needs and desires and the demands of living in the world. Because of this reality of life, each person must adapt to the outer world and, to do so, control certain inner impulses. As a consequence, most people carry some armoring. Two critical factors determine the type of character structure that is formed. One factor is the *timing* of the emotional stress relative to the stage of personal development. For example, character formation takes on a different pattern if it forms in the first 6 months of life when an infant is in the stage of being accepted than if it takes place at around 3 years of age when autonomy issues are foremost. The second is the *degree of intensity and frequency* of the stress. A single stressful developmental or emotional event might not lead to character formation, but if the intensity and frequency are greater, it could.

The child's defense against the emotional stress can eventually create a pattern that, in a sense, is devoted to coping with a particular set of problems. Rather than being a collection of diverse defenses, character and armor become a unified system of defenses that encompasses both mind and body. As a result, this unified defensive system necessarily combines a psychological pattern with a physical pattern that manifests in psychological defenses and chronic muscular tension. In this sense, the patterns develop cognitive, emotional, and physical structure. The structuring of psychological defenses—character—and physical muscular tension—armor—together can take different patterns. We have selected the four structures that stand out and also correlate to the major developmental stages.

In practice, most people do not have a pure character structure, but some form of combination. At the same time, most people, perhaps around two thirds, have a predominant character structure. The type that predominates usually has something to do with the stage of development with which a person ends up having the most difficulty. As in many things in life, timing affects character formation, that is, the time of life in which stress takes place.

As each character structure is described, the reader may find him- or herself identifying with each one. The reader may even feel he or she fits each type. This is a form of "medical student's disease" in which one identifies with the conditions one is studying. Being able to imagine oneself as each type is a form of learning. However, there is a deeper meaning to this and why this happens. All of us pass through the same "way stations" in childhood. We all need to feel accepted and wanted, to be nurtured, to develop a sense of autonomy, and to have the right to feel and want. We all can recognize the pain of not having these needs satisfied. We have all journeyed along the same human path on the way to physical and psychological adulthood.

If we successfully have these intrinsic needs fulfilled, we become equipped to have emotionally healthy lives. If not, we get "stuck" at that particular "way station" and have difficulty moving forward until we "solve" the problems presented by that particular stage in which we are stuck. More formally, being stuck is termed *arrested development.* Because we share this developmental commonality, we can identify with all the character structures in some way.

Another common response to learning about character structures is that they can seem to give negative portrayals. To an extent, the negative flavor comes from looking at what results from negative outcomes in human development and from the focus that psychology, psychiatry, and psychotherapy have on psychopathology. However, the character structures are also portraits of *survival-motivated adaptations*, and in that sense they are positive in that *they reflect the human desire to live and thrive to the extent that is possible for each person.* Indeed, as a character structure develops a survival-oriented solution to the problems confronting an individual, the solution involves emphasizing the development of certain attributes that can also be seen as gifts or strengths. For example, character structures may develop strengths in a similar manner to how people who lose their sense of sight may develop a heightened sense of hearing and touch.

These character structures are presented as a tool for gaining greater insight into the psychology of the body, a deeper understanding of your clients' responses to your work, and forming effective therapeutic strategies. They should stimulate readers' thinking and awareness, which is more the intent than presenting an exhaustive discussion of character analysis. Critiques of character typology have stated: (1) Character typology is more accurate the closer a person fits the description of a structure, but less accurate the more someone is a mixed or "in between" type; (2) because our bodies are highly complex, each person possesses many idiosyncratic nuances, some of which can be psychologically significant, and character reading sometimes leaves the subtleties of body structure aside; and (3) in terms of etiology, character tends to emphasize the relationship with the mother, while not looking as much at the father, other people, and the family system, with the result that the conflict between mother and child is sometimes distorting in its emphasis and accent. Furthermore, character analysis is not the only psychological system for understanding people, and the authors make no claim as to which is *the* best.

However, having said this, our experience has been that these ideas about character are enormously useful and practical. We have found in our teaching and practices that understanding character is an effective way to gain a better understanding of the psychology of the body. In practical terms, understanding character structure is a good way to get hold of the relation between body structure and personality, to learn how to apply that insight to how and why people respond differently to different kinds of touch, and to know what kinds of touch to use with different clients. Understanding character also helps us to understand better the limits imposed on clients by previous life experiences. At the same time, any system of psychological classification is bound to be limited to some degree and reductionistic. *Nobody can be reduced to a label and a precise set of traits.*

We are describing a systematic method of defending oneself when we describe character, rather than actually describing the "self." These labels should not be offered or presented to clients. In our practices, we rarely discuss these labels with clients. We use them primarily for our own guidance. When kept in respectful perspective, understanding character can be very rewarding and immensely effective in deciding how to work with and respond to a client. Please keep this "grain of salt" offered here in the back of your mind while reading on.

The discussions about character in these chapters are based primarily on the theories and writings of Wilhelm Reich, Alexander Lowen, Malcolm Brown, and David Shapiro, along with the writings of Stephen Johnson and Edward Smith and our own experiences from our work with clients. We have sought to minimize jargon when possible and avoid using psychopathologizing language, so we have accordingly used terms that in some instances differ from the terminology used by these writers.

THE DISEMBODIED STRUCTURE

The primary traits of the *disembodied* structure are to dissociate thinking from feeling and to withdraw inwardly, and to break or lose contact with the world or external reality, especially when such contact is threatening. Contact with the body is also greatly reduced. People with this structure tend to "live in their heads." Very early in life they experienced rejection by their main caregiver, which was felt as a threat to their very existence. To survive, especially to deal with such intensely terrible feelings, as children they cut off all feeling and split from their bodies. As adults, intimate, feeling relationships are both difficult to establish and avoided. The disembodied structure is overcharged, undergrounded, and underbounded. The holding pattern is held together (Lowen 1971).

Psychological Dynamics

People with a disembodied structure exist in a fundamentally extreme state of chronic dissociation, divided between the head and body. They are *literally living in thought or fantasy and not in their body* (Smith). Their sense of self is located exclusively in the head, as if the head were floating above nothing, or directing the body as if it were a machine. As a result, such people literally do not feel their body. This is why the term *disembodied* is used to describe this structure.

The head-centered orientation may manifest as detailed self-observation and self-direction through thought. People with a disembodied structure may be acutely self-conscious, observing every minute action they do as if they were observing someone else. Movement is often initiated and guided by their head, which gives their body verbal mental directions. For example, to brush their hair, they might tell themselves (silently to themselves as thoughts) to put their feet on the floor, to stand up to walk across the room, to pick up the hair brush, and then draw the brush through the hair.

Sensation stimulated by outside events, such as being touched, may also be mediated through this kind of mental running commentary. For instance, our clients living within this structure have reported that sometimes the only way they can begin to feel a massage is through an internal voice pattering something like, "Now he is touching my ankle; now he is touching my shin." The tone of this internal voice is often monotone or flat. A client with this structure may even report feeling "flat" or "one-dimensional." This disconnectedness accounts for the lack of spontaneity and awkwardness that one can observe.

The profound *disconnection* of thought, action (if it occurs), and feeling has powerful existential impact. People living within this structure not only experience a deep disconnection within themselves, but also between themselves and the rest of the world. Clients with this structure often describe their disconnection from the outer world as "living behind a glass wall" where they can see everything, but cannot feel anything. A sense of alienation results, leaving the person locked within a structure that generates crushing loneliness.

Although they are lonely, contact with others presents a paradox for people with a disembodied structure. They long for contact with others, but they also fear it because contact exposes them to rejection. *Rejection is a central issue of this dynamic.* They feel fundamentally rejected and subsequently reject themselves and their own body, frequently reject others, and fear rejection by others. Feeling so intensely vulnerable leads to a strong defensive need to guard against contact. The conundrum they face is if any contact somehow gets through, they will be nearly defenseless.

People with a disembodied structure are vulnerable in relationships to a sense of betrayal. They do not open up to others very often, but if they do, the trust they then place in another person is nearly absolute. Such absolute trust can lead them to expect that the other person knows and understands them better than they really can. When the other person begins to show that he or she is not all-knowing, the person in the disembodied structure may feel betrayed (Lowen 1975). A hallmark phrase of people with a disembodied structure is "You should know, and if you don't, you've betrayed me." As a result, the paradox of contact *with* others extends to living in paradox when *relating to* others. Although they are often hypervigilant, perceiving and noting the emotional atmosphere around them in great detail (Johnson), at the same time they may be completely unaware of and insensitive to the needs and feelings of others around them.

For the most part, however, contact is avoided. *Withdrawal* is a primary survival strategy for the disembodied structure. Other survival strategies include becoming superior to others, "rising above" situations and other people, or becoming hypercritical. However, being dissociated from almost all feeling, using aggression as a defense is difficult and rarely used.

Because people with a disembodied structure often have no bodily sensation, they also cannot sense where they begin and end, which reflects being highly underbounded. They also often have distorted sensations of how big or small different body parts are and frequently believe their head is much bigger than it actually is. The lack of bounding results in people with a disembodied structure being engulfed by the relatively unfiltered input streaming in from the environment. They are also prone to project their prolific fantasies onto the outside world.

The disembodied structure is highly defended against feelings. Feelings that are able to break through into awareness often include or consist of terror, extreme anxiety, and a pervasive feeling of being "bad." To keep these feelings out of awareness, people with a disembodied structure may be "spaced out" for substantial amounts of time, construct elaborate fantasy worlds, live in books, play complicated computer games, or work out patterns of abstract thought.

The intellectual defensive style often cultivates highly sophisticated cognitive abilities (Johnson). As a result, people with a disembodied structure tend to be drawn toward careers and activities that emphasize using the intellect and imagination. Such work also provides a comfortable refuge, allowing them to operate within their "safety zone" of being in their heads. Such activities also allow them to be socially isolated and remain out of feeling contact with others, since social contact may create too much anxiety. Examples of such careers would be computer-oriented jobs and jobs in physics, mathematics, philosophy, ministry, writing, and art. All of these also often center on thinking abstractly, theory, and intellectual creativity (Johnson). The absent-minded professor is a classic stereotype. This is *not* meant to imply that *all* people who are in these occupations have a disembodied structure.

Although people with this structure may feel "bad," they may also have a grandiose ego ideal in which they feel "special" (Johnson). This sense of specialness, which often manifests in fantasy, offsets feelings of rejection, alienation, and nonexistence that lie beneath the surface.

Each character structure has comparative degrees of severity; therefore, the disembodied qualities of some clients will not seem as evident or severe as others. In some cases, the disembodied characteristics do not seem so evident because the people with this structure developed the ability to *compensate* for or disguise their disembodied characteristics. As a result, they learn to use their highly developed head-centered thinking abilities to figure out social reality and convention to overcome their lack of relatedness (Lowen 1971). In general, regardless of character structure, when a person makes adaptations that help him or her function but do not fundamentally affect the person's character structure, it is called a *compensation* and the person may be referred to as *compensated*. As an illustration of a compensated disembodied structure, consider Louis.

Louis

Louis is a very energetic and extroverted person with a high degree of curiosity about other people. Initially, Louis comes across as affable and easy to know. However, one day after a workshop, Louis's children came to meet him. Louis picked up his children to hug them, and, in doing so, his chest, head, and neck never yielded to the embrace with his kids. Louis clearly loves his children very much, but his body could not respond to the bodily contact and feeling. Louis does not appear outwardly disconnected from others or his own feelings, but his responses are mediated and buffered by his head, that is, his mental process. He has learned to be a social person and to make social gestures. He may not be "in" the gesture in the moment, and this is how the disembodied quality manifests, in Louis' case, subtly.

Even though people with a disembodied structure often think rather than feel, they do experience *intolerable* anxiety. They may not be able to experience it directly, but they know they "have it." It may be experienced as distress, anguish, desperation, or, very often, existential angst. This anxiety can build until it reaches an excruciating state and becomes difficult to bear. This is the point at which people with a disembodied structure disconnect or dissociate from their bodies with even greater intensity, because they perceive their bodies (consciously or unconsciously) to be the generators of the anxiety. By going into their head, they literally "rise above" the anxiety. This is a defensive strategy to avoid disintegration or annihilation, which the person living in a disembodied structure fears above all.

Etiology

To understand the cause of the disembodied structure, we must go to the time between prenatal existence (Smith) and the first 6 months of life and recognize the *absolute existential dependence for survival the newborn has on those caring for him or her.* The newborn normally is assured of continued survival and a feeling of security by feeling welcomed and loved by those around him or her. This feeling of welcome and acceptance cannot come through words or thoughts because a newborn is not developed enough to process this form of communication, but it can be communicated to the newborn through touch, attention to needs, and the energetic perception of the caregivers by the newborn. *The connection with his or her caregivers represents life itself for the newborn and establishes a foundation of existence and identity* (Lowen 1971). However, if the newborn is thrust into a hostile physical or emotional environment, he or she will feel mortally threatened. To disconnect with his or her caregiver means to be rejected *to the core, to be nothing.* This feeling is *unbearable* for almost anyone in such a predicament, especially a completely vulnerable infant who has no defenses.

This unbearable feeling is in the body. To survive the intolerable situation, the infant *must* escape the body. The infant experiences fragmentation and atomization, that is, breaking apart into bits. The infant must simultaneously hold him- or herself together, which is done at the joints, but escape the body entirely because the infant's body is the locus of pain and anxiety. The infant flees to the head—that is, the mind.

Cognitive functions develop prematurely when anxiety causes a split between the head and the body (Brown). At the infantile level, these cognitive functions are not performed through words. Instead, the infant nonverbally "figures out" how to survive a hostile environment by developing a set of responses to that environment. The infant can figure out, for instance, when crying will generate a hostile response from the caregiver. Even though an infant may not be able to stop crying in certain circumstances, he or she may be able to modify or curtail it. We can observe that certain immature domestic animals modify their behavior in response to their caregivers. Human newborns also display this ability.

What constitutes such a hostile environment that can lead to the development of this structure? Sometimes, it is a situation that has more to do with circumstances than human fault, such as premature birth with extended periods spent in incubators with inadequate human contact, severe long-term illness after birth during which the child is close to death, death of the mother or primary caregiver, illness of the mother that results in prolonged separation of mother and infant, or hospital restrictions that do not allow mother and infant enough physical contact to bond.

At the relationship level, this existential crisis occurs when the primary caregiver does not bond with the infant or, more severely, feels hostile—consciously or unconsciously—to the newborn. (Lowen 1971). This is not set into place by being angry at a squalling baby for a short time, but by a continual situation of hostility and disconnection at a human level. This often leaves the infant with a feeling of being cast out into outer space without a tether, since the primary caregiver is the anchor in the infant's world.

Some people with this structure describe themselves as being the "hated child" (Johnson). More than being not wanted, they are often hated simply for their existence (Smith). To complicate matters further, this hate may never be openly expressed, but is acted out in subtle and unspoken ways. The "hated child," however, is living in a poisoned atmosphere that he or she perceives, even though the child may not be able to articulate what it is. This is most likely to occur in families in which the hatred is manifested as a prohibition against feeling and transmitted with an underlying pervasive sense of coldness.

This rejection is a shock to both body and soul. People with this structure sometimes report the sensation of being "electrocuted" as infants. They do not mean this literally, but are reporting that the *rejection is shocking.* Sometimes, they actually appear as if a jolt shocked them. Their eyes are wide open, joints are rigid, shoulders raised, and back stiffened.

The first 6 months of life establish the foundation for relatedness, safety, security, acceptance, and belonging. If the infant is wounded around these issues and during this particular time, future developmental stages also become harder to complete. Because this wounding is so early, the person is imbued with a sense of anxiety that seems to have no source. From the moment the person is conscious, he or she feels that something is "wrong" with him or her or that he or she is bad at the core, which adds to any sense of alienation. Physically, this kind of alienation is established through lack of touch, touching with an absent quality, or touch that carries a hostile feeling. *To be in touch becomes a negative thing.* Here is an example of someone who was threatened by touch.

Roberto

Roberto was a client who was aware that he had little bodily feeling. He had been born into a wealthy family that turned over taking care of the children to hired help almost immediately. Roberto had little contact with his parents and developed the attributes of the disembodied structure. When Roberto became an adult, he married and had children. His family physician, who was aware of Roberto's limited emotional range, told Roberto that it was important that he hug his children and give them affection. Roberto carried out the instructions dutifully. However, after he hugged his children goodnight each evening, he actually had to vomit because of the extreme discomfort and anxiety he felt from touching his children. Although he loved his children, for Roberto, touch had become sickening early on in his life. To be more precise, touch brought Roberto into his body, and his body was a place of discomfort. It did not feel good to be there.

As Roberto grew older, he retreated even farther from feeling. He shut down his senses. He could not smell or taste much anymore and was beginning to lose his hearing. He was abandoning his body, a carrier of pain and anxiety for him.

Roberto's case is extreme, but serves as a good example of how touch and being embodied can be threatening. Touch serves as a connection to the body and to other people, which stimulates anxiety in the disembodied structure. Since touch is the main medium of massage, therapists need to consider this in their work with clients with a disembodied structure.

Appearance

Disjointedness and disconnection distinguish this character structure in the body, as well as the psyche. People with this structure may appear to move mechanically at the joints. Movement often has a marionette-like quality, with extreme stiffness, woodenness, or frozenness seen in the body. The body may appear lifeless and like an object. People with this structure often report that at times in their life they have felt like dolls, machines, robots, computers, or other mechanical objects. They also may describe feelings of being "not real" or feeling like an alien. They are often, but not always, ectomorphic (Smith, 1985), that is, elongated, thin, bird-like, rail-like. They are frequently physically awkward, but some people living in this structure have had dance or other forms of body-related training and have learned to move more gracefully. However, the training is not integrated in the body, so they are actually mentally directing themselves rather than simply moving. Even with the grace that may result from training, a lack of fluidity and an echo of the stiffness may remain (Lowen, 1971).

Disembodied structures have knotty armoring. The knots tend to be present in most places in the body, but especially around the joints, which accounts for the stiff, even disjointed appearance often observed. The holding around the joints is an indication that they are *holding themselves together*. The armoring is an attempt to defend against a feeling of disintegration or flying apart. As explained in the etiology section, people with a disconnected structure faced overwhelming feelings of rejection. This is experienced as a shock to the body. The tightening around the joints seeks to counteract this shocking effect and hold the person together. For someone who has never experienced this structure or such a threat, imagining what the terror is like and what it is about can be difficult. However, if you have had nightmares about falling into little pieces or becoming atomized or can imagine it, you can begin to understand this fear.

High levels of knotty armoring in the occipital area of the neck reinforce, on the bodily level, being in the head (Lowen, 1971; Smith, 1985). The tension in the occipital area forms a "ring of fire," which discourages any forays from the head into the body. This is why disconnected people at first tend to fear massage in the neck area and feel fragile. Later in the therapeutic process, they may come to crave being worked on deeply in that area. The armor band at the base of the skull keeps the charge extremely high in the head and possibly low in the body. However, hidden deeply and walled away within the endoderm is another high charge that fuels the anxiety felt by people with a disembodied structure (Lowen, 1971). In terms of body structure, the strong band of tension at the occiput can lead them to hold their head in a position that is tilted back so that they appear to be "looking down their nose," aloof, or superior. The blocking at the base of the neck can also lead them to tilt their head to the side (Lowen, 1971).

People with a disembodied structure may have difficulty making eye contact, which may come across as shyness or cold rejection. They may habitually turn their head slightly so that they look at others out of only one eye. Tension located around the temple, as well as the occiput, sometimes affects the appearance of the eyes, which in some individuals may appear absent or vacant and in others too intense and burning.

The faces of people with a disembodied structure can appear drawn, expressionless, and mask-like (Lowen, 1975). They frequently speak in a monotone except when very agitated. The vocal tone accompanies the mechanical quality seen in the body.

Other identifying features include raised shoulders such that their body seems to be "hung from a coat hanger," rather than standing on the ground. At the same time, they may actually be gripping the ground with their toes as if to hang on. People with this structure tend to have exaggerated high arches in their feet. The shoulders may also curl forward, as if attempting to protect the chest, while the scapulae are immobile (Lowen, 1971).

The chest is usually deflated in the upper region with little muscular or fatty tissue protecting the ribcage, giving a sense of vulnerability. Some people with this structure are very sensitive in the sternum area and cannot bear to be touched there, even by themselves or clothing. The lower half of the rib cage is often flared outward owing to a holding in of the diaphragm. People with a disembodied structure usually have great difficulty breathing in: "The expansion of the chest cavity is accompanied by a contraction of the abdominal cavity. This prevents the diaphragm from descending . . . so that a downward movement of the lungs cannot occur" (Lowen, 1971, p. 375). This type of breathing is called *paradoxical breathing.*

Because people caught in the disembodied structure live in a state of unconscious fear, the body chronically expresses this intense fear and anxiety through signs one would see in an acute fear situation, such as shallow breathing, and energy drawn away from the limbs and into the center of the body, leaving the hands and feet perpetually cold (Lowen, 1975).

Finally, the disembodied structure is undergrounded, underbounded, and overcharged. The undergrounding is accounted for by the head-body split and general disconnection, underbounding by the high level of vulnerability and expectations of

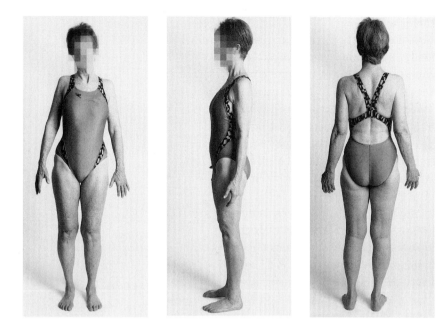

Figure 8.1
Disembodied structure. Front view: *Note rolled forward, flared lower rib cage, bird-like, elongated appearance, holding at joints, tilting of head, and lack of contact with the ground.* ***Side view:*** *Note contraction around occipital area and extended neck, holding of diaphragm.* ***Back view:*** *Note the "hung-up" or hanger-like appearance of shoulder and upper back, and lack of contact with the ground. All views show the general disjointed quality of this structure.*

others to know how they feel, and overcharging in the head, around the joints, and deep in the core, although the rest of the body is undercharged.

Therapeutic Strategy

In a sense, seeking out a body-centered method like massage therapy is a big step for people with a disembodied structure. After they become aware of their need to become more embodied, they are very motivated, increasing the chances of therapeutic success.

In the first several sessions of massage therapy, the person may not feel very much in response to touch. Because the knots are so hard and tenacious and the client has a relatively low level of feeling, the massage therapist may be tempted to work aggressively to "break open" the armor. However, doing this would ignore the very purpose of the armoring, which is to *keep the person away from any source of anxiety*. In the case of a client with a disembodied structure, *the source of anxiety is the body itself*. Opening the body too rapidly can flood the individual with the very feelings he or she is trying to avoid and defend from experiencing.

The key is to *invite* disconnected people into their bodies rather than break them open. The massage therapist often faces a therapeutic conundrum when working with clients with a disembodied structure. The massage therapist's usual goal of loosening tension to create a more pleasant relaxed state sets up a paradoxical result. Helping clients with a disembodied structure "be in touch with their body" can turn out to be a scary experience for them because the body is the repository of the excruciating pain that their defenses are designed to keep out. For people with a disembodied structure, to be in the body means to face the pain of rejection and all the awful associated feelings. Therefore, inviting this type of client into their body means facilitating a gradual "putting one's toe in the water" progression of bodily feeling, so that they are not taken to the point of being overwhelmed. The challenge is to allow some opening and let it be tolerated before going further (Johnson). Clients with a disembodied structure must discover for themselves, through their own experience, that they can tolerate feeling their body *and* feeling their feelings. They also need to learn to tolerate the surges of anxiety that may come upon them when they begin to feel, and then let themselves feel safe and comfortable with the experience. Once they begin to request more pressure and more depth while being touched, *then* the massage therapist can comply.

An important direction here is that the work must be done incrementally so that sensation is built upon sensation (Johnson). If the therapist goes too fast, the client will retreat back into his or her head. Therefore, any indication of dissociation or splitting is a sign that the pace of the work is too much for the client to tolerate. Starting with parts of the body that already contact the world is usually safer, such as the head, hands, and feet. These areas usually feel less vulnerable. Therefore, a session with this type of client may begin by simply touching the hand at the fingertips and waiting for a signal that moving beyond this area, such as the back of the hand, is okay. An example of incremental pacing is that the person with a disembodied structure may be able to feel a toe, then the outline or edges of the foot. Feeling only the outline may last for quite a while, but then the outline might begin to "fill in" and become an experience of a three-dimensional foot. People with a disembodied structure feel flat and two-dimensional to themselves—cognitively, emotionally, and bodily. As the body begins to be experienced three-dimensionally, a foundation is made for feeling in general to be experienced more fully.

Massage can also bring both a sense of connection *to* the body and connection *between parts* of the body that the client may never have experienced. Because *disconnection* is a trait of the disembodied structure, facilitating connection can be quite beneficial. A great deal of disconnection occurs at the joints in the disembodied structure; therefore, working with the joints can substantially increase connection and awareness. Holding joints between your hands firmly for several minutes can bring about both connection and relief. In essence, with the therapist holding the joint together, the client no longer has to create the excessive tension needed to do so. A second technique consists of gently "pressing" or pushing bones toward each other in the joint area.

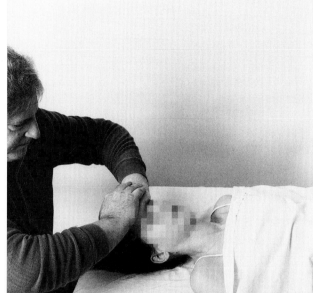

Figure 8.2
Technique of applying pressure to the forehead. *Applying a moderate to heavy amount of pressure to the forehead. This pressure is held without movement of the hands for quite some time.*

After the body begins to feel safe and "thaw out," clients with a disembodied structure develop a delightful insatiable need for massage and begin to crave ways to feel their body. When the client reaches this point, the enthusiasm and child-like discovery of every new body sensation that the client experiences can be inspiring. As massage progresses, this client may ask for seemingly painful amounts of pressure, especially in the area around the head. This amount of pressure may be necessary now to bring feeling into the numbed areas. What might be painful for another person who does not have a disembodied structure has become pleasurable for the client who does, so any reluctance that the massage therapist may have to applying such pressure at this point in the process must be suspended. In contrast to the beginning of therapy, the client now *needs* to break through.

When the client is ready, apply moderate pressure to the forehead, increasing the pressure gradually if the client tolerates it. Sustain the pressure without movement of the hands for several minutes. An added benefit of this technique is that it calms mental activity, especially the mental chatter and images that are manifestations of the extreme anxiety typically generated by disembodied structures. If the client reports physical rather than mental sensations, then the technique is working well (Figure 8.2).

Working to bring more energy into the body, particularly the legs and feet, will benefit the client in two ways. First, the disembodied structure maintains a high charge (an overcharge) in the head, and a much lower charge (an undercharge) in the rest of the body. Increasing charge in the rest of the body lessens the overcharge in the head. Second, this also increases grounding, which benefits the undergrounded disembodied structure by bringing the client into a greater sense of here and now, concrete reality. Therefore, as the client's tolerance for touch increases, invigorating work can be done on the legs and feet.

Bounding is a challenge for clients with disembodied structures because they must have "enough body" to build boundaries. Therefore, bounding will improve when they are more able to be in their body. One simple way of improving body boundaries, after trust is established, is to firmly apply broad pressure to each body

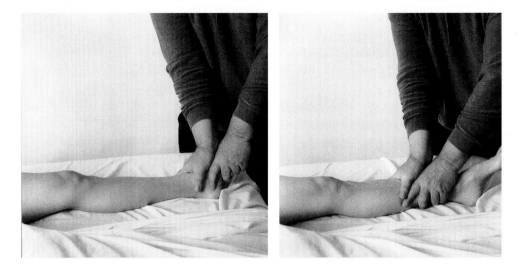

Figure 8.3
Technique of applying pressure to each body part. *One simple way of introducing body boundaries, after trust is established, is to firmly apply broad pressure to each body part for a moderate amount of time.*

part for a moderate amount of time. This helps clients with a disembodied structure to feel their boundaries (this technique also works for any underbounded clients (Figure 8.3).

The therapeutic relationship with clients with a disembodied structure must be monitored carefully by the massage therapist. As explained earlier, these people are prone to mistrust and feeling betrayed; therefore, being scrupulously honest about communications is vital. This does not mean that the massage therapist must disclose his or her personal life or every thought. It does mean, for example, that if you cancel a session because you are ill, you need to explain why you are canceling.

THE COLLAPSED STRUCTURE

The primary traits of the *collapsed* structure are a tendency to be dependent, low aggressiveness, and an inner feeling of needing to be supported and taken care of. People with this structure experienced a lack of fulfillment in infancy, leading to an underlying experience of deprivation. Having difficulty standing on their own feet literally and figuratively, they tend to lean on or cling to others to prevent their collapse. Some people may adopt a compensating pattern based on exaggerated independence, but this fails to hold up under stress. Energetically, this structure is undercharged and is also underbounded and undergrounded. In contrast with the disembodied structure, energy flows out to the periphery, although weakly, rather than being frozen at the core (Lowen, 1971). The holding pattern is held down.

Psychological Dynamics

People with a collapsed structure have a strong need to be *dependent,* and they feel profoundly powerless. They seek rescue and fear abandonment (Keleman), which they try to deal with by ascribing a powerful role to select others, relating to them on a "big one, little one" basis. The big one is their designated rescuer. This means the other person is cast into the "big one" role of being powerful enough to provide for their needs, while they have the "little one" role of being taken care of. By inflating (i.e., building up) a person upon whom they want to depend and giving the

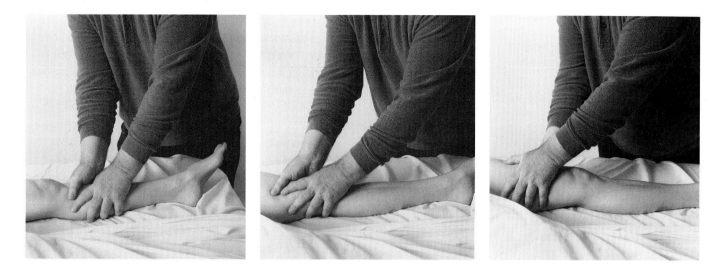

potential nurturer a lot of power, they are unconsciously attempting to satisfy their need to find someone able to provide the love, warmth, and nurturing they did not receive as a child. Inflating the person cast into the "big one" role makes that person fill the part. The person might be a lover, but could just as well be a minister, teacher, psychotherapist, or massage therapist.

The inflation of others comes at the price of deflation of their own ego, which is reflected in their bodies, particularly the chest. Just as people with a collapsed structure are constantly inflating others, they are also looking constantly to others for inspiration as they do not have enough energy to sufficiently stimulate inspiration on their own.

Inspiration, inflation, and deflation also are metaphors related to breathing. Similarly, the breathing capacity of the collapsed structure is diminished (Keleman). The individual's emotional collapse is reflected in the collapse of the chest, which in turn depresses breathing. The depressed breathing lowers energy levels, which in turn makes it more difficult to breathe.

This vicious circle is characteristic of the dilemma presented by the collapsed structure. Deprivation leads to an inability to sustain energy, feeling, and function. Difficulty in mobilizing energy, feeling, and function leads to greater depression and a sense of *helplessness and hopelessness* (Keleman). A sense of helplessness and hopelessness discourages actions that could counteract deprivation, which leads to further *collapse*. Seeing how to break the cycle is difficult frequently for both the person with a collapsed structure and for whomever is working in a therapeutic role with the person

The motto of the collapsed structure is "I can't." This leads to frustration for both the person in the collapse and others who interact with him or her because efforts end up easily aborted. The "I can't" is both a reflexive and immediate feeling and is not thought out. Later, the "I can't" may become elaborately rationalized and justified. Sometimes, the excuses are outlandish, such as "I can't look for a job today because this is the day I need to volunteer at the animal shelter," while at the same time the person does not have enough money to pay rent. The "I can't" position keeps them down, so in this sense this person is *held down* by the collapsed structure. Their existential predicament is as if they feel they must "pull themselves up by their bootstraps," but they cannot find their bootstraps.

The need to be dependent of people with a collapsed structure also causes them to want to be in a passive position to receive nurturance. They want to be taken care of, which is why they firmly believe, "if you have to ask for it, it does not count." Reaching out for what one wants, grasping it, asking for it, or demanding it cancels or diminishes whatever return is forthcoming (Johnson). Consequently, they operate interpersonally by the principle of attraction. One must figure out how to *attract* attention and love, rather than deliberately going after either. This principle reinforces the passivity of the collapsed position. One is allowed to manipulate to get attention and love because the manipulation is disguised, whereas open aggression is too obvious. Others usually experience the refusal to ask for what one needs as burdensome and tiring.

Not only do people with a collapsed structure not ask for what they need, they expect the other person to figure out in detail what their needs are. After all, as the "big one" they are assumed to have the power to do so. If the other person does not do this, he or she ends up being seen as mean, withholding, cold, or bad.

Within the psyches of people with a collapsed structure, getting the world to give to them is often the only thing that counts. Taking action of any kind cancels the benefit and nurturing value of what is given. What sets up this dynamic is that the most important moments in the person's life happened when nurturance came in a seemingly random or magical manner (this is discussed in more detail in the etiology section). Another paradox exists for this person as a result. *The very attributes a person needs to survive, function, and hopefully thrive within the adult world are those that people with a collapsed structure believe will not work.* Their dilemma is that they are attempting to exist in an adult world by playing according to infantile rules. The fact that this subjects them to much frustration, misery, and pain does not motivate them to change because they are accustomed to waiting and enduring the pain—and collapsing—until the hoped for love and warmth appears eventually.

Furthermore, people with a collapsed structure have an unconscious need to *remain* needy and dependent. The reason for this will become clearer when we explain the cause, but it is basically because they believe unconsciously that this is the *only* way they can attract caring. As much as people with a collapsed structure want love, warmth, and nurturance, once they receive it, they cannot hold onto it. Any sense of fulfillment quickly disappears and is replaced by need and longing again. This dynamic has a sieve-like quality in that whatever energy is poured into them does not seem to be enough, so it seems to go right through them. In addition, people with a collapsed structure tend to discount or "wipe out" warmth and nurturance that is offered. They may experience sincerely made compliments, acknowledgments, offers of love, and support as not enough, not quite the right kind of help, not believable, or too easily given. Both the "sieve" and "wipe out" dynamics can be very discouraging or even alienating to whomever is trying to give to them.

The sieve and wipe out dynamics reinforce the undercharged state of this structure. In turn, the low level of energy causes people with a collapsed structure to tend to globalize physical and emotional pain. Because of this amorphous generalization of aches and pains, the reports by a client with a collapsed structure may seem so exaggerated that they may not seem real. The client may even seem hypochondriacal. However, all of the pains of people living in a collapsed structure express are *real* (Lowen, 1971*)*. They are trying to accomplish adult tasks as if they were living in the body, particularly the musculature, of an infant or very young child. Their musculature does not support adequately their ability to stand on their own, much less carry weight, run, and move objects. Imagine the pain in a small child's body if he or she were forced to live the bodily life of an adult. If we watch children, who do have limited muscular development, the organization and coordination of their movements breaks down at some point, and they become frustrated, cranky, and upset. This is similar to what happens to the adult with a collapsed structure.

Having a developed musculature allows us to sustain an energy charge. Because collapsed structures are underdeveloped muscularly, maintaining a charge for any length of time can be difficult. People with a collapsed structure may experience short bursts of energy, particularly in emergencies, but find they cannot maintain their energy over a length of time. This leads them to regard their energy as mysterious and capricious, as if it were something coming from a source outside of them (Keleman). This is the somatic aspect of why people with a collapsed structure *psychologically do not depend on themselves, but look to form dependencies with others for both human and material needs*. This dynamic is sometimes called the Manna complex because of the tendency to want or expect something good to "come from the sky." C.G. Jung described Manna as a symbol for the psychological desire to be automatically fed and taken care of by a benevolent source or the power of such an individual to provide whatever is needed (Knapp). The concept is derived from the biblical story of Moses and the flight of the Israelites from Egypt, in which the Israelites are condemned to spend 40 years wandering in the desert before they reach the Promised Land. Unable to feed themselves in the desert, Jehovah has a sweet foodstuff called Manna appear from nowhere, that is, the Heavens, each day to nourish the children of Israel.

The inability of people with a collapsed structure to find consistent resources within themselves leads them to form self-judgments, such as being lazy or feckless. The outside world also may view them in these negative terms, since their energy tends to be low and they often avoid or are unable to sustain an effort in difficult tasks. In part, this happens because their energy system is *so* undercharged (Keleman) that they cannot get a sense of the steps needed to get themselves out of a negative situation and into a more positive one. The word "steps" is an operative one as the origin of their collapse occurred before they could take their own first steps.

In addition, the organism of the person with a collapsed structure does not feel capable of enough aggression to be able to get what he or she needs, to protect him/herself, or to fight off enemies. There is a feeling of having no "backbone," of being "spineless," and of always giving in or caving in (Keleman).

The existential condition of people with a collapsed structure is also important to understand. They live a life filled with conditionality and contingency. Actions that would benefit, support, or sustain them are often not taken because the conditions do not appear quite right. An example of conditional thinking would be, "When I can afford an exercise machine, *then* I'll begin to exercise," or "When I can afford to buy a car, *then* I'll look for work." They believe (unconsciously) that something they do not control must happen for them to get their desired results. For example, happiness or contentment is delayed until certain conditions are absolutely fulfilled, such as "I won't be happy until . . . I'm married, or I have a Lexus, or the porch is fixed, or I get a job working for the president." However, the excuses are not manufactured. People living in collapsed structures *truly believe* they cannot be happy without certain preconditional events taking place. This belief reflects an unconscious need to be dependent, thereby acting out of the unmet need to depend on someone or something to provide for them and that it cannot be the result of their own effort.

Another set of conditions is an "only if–then" situation, which is frequently attached to other people. For example, "only if my friend has her hair dyed blond, then I can dye my hair blond also," or "only if a prospective therapist is near public transportation, will I then go to her." The "only if–then" also can be reversed to "if only–then," in which the person falls or collapses into a state of misery thinking about what might have been if only they had made a different choice or if the universe had provided different conditions. For example, "if only I had married the boy next door, I would be happy now." Not surprisingly then, regret also preoccupies the emotional life of people with a collapsed structure. The fear of regret or making the wrong decision often paralyzes them and reinforces their tendency to assume a passive position.

People with a collapsed structure are caught in a dilemma of wanting and wishing to feel good, but not actually knowing what to do to create good feeling. Their belief that feeling good is something that happens *to* them, rather than being a result of *their own actions*, is part of what blinds them from seeing how their actions have something to do with gaining the good feeling they crave and that action is a manifestation of that desire. In other words, *they fail to see that actions rather than fantasies fulfill desires*.

Wishing, a mental activity and often a form of fantasy, replaces the bodily activity of doing. Wishing then becomes part of the elaborate system of conditionality. For example, "I hope my ship comes in" actually means, "I can't do anything until my ship comes in, so there's no sense in trying for now." Thus, wishing can actually become an ironic form of *preventing* any action toward any goal.

Being overwhelmed is another common experience for people with a collapsed structure and is also associated with the complex system of conditionality and contingency. From the position of collapse, they are unable to envision endeavors being completed in small steps or in bite-sized chunks. They approach a project in an undifferentiated manner, meaning the project is seen only in its totality, without any sense of the process of how it will be accomplished. They do not see the *steps* (Johnson), only the end. As a result, they are easily overwhelmed by the undifferentiated enormity of a project and prefer to give up—*collapse*—rather than persist with what appears to be an impossible task.

One common phrase that describes this sense of being overwhelmed or having more than one can handle is, "biting off more than you can chew." Metaphorically speaking, people with a collapsed structure have not yet reached the developmental stage of chewing (Perls, Hefferline & Goodman). They often swallow things whole. Like young babies who can eat only soft foods because they lack teeth, they want to take in without having to process. They have difficulty chewing up, breaking down difficult ideas, concepts, or situations so that they can be digested in the service of making decisions.

Feeling their own helplessness can make people with a collapsed structure be more sensitive to other people's helplessness and vulnerability. They are frequently attuned to issues of closeness and distance, warmth and coldness, hurt and sadness in others in a way that other people might miss. Despite the low energy that plagues their structure, they can summon up energy for a friend in a crisis and be quite giving (Johnson). Because of where they are "stuck" in their development, people with a collapsed structure have often preserved many of the positive qualities of childhood—playfulness, openness, warmth, creativity, and a capacity for joy.

Etiology

The origin of the collapsed structure is centered on the first 18 months of life and how the child is *both physically and emotionally* nurtured. The lack of nurturance is a crisis for the child, which results in *deprivation*. This rarely involves total deprivation, for the child gets something, as evidenced by the child's survival. However, the child must find a way to survive without enough—enough love, food, support, contact, attention, or other resources.

Studies have shown that humans have a strong biological need for touch and contact that may even be greater than the desire for food. For example, the famous Harlow monkey studies showed that touch is as important as food. Baby monkeys separated from their mothers surprised researchers by preferring a soft, fuzzy surrogate mother without a bottle, rather than a wire surrogate mother with a bottle (Montagu). These experiments were the beginning of a long line of studies that have consistently confirmed the imperative need for touch and touching. The proper development of our nervous system depends on this contact, and the child continually seeks it from caregivers. Other studies have found actual brain damage related to touch deprivation. Not being touched and not being emotionally nurtured are akin to devastation and death.

Contact and connection with the caregivers therefore assure the child of continued survival. The child is severely threatened without such contact. This is not quite the type of threat of *rejection* that the person with a disembodied structure faces, but it is one of *deprivation*. The bodymind of the well-cared-for child knows when he or she has received sufficient nurturance through food and contact. The child is left with a sense of contentment and satisfaction and is usually calm and peaceful. However, when nurturance has stopped short of being enough, the organism feels pain, frustration, anger, need, and even agony. This shocks the body. In contrast to the disembodied structure, the person living in the collapsed structure has *just enough* embodiment *not* to experience this threat to survival as annihilation through fragmentation (Lowen, 1971). The threat to survival for the collapsed type is being starved through neglect; that is, being inadequately nurtured.

The child feels needy and powerless. The child may cry or cry out, but such entreaties do not help and may even attract negative attention. Since people with collapsed structures are deprived, they must learn to operate with a limited energy supply if they are to survive (Johnson). They have a limited energy supply because they are not getting sufficient input of food and love, but yet are expending energy to try to get it.

This leads to a pattern in which the child cries out and either gets nothing or gets an insufficient or intermittent response. Then the child becomes exhausted and collapses, either from depleted energy or giving up to conserve a sliver of energy (Lowen, 1971). It is often at this point—*collapse*—that the caregiver eventually takes care of the child. *This "teaches" the child that he or she has no effect on the world and that nurturance comes when they are collapsed.* This suspension of cause and effect happens when the child cries, no one comes, they stop crying, and *then* something happens. Finally, receiving care does not seem to come from their effort, but as if "it" came from the sky—like Manna from heaven, it just appears. If there is any sense of cause and effect implied, it is *that by being collapsed, they can be saved.* This sets up a reward for remaining passive and not initiating action or making an effort. This can become a deep underlying problem in therapy because people with this structure may unconsciously fear that by working hard to "get well," they will no longer be eligible for supplies and rewards.

The child, and later the adult with a collapsed structure, may begin to make unspoken deals with whomever is seen as the "big" nurturer. The nurturer seems to the collapsed child to be like a powerful and unpredictable deity whom the child must figure out to get the needed supplies and rewards. The child puts an immense amount of thought and awareness into what will please the nurturer to gain love, affection, and support. From the child's perspective, this must be done "under the table." The nurturer must not know that the child needs or wants anything, but must be tricked or manipulated into giving it. However, people with a collapsed structure do not experience themselves as manipulative, but as attempting to make themselves more attractive to the nurturer. In this sense, they are playing the "attraction game," which is based on getting what one wants without asking for it by being attractive (this means emotionally attractive rather than physically attractive) in some way to the nurturer. Only by giving the "supplies" does the nurturer assure the child, and later the adult, that the collapsed person has any value.

Many reasons exist for why caregivers may not provide adequate care. Caregivers may be depressed, chronically ill, or preoccupied with problems and may have difficulty in being consistently nurturing to a baby. Or, the caregivers may have little education or understanding about how to care for a child and not comprehend that many of the child's needs must be met within a certain amount of time. Caregivers who are beset by financial problems and must work long hours may be too exhausted to give the necessary attention to the child. Some babies live in orphanages and foster homes, where the care is well intentioned but scarce, so they survive but do not thrive. Caregivers may practically be children themselves (chronologically or emotionally) and have immature attitudes about caregiving (Johnson).

In some situations, the child compensates for the caregiver's shortcomings and becomes a "little adult" by being forced to care for himself, and perhaps others, too early. For example, a caregiver may be too needy, overwhelmed, or otherwise not very functional to give much to the child, so the child finds him- or herself taking on adult responsibilities too early in life. Sometimes, this child also ends up taking care of the caregiver and younger siblings (if there are any), particularly in cases in which the caregiver has a problem with substance abuse. Ironically, people with a collapsed structure are forced to grow up too fast, which leaves them as children internally when they become adults (Johnson).

The more the person is forced as a child to take on adult responsibilities, the more likely they are to form a *compensated collapsed structure*. They resist collapse in order to carry out their responsibilities; however, they do so without adequate resources to sustain them. This type of person often shows a tendency toward overwork and giving too much. Although they do not collapse, they tend to drag themselves along despite their difficulties. Although they often act responsibly, they are not thriving.

Appearance

Collapsed structures appear in two patterns, either apparently collapsed or resisting collapse. In a *collapsed* position, the head is displaced forward, the shoulders are rotated forward, and the chest is rigid with a flattened, or even concave, appearance. The pelvis is tilted anteriorly slightly, giving an S-shaped appearance to the posture (Lowen, 1971). The knees are hyperextended and tend to lock. The feet do not appear to be well connected to the rest of the body (figuratively speaking) (Figure 8.4). The most common description given for this stance is depressed. Because of a hypotonic musculature, they do not have enough energy or musculature to hold themselves up well. Experientially and metaphorically they are "down." They live in a pattern of up-and-down moods and are unable to sustain effort very long before giving up.

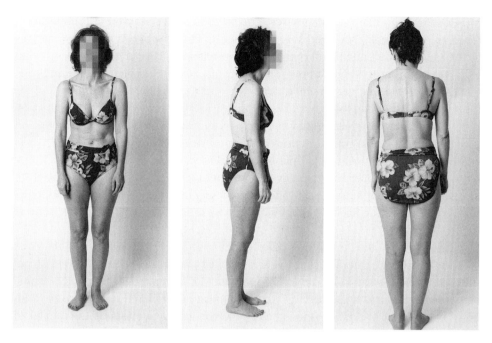

Figure 8.4
Collapsed structure. Front view:
Note deflated chest, forward dis-
placed shoulders, locked knees, and
*lack of grounding through feet. **Side***
***view:** Note the S curve formed by the*
forward displaced head and posteri-
orly tilted pelvis, collapsed chest, and
*hyperextended knees. **Back view:***
Note general lack of muscle tone.

When the structure is *resisting collapse*, the appearance is largely similar, although there are some significant differences. The stance is subtler, because the collapse is *compensated* and hidden by that compensation. In contrast to the collapsed pattern described above, the person with a *compensated collapsed* structure makes a strenuous effort not to collapse in their body or in their lives. The holding up against collapse often appears in the shoulders and upper back (Lowen, 1975). Some tension develops there to resist the tendency to collapse. The collapse in the chest is compensated for with considerable hardness in the chest area, which is one of the structure's telltale signs. A subtle expression of low energy in the eyes and mouth is often seen. Frequently, the jaw is retracted, giving the appearance of being "weak" (Figure 8.5).

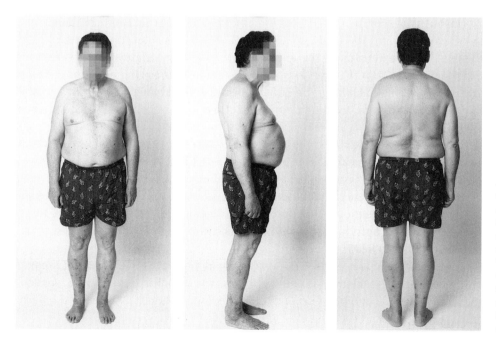

Figure 8.5
Compensated collapsed structure.
***Front view:** Note the chest of the*
compensated type does not appear
as collapsed, but is undercharged
*(still undernourished looking). **Side***
***view:** Shows both the tendency of*
collapse (as shown in Figure 8.4) and
*tension resisting collapse. **Back view:***
Note that the upper back holds rela-
tively more tension, which gives a bit
more resistance to collapse.

People with collapsed structures tend to look either starved and undernourished to some degree or overblown (Keleman). The overblown condition carries fatty tissue without much underlying muscular tissue, as if in an attempt to store up what seems to be in short supply. The flaccidity and hypotonicity of the muscles make it hard to retain very much charge in the tissues. This reflects and reinforces the tendency of collapsed structures to have to struggle with low energy, exhaustion, and chronic tiredness. They may experience brief bursts of excitement and energy that are quickly spent, followed by a return to the low energy state. This is confusing and frustrating to people living in this structure because they feel they have little control over their energy and frequently do not know how to generate more. A mistake that massage therapists frequently make in working with this structure is confusing the flaccidity they find for relaxation. The *lack* of muscle tone is the problem!

There *is* some tension in the bodies of collapsed structures. One notable place is in the muscles located around the arm and leg joints. Although collapsed structures do not carry the more obvious appearance of being shocked as much as disembodied structures do, collapsed structures also experienced shock to their bodies at some point in time. The tension around the joints counteracts the impact of being shocked early in life by the lack of nurturing that is so threatening. The tension provides a feeling of withstanding the explosive, life-obliterating quality of the shock. Keeping in mind that this is not a one-time event, but the result of a chronic repetition of physical or emotional deprivation, is important.

The chest tends to be collapsed and deflated. The deflation in the chest keeps breathing minimal. Because breathing is a critical part of energy production, this keeps energy low. *Minimal* breathing is part of the energetic vicious circle that collapsed structures endure.

The shoulders follow the collapse by becoming rounded and curled forward as if trying to protect the chest. The collapse in the shoulders gives the appearance of weakness, as if being unable to "shoulder" much weight. However, if a compensated pattern is present, the shoulders try to hold up the weight. Because there is minimal support in the back and the legs, the upper torso collapses too around the area of the diaphragm. In the compensated pattern, the lack of support in the legs is compensated for by tension in the upper back.

In both the compensated and noncompensated structures, the knees are hyperextended and the legs appear stiff. Because there is little muscle tone in the legs, hyperextension of the knees is the only way collapsed structures can get a feeling of support in the legs. (Lowen, 1971) This feeling of support easily disappears with a push from the outside because the stance is inherently unstable. From a side view, the body appears to take on an S shape (Keleman) (see Figure 8.4).

Because there is no support in the back and legs, the neck is often flexed, which gives the head an appearance of being thrust or tilted forward. This head-down position both externally and internally gives an impression of low self-esteem, lack of pride, and depression. In addition, walking around with the head down significantly reduces perception of the outer world. The holding at the base of the neck, which thrusts the head forward or down, makes the person in the collapsed structure susceptible to headaches (Johnson).

The compensated collapsed pattern also may have additional areas of tension in the neck and shoulder areas and the intercostal muscles. This tension, particularly in the scapula, inhibits reaching or striking out (Johnson). Although the body is generally undercharged, the upper half of the body tends to carry more charge that greatly diminishes in the lower half. If this pattern is present, it tends to be a compensation for the lack of support in the rest of the body.

Therapeutic Strategy

Clients with a collapsed structure often come into sessions complaining of various aches and pains, but on questioning are unable to locate them. When asked what is wrong, they tend to say "everything." When asked to be more specific, they seem to ignore this question and repeat some variation of the expression "everything." Similarly, when asked where they hurt, they tend to respond "everywhere." In other words, people living in this structure experience globalized pain. A more specific answer is not accessible to them because they experience their body as out of focus.

The typical flaccidity of the structure is the cause of the aches and pains *and* the inability to locate them. The person with a collapsed structure, who lacks a developed musculature and a well-charged mesoderm, literally has no barrier against these pains, and consequently feels them more intensely. One way to imagine being in this person's skin is to remember when we were children and physical pains that would seem insignificant to us as adults were more painful to us as children. Not only do our adult attitudes help us cope with these pains, a developed body, especially a well-charged mesoderm, provides the containment needed to control the feelings on both the emotional and sensation levels.

A similar process happens with psychological pain. Sometimes these pains become submerged in the consciousness of people with collapsed structures. As a result, a generalized sense of misery and suffering becomes a reinforced experience in the bodymind. This accounts for why they often respond "everywhere" when asked where they hurt, and when asked to become more specific, become frustrated.

One very important intervention the massage therapist can make is to help the client be able to *specifically* locate pain. This intervention serves several purposes. The massage therapist needs to know where the client hurts to be able to work effectively. In helping the client learn to feel and communicate this type of information, the massage therapist is making the work be more effective by working more specifically. By helping the client locate pain in specific places, the massage therapist is working on a micro-level to help the client feel less overwhelmed and emerge out of the generalized swamp of pain (Box 8.1).

Both physical and psychological pain are so globalized in collapsed structures that people with them tend to also deal with much in their lives in a globalized manner, which is a coping strategy that is seldom effective. Imagine trying to solve all your problems all at once! By locating or "corralling" pain in the body, the client can learn to deal with each pain more discretely, one at a time. This can begin a process of more effectively coping with pain, discomfort, and unpleasant events, rather than being overwhelmed by them.

Lack of differentiation of sensation in the body also leads to lack of differentiation in perception of oneself and perception of the world (Johnson). The feeling of indistinct "blobbiness" and wishy-washiness comes directly from a lack of differentiation. One way that massage can greatly help people with collapsed structures is by making the musculature more alive, perceivable, and distinct. This becomes the

Box 8.1

CORRALLING THE PAIN

When a client has globalized pain, the therapist can train the client to corral the pain.

Therapist: "Where does it hurt?"

Client: "Everywhere!"

Therapist: "Okay, I'm going to help you be specific by asking some questions. Let's go through your body one part at a time and see just where the pain is. Let's start with your neck. Does your neck hurt?"

Client: "Yes!"

Therapist: "Okay. We've located one part of what seemed like everywhere . . . that's good. Does it hurt where your head connects to your neck? On the ridge of the back of the skull?"

Client: "Yes . . . and everywhere else, too!"

Therapist: "I know that and we're going to do a good general massage, but we're also going to concentrate on one part. I'm going to give you a pain scale. Can you remember the worst pain you ever felt?"

Client: "Yeah, when I had appendicitis!"

Therapist: "Okay, that's a 10. Zero is no pain at all. Under 5 is uncomfortable. Five is pain that's really starting to hurt. Can you tell me what number this is?"

Client (with a whining tone): "I don't know. Everything hurts."

Therapist: "Wait, this is important. Knowing this will really let me help you. Try to focus and tell me what number it is."

Client: "Do I have to? Why don't you just find it and fix it."

Therapist: "Because learning this scale is an important way to help me and eventually for you to help yourself when I'm not working with you between our sessions."

Client (reluctantly): "Okay . . . it's a 4."

Therapist: "Good job! Is there anywhere else in your body that's more than a 4?"

Client: "I don't think so, but I think there's lots and lots of 4s."

Therapist: "Okay, that's another great piece of information we're going to use. Let's focus on this pain now. Look inside yourself. What shape does the pain have?"

Client: "What?"

Therapist: "I mean, does it look like a golf ball, an octopus, a pellet, a rock, anything . . .?"

Client: "It kind of looks like a little rock that's been heated up."

Therapist: "Okay! Great! Now I'm going to work on that little hot rock, and as I do it you can tell me if anything is changing and how it's changing."

In corralling the pain, the therapist trains the client how to focus, differentiate, take power and responsibility, and observe change.

---

foundation for building an internal structure for the first time. People with collapsed structures often perceive themselves as a nobody because they feel they have no body.

The massage work should at some point include invigorating work on the back, legs, and feet. This increases the client's ability to hold and contain any good feeling from the massage. The back and legs are the support system of the body. For people with a collapsed structure, the back and legs tend to be fatigued since they are working with insufficient tone to hold the person up. Bringing awareness and energy into these parts allows the person to somatically experience the possibility of supporting themselves, of "standing on their own two feet" (Johnson).

Invigorating massage of the musculature also gives a client with this structure a sense of boundary and containment. The sense of aliveness generates wanting to be more alive. Bringing sensation into the musculature in general gives a heightened sense both of having a body and being somebody.

To raise their energy level, clients with collapsed structures must increase their breathing. However, because their energy levels are so low to begin with, this increase in breathing is highly uncomfortable because they have no energy to accomplish it (Lowen, 1975). Opening the chest with massage is one step toward increasing breathing. However, the low energy state is so ingrained that a spontaneous and sustained increase in breathing may not happen immediately. This kind of client may need coaching and support in real time within the session to increase breathing. Telling such a client to practice breathing exercises on his or her own can be a setup for failure. Chronic low energy overwhelms most desires to do this type of exercise even though the client may know it is to his/her benefit. The repetition within sessions of opening the chest and encouraging breathing has a gradual benefit of developing a new somatic pattern over time.

The greatest physical need for people with a collapsed structure is to literally develop the body and begin to build more physical structure to counteract the tendency toward weakness and collapse. This means they need to develop their musculature and increase strength through exercise. The massage therapist can play an important role in this quest by offering encouragement, support, and direction. However, the therapist cannot simply tell the client to exercise. This also can be a setup for failure. The therapist needs to keep in mind the chronically low energy (undercharge) in the client and the psychological tendency to collapse and declare "I can't." The therapist can help the client by giving exercises that start slowly and are basic and by increasing these in small increments (or referring to a trainer who will do this). By basic, we mean that the therapist may ask a severely collapsed client to walk around the block once a day for a week and increase it by half a block each succeeding week. It also means that the therapist must "lend the client a backbone" by helping the client get back up on their feet again after a collapse. For example, if a client reports not walking around the block for a week, then accept this without judgment and at the same time insist that the client stick to the program.

One behavior the therapist may encounter with clients with a collapsed structure who have agreed to a fitness plan is complaining. This is an unconscious behavior that is endemic in people with a collapsed structure. Essentially, complaining "lets steam out of the pressure cooker" so that energy cannot build toward action. Complaining may also have served the purpose in the past of getting them off the hook or attracting sympathy.

Understanding the dual nature of the complaining is important for the massage therapist in order to understand what the client with this structure is doing. The pain and discomfort that the client is feeling are very real. At the same time, the complaining can come across as exaggerated, manipulative, and unrealistic. The inherent duality that can be difficult to discern is that the feeling is real, but the *expression* of it is affected. People with a collapsed structure *really do feel pain*, but they also use the expression of pain to engender a response from others (Johnson). They seek to both express the feeling and simultaneously elicit a caregiving response from another person. The therapist needs to accept the expression of pain as real, but not be drawn in to let the client off the hook and let him or her collapse. The therapist also needs to maintain the role of providing backbone and to find ways to support the client to persist in the activities that will lead to change, *despite the anxiety that always accompanies change.*

In working with clients with a collapsed structure, the massage therapist must become clear about goals for the client. They come to massage, as does everyone else, to feel better, benefiting from the soothing effects of massage. Clients with a collapsed structure often seek that soothing exclusively, craving it above all. They tend to give the therapist positive reinforcement to do only soothing and nurturing massage, often by making the therapist a great healer who is wonderful, wise, and powerful. This is fine if maintaining the status quo is what has been agreed to within the therapeutic contract. If not, the work will tend to reach an impasse or plateau.

Changes made by one massage may not endure until the next one with clients with a collapsed structure. Even though this happens with many other clients, it is more pronounced with them. It can be as though each massage starts over from the beginning. Because of their psychological underpinnings, people with a collapsed structure tend to look for situations in which they can be soothed within a dependent relationship. This means their idea of success, which is usually unconscious, may be different from what the massage therapist assumes. For them, the need to feel soothed wins out over having to tolerate any discomfort that may be experienced to build up the body. Above all else, they want the therapist to make them feel better. Therefore, collapsed clients can be rather discomfort avoidant and seem resistant to "paying their dues" of enduring the physical and psychological discomfort that accompanies a fitness program. The therapist needs to see them through this and avoid becoming frustrated with the client (which is a typical countertransference situation).

Even with an agreement to maintain the status quo, clients with a collapsed structure tend to expect to progressively feel better. However, their sense of feeling better is a global one that is akin to being in a paradise of good feeling, but without changing their personal status quo. Even though clients with a collapsed structure supposedly just want to feel good, they will nevertheless at some point begin to let the therapist know they are not getting enough. This means the therapist may end up feeling in a frustrating bind in which the client has unrealistic expectations accompanied by unrealistic personal effort. This is another frustration the therapist must be careful about so that it does not drive the therapist to react negatively toward the client.

If the client begins to question progress, discussing what is necessary at a body level for progress to happen is important. Few clients walk into the therapy room with full knowledge of what is necessary for change. The therapist must discuss in an objective fashion how hypotonicity affects the client's body. If the client feels unwilling or unable to enter a fitness program or increase exercise, the therapist must accept this without judging the client. At the same time, the client must accept that the massage work has limits. The client may accept this idea at the moment, but because of his or her character structure, may forget and begin complaining. The massage therapist must gently remind the client of the limits of massage on a hypotonic body. This reminder must not be a disguised chastisement or nagging. When a client with a collapsed structure cannot or will not choose to work on toning and strengthening the body, the massage therapist must walk a narrow path between the client's complaints and not blaming the client for failing. The therapist may find this requires great patience and may even need help in supervision to deal with the countertransferential feelings stirred up by working with a client with this structure.

This intense focus on feeling "good" or "better" through being taken care of in a dependent relationship that is typical of the collapsed structure may manifest as inflated, unrealistic expectations placed on the therapist. For example, the therapist may be expected to have *a priori* knowledge of what the client's physical and emotional needs are at any given time and satisfy them. As a result, the therapist also may be expected to meet the client's needs despite whether these are appropriate or within the boundaries of the therapeutic frame; that is, despite the time limits of a session, accepted hours for phone calls, agreed-upon methods of payment, or beyond the therapist's physical, emotional, professional, or ethical limits. Acting out of their character structure, they attempt to get more and more without a natural understanding that the other person may experience this as invasive or burdensome (Johnson).

More examples of acting out by clients with a collapsed structure are seeking to extend their time by complaining of one last little pain that needs some attention, asking one last question, or dressing slowly when it is time to end the session. Their acting out often eventually triggers rejection by others resulting from their slow but steady incursion on others' boundaries and the other person eventually reaching a limit and feeling "they can't take it anymore."

Massage therapists can be drawn into this pattern. Because many massage therapists overdo caregiving, they tend to overextend giving to this type of client. The therapist may feel unloving or like a bad or selfish person for not giving just a little more. Only after weeks, months, or years of doing extra services will such a massage therapist finally become angry and push the client away. This result becomes a repetition of a childhood situation that the person with a collapsed structure unconsciously recreates.

To avoid repeating and reinforcing this pattern, making professional boundaries clear from the outset, holding to them firmly, and saying no to uncomfortable, unrealistic expectations—even when it is difficult to do so—is critical for the massage therapist to do. The boundaries need not be rigid, but they do need to be firm.

If the therapist is getting hooked by the client, distinct signs of countertransference eventually develop. Some classic signs are finding oneself trying harder and harder to satisfy the client, not holding frame boundaries, dreading the client, resenting the client, and giving lots of advice (Johnson). Such relationship issues are often more prominent than the actual massage work in working with clients with a collapsed structure.

Finally, the massage therapist can make two important types of interventions on the relationship level that will help the client grow by countering the drive to be dependent. One is what we call "giving the power back to the client." As part of the "big one-little one" dynamic, the client may tend to praise and credit you for progress made. Whenever the client does this, it is an opportunity for you to point out what the *client* did to make accomplishments happen and praise the client. This reinforces the notion that good things happen because of effort by the client, not by the client being a passive, dependent recipient of the fruits of someone else's power.

You can also reward the client whenever he or she does something positive. Any accomplishment by the client is an opportunity to offer praise and positive feeling. This counteracts the pattern of receiving at a random moment after being collapsed. This teaches the client that it is not necessary to be collapsed to be rewarded with nurturance and that if the client feels good, he or she will still receive caring and support. The following case study is an example of "giving back the power" and supporting the client's active participation.

Theo and Mel

Mel is a client with a collapsed structure. Theo is his massage therapist. They have been working together for about 6 months. The massage session is just beginning.

Mel: Theo, that was the greatest massage last week! I've felt really good almost all week. You're really amazing. I don't know how you do it, but I sure like it.

Theo: Thank you. By the way, how did your walking go this week?

Mel: Well, I somehow managed to increase my walks another couple blocks, just like you suggested.

Theo: That's great, Mel! You are really making progress. I think you are doing a fantastic job of hanging in there and going out walking even when the weather's been a bit dicey this week.

Mel: Gee . . . though it's thanks to you, really.

Theo: Uh-uh. It's thanks to you. *You* did the walking, not me. You know, another thing is that because you've been doing your walking and building up your legs, that is why you kept feeling good this week after the massage . . . and for much longer than before.

Mel: Hmmm, I didn't think of that . . . guess that's true. Thanks.

Theo: Keep up the good work! Let's go over the workout plan for this next week and then let's start the massage.

THE COMPRESSED STRUCTURE

The primary traits of the *compressed* structure are an outward submissiveness and desire to please, an internal resistant attitude, and a deep fear of inner impulses and their assertive expression. These threatening inner impulses are held in by thick, muscular sheath armoring that compresses the body. People with this structure were cared for materially as children, but with severe pressure, usually in the form of being made to feel extremely guilty for any attempt to assert autonomy or negative feelings. As adults, aggression and self-assertion are greatly limited (Lowen, 1971). The compressed structure is undercharged, overgrounded, and underbounded. The holding pattern is held in.

Psychological Dynamics

People with a compressed structure often experience themselves as submissive, accommodating, and servile. They please others more subtly than people with a collapsed structure, usually doing so through self-sacrifice, providing others' needs, and being overly responsible. They consistently place their own needs last and are sometimes proud of doing so. A high premium is placed on being a "good person," that is, not morally good, but by being a giving person . . . even to the point of not saying no. Indeed, they often feel that they cannot say no or expect acknowledgment. They give to the point of self-sacrifice because they feel as if they should not have limits. Sharply attuned to the needs of others, they are often able to anticipate and meet such needs even before the other person asks.

Because they give in such a self-effacing and low-key manner, they are faced frequently with the dilemma of choosing between meeting the needs of others and meeting their own needs. Practically compelled almost always to choose the needs of others, they suppress their own impulses to express or take care of their own needs. This self-sacrifice leads to resentment, which is seldom expressed outwardly, and a pervasive underlying attitude of resistance.

Because of their fear of demands and sensitivity to the will of others, people with a compressed structure are highly attuned to any agendas that another person may overtly or covertly have. What a noncompressed person may consider reasonable, or even hardly noticeable, can become a glaring demand for the person with a compressed structure.

Resistance to the perceived will of others is the hallmark of the compressed position, and this resistance is experienced as a survival tool. People with a compressed structure feel easily bullied. In reaction, they often become overtly or passively resistant, withholding, and spiteful. People in a compressed structure often see others as authorities and feel compelled to rebel even if it sabotages their well-being.

People with a compressed structure are burdened with a constant feeling of demand and consequent resistance, often accompanied by guilt for doing so. This feeling of being demanded upon may intrude on even the most basic survival needs. For example, they may even experience being required to support themselves financially as an unreasonable demand.

They often get locked into two equally unrewarding responses with regard to interaction with the outside world—*compliance and defiance* (Lowen, 1971). *Both positions are reactive to the outside world rather than responsive to the inner needs and desires of the individual.* The tragic situation of people with a compressed structure is that while they long to feel their own impulses, desires, and autonomy, instead they are attuned to the will and needs of others. They either fulfill that will or they resist it, but they cannot feel their own.

People with a compressed structure are commonly faced with friends, lovers, and other intimates who perceive them as unfeeling and withholding sometimes. Although they are definitely withholding, they are not unfeeling and frequently feel baffled by this perception. However, attempts by an intimate to get them to talk about or show their feelings is experienced as an unreasonable demand to "produce" feelings and is met with withholding. This is often a source of constant struggle in the relationships into which people with a compressed structure enter.

As with the other character structures, the compressed structure presents a paradox in which a person with it lives. The only way to own oneself is to *oppose any* ownership of oneself, even by the individual him/herself (Lowen, 1971). As a consequence, people with a compressed structure avoid taking responsibility for their feelings and emotionally based actions. They tend to blame others and perceive themselves as having been forced into actions or feelings by others, rather than by personal choice. For example, a classic pattern is to wait until the other person has committed some actual or perceived transgression, which then permits the compressed person to blast them with stored-up resentments, rather than aggressively assert his or her feelings for their own sake (Lowen, 1975). This allows the person with a compressed structure to see himself as "good" and not aggressive and the other as "bad" and aggressive.

Since aggression is a forbidden feeling in the compressed person's childhood, he or she must avoid ownership of such a feeling at all costs. Therefore, the only way aggression can come out is if the person with a compressed structure experiences being "pushed into it." People with a compressed structure unconsciously seek out situations in which they will be pushed to the wall and can finally have the release of getting angry as a payoff. Noting that people with a compressed structure, because of the prohibition against aggression of any kind, cannot assert annoyance or request a change in behavior on a smaller scale is important. Only a monumental transgression is big enough to allow, that is, to justify, them to become angry or otherwise assert their needs. They may collect slights or, as Eric Berne, a psychotherapist and developer of Transactional Analysis, described such behavior in *Games People Play*, collect "brown stamps."

In the brown stamp game, the "player" gets a brown stamp every time he stores a resentment rather than expresses one. When the player has saved up enough brown stamps, he can redeem them to collect the prize, which is a "free" explosion of anger. At an organismic level, an accumulation of aggressive energy is necessary to break through the armoring of the compressed structure. Small annoyances cannot generate enough energy to break through the defenses against feeling and expressing displeasure. Only the collected energy of many annoyances, with the addition of the person's own righteous internal feelings about how he or she has been unjustly treated, can generate the energy needed for release. It is this lively release that the deadened compressed person craves, but of which he or she also is terrified. The following case study is an example of playing the brown stamp game.

Richard

Terry had been working with Richard in massage therapy for 2 years, every Saturday morning at 10:00 A.M. Terry liked Richard, a soft-spoken and mild-mannered man. The massage worked well for Richard, and the therapeutic relation-

Richard

ship seemed to be easy and friendly. At the beginning of the third year, Terry entered a training program that caused her to rearrange her time schedule. In fact, she had to reschedule nearly all of her clients. Because of the nature of the training, she could not make a consistent schedule, even though she was able to fit everyone in every week.

The first time she called Richard to reschedule, she explained the situation to him and asked him if he could come for his appointments Tuesday evening. Her request to Richard was polite, professional, and acknowledged that her rescheduling might be inconvenient to Richard. "No problem," said Richard.

Terry had to reschedule Richard five more times over the next 7 months. Each time Terry called, she was polite, professional, and concerned with the possible inconvenience to Richard. The sixth time that Terry rescheduled, Richard did not show up. This was very unusual for Richard. Terry was worried. She called him and said, "Are you okay? You didn't show up and you always show up. I was worried that something may have happened."

"I just decided I needed someone more professional," Richard spit out, "Maybe you should go back to school for more training."

Terry, taken by surprise, blurted back, "Richard, I don't know what to say. What's this about?"

"You don't know?" Richard said, "You should, you know. Well, I've found another massage therapist who is less flaky than you are . . . someone who can keep their word, someone who can keep a schedule. I thought you were more together than this. Physician heal thyself. Goodbye. Have a nice life."

Terry was shocked and felt very bad. She went for supervision. The supervisor asked Terry to describe Richard's body, his interactions with her, and the circumstances of termination. "Hmm," said Marla, the supervisor, "I can't be absolutely sure, but I can make an educated guess about what happened. The first time you asked Richard to accommodate a change, he may have been mostly okay with it, but after that he must have really resented it."

"Then why didn't he tell me?" Terry wondered.

Marla figured, "I don't think he can allow himself to say he doesn't want to do something or to tell you he was irritated and inconvenienced by the series of changes. He may have felt like you thought he was unimportant. You know, good old Richard. He'll do anything."

"I told him I knew this might inconvenience him," noted Terry.

"I know," nodded Marla, "For another person, that might have been just right the right thing to say. It's not a question of your being a professional or acting correctly. It's more a question of how Richard experiences things. I know you really wanted to do this training, and rescheduling people wasn't wrong. Here are a couple of things I might have done differently. I might have told Richard in advance that I was going to have to reschedule him several times, asked him how he felt about that—and this is the important part—asked him what he wanted."

"What if he didn't know?" asked Terry.

Marla replied, "Then I might have thought up some choices and offered him a choice. Then he might not have felt so forced and taken advantage of. He might have felt the respect that you actually do feel for him."

"Okay," said Terry, "I just hated how this ended."

"I know," sympathized Marla, "You didn't do anything wrong, but now you know more about how people in a structure like Richard's might perceive things."

In the brown stamp game, Richard reacted to feeling constantly compelled to give in to the needs of the other person. He was accommodating to a fault to maintain a connection with Terry. The central conflict that people with a compressed structure face is that of *love versus autonomy*. The armoring is such that if they are in relationship, they are completely attuned to the will of the other person and cannot feel themselves. To feel themselves and their own autonomy, they cannot be in relationship, which leaves them in isolation. This also leaves them in a frustrating lose-lose dilemma—they either lose themselves or the other person.

This can be highly confusing to someone in relationship with a partner with a compressed structure. Often, partners in intimate relationships *do not want* the person with a compressed structure to give himself or herself up, but the compressed person does so almost automatically *as if* the other partner wants it. In this way, the person with a compressed structure is recapitulating a childhood situation in which the parent wanted the child to be an extension of the parent's will.

People with a compressed structure are overbounded, and their bodies show this in a certain density in the tissue. However, the overboundedness is a compensation for a severe underbounded quality just beneath the surface. Feeling underbounded, people in the compressed position feel easily smothered, invaded, and trapped in relationships. A related effect of their underlying underbounding is that they often need to have immense amounts of physical space just to feel what they feel. Without the buffer that such space provides, their boundaries are too vulnerable to being penetrated; even another person's physical proximity may lead them to tune into the other person's feelings.

People with a compressed structure, out of necessity, have crushed, numbed, and muffled their feelings. Not only do they need space, but it sometimes takes them long periods of time to be able to feel and then articulate their feelings. As a result, they often have markedly delayed reactions to events and people.

Although it is true that people with a compressed structure should not have to produce or perform their feelings, they take this to such an extreme that their intimates may never experience their feelings directly. People with a compressed structure are more likely to show love and caring by providing support, loyalty, service, and material goods. In this way, they unwittingly recapitulate their childhood by providing physical care, but not direct emotional or spiritual contact.

In addition, people with a compressed structure may experience opening up emotionally as being exposed, and sometimes even an occasion for humiliation. Fear of humiliation haunts people in the compressed position, and they may avoid many activities because of possibility of humiliation (Lowen, 1971). They are so sensitive about humiliation that they may feel acute humiliation in situations that would barely cause a ripple in another person's awareness. This is one of the reasons that they avoid the spotlight, taking center stage, and taking charge as the leader, even though they might have excellent capabilities.

One often finds people with a compressed structure in secondary positions because they are more comfortable as the "power behind the throne." They function very well as vice presidents, aides de camp, executive secretaries, and other support positions (Keleman). Although they may be comfortable in the role of "loyal servant," they may silently want the boss or some other authority to acknowledge their skill and promote or reward them. In lieu of such recognition, they may stew in resentment about all the work they are putting in without the rewards.

The low profile that people with a compressed structure keep can often lead others to think that they are less intelligent or talented than they actually are, often acting "stupid" or awkward and clumsy (Smith). This is an unconscious mask that frequently belies a keen intelligence and vivid imagination.

Martyrdom, which combines the psychological dynamics of the hero and the victim, plays a role as a psychological pattern in the work and personal relationships of people with a compressed structure (Keleman). Their feelings of martyrdom may remain completely unstated, but friends, lovers, and acquaintances often end up feeling vaguely guilty around them without being aware of the source of the guilt.

People with a compressed structure frequently feel depressed, though not necessarily clinically depressed—more like "feeling blue." The quality of the depression is swampy and morass-like (Lowen, 1971). They struggle, but the struggle takes them even deeper into the swamp. They also tend to experience chronic suffering (Lowen, 1971), often with a tortured quality to the depression. Indeed, they often report having an inner voice that tortures them. The depression can lead to low self-esteem and a feeling of worthlessness that is often expressed as "feeling like a piece of crap." When they are able to lift out of the depression, they often do it through having a secret sense of superiority (to counteract the low self-esteem) and contempt for others (Smith).

Ironically, the swampy depression is often amplified by a capacity for endurance. The bodymind of people with a compressed structure has learned to endure discomfort, pain, and insult without protest or without moving. Part of their survival strategy is to "hunker down," resist, and wait until the situation has passed. This waiting tactic does not allow them to initiate fight or flight as options, either of which might be more effective responses in certain situations.

Etiology

A compressed structure is most likely to form in the developmental period of between 18 months and 3 years old (Johnson). This period is when the child is on his or her feet, toddling and walking. Independence and autonomy begin developing during this period. Some of this independence is displayed in the infamous automatic "no's" and tantrums of the "terrible twos" stage. Toilet training and socialization begin at this time. The dance between allowing the flowering of healthy assertiveness, exploration, and autonomy and creating good boundaries and limits for impulses is a difficult one for parents and child.

People with a compressed structure may experience a sensation of suffocation that relates directly to emotional experiences in childhood. On rare occasions, they actually have experienced suffocation either by accident or as a punishment. The primary experience of suffocation, however, mainly reflects the emotional quality of early relationships. What is suffocated—smothered—is the *individual impulses and autonomy* of the child (Lowen, 1971). The child's caregivers are often too attentive or controlling. In other words, their will and needs dominate. The caregivers often believe consciously that their actions and feelings are in the best interest of the child, that is, "for her own good." They are frequently overprotective and watch the child's every move (Lowen, 1971). However, unconscious needs to shape and control not only the child's behavior, but her *being*, belie the idea that they are acting in the child's interest. By this we mean the caregivers want (unconsciously) to control the child's thoughts, feelings, and beliefs, as well as actions. Whether caregivers do this benevolently or punitively, the child experiences the caregivers as being intrusive and invasive (Keleman).

The caregivers usually put a high premium on the child being a "good boy" or "good girl." Getting angry, saying no, or any kind of overt rebellious behavior is stifled. Disappointment, shame, humiliation, and guilt are tools the caregiver uses to smother the fires of independent impulse (Lowen, 1971). If the caregivers are violent, they use physical and verbal punishments, such as beatings, physical restraints and imprisonment, physical and emotional humiliation, continual denigration, and even torture.

Much of the control exerted by the caregiver is accomplished through being indirect, such as implying expectations. The caregiver may tell the child what the child feels and thinks, particularly when he or she is upset or angry. "You don't really feel that way, do you?" is a phrase heard often in the families of people with a compressed structure. Statements like, "You want to play the piano for Aunt Martha, don't you?" are used to get the child to do what the caregiver wants without directly asking the child what he wants or not leaving the child any room to say no. The caregiver may act in a way that assumes the child feels as the caregiver feels, as if the child were an extension of the caregiver, by saying, for example, "I'm cold, put on your sweater." Children growing up in this situation become so well attuned to the feelings and will of the caregiver that the caregiver may eventually need only to shiver a little for the child to go to get a sweater for both of them.

Dominance and submission are always present in families of people with compressed structures. However, sweet, apparently benevolent forms of dominance can be just as effective as nasty, cruel, and punishing behavior by the caregiver. The child often receives adequate—sometimes even more than adequate—physical care. However, the care is not *emotionally* sufficient, often having an invasive quality based on what the *caregiver* thinks the child needs, not what the *child* feels he or she needs. The child's needs do not count.

Outright expressions of love and affection are typically lacking, although the child knows that the caregiver loves him/her (Lowen, 1971). Indeed, the caregiver may substitute physical care for contact to show love. The fact that the caregiver gave adequate, or even excellent, *physical* care often leaves the adult person with a compressed structure feeling confused and guilty about having negative feelings. Sometimes the person even wonders if he or she made up memories of being ill treated.

People with a compressed structure are caught in the dilemma of choosing *love or autonomy* in almost all relationships. To be in a close relationship is not to be free. To be free is to be unloved and alone. The genesis of the dilemma is that *the caregiver uses the relationship itself as a weapon against the autonomous impulses of the child.* The child who acts on his or her own impulses or feelings is faced with guilt, disappointment, or disconnection from the caregiver. Just as the child fears losing the love of the caregiver if he or she is autonomous, the caregiver implies that independent action, in itself, is unloving. Therefore, the only way the child can manage to relate to and be loved by the caregiver is to be and do what the caregiver wants. The child is faced with an untenable, unbearable dilemma: freedom to be oneself *or* love and approval from the caregiver. *The child cannot have love AND freedom.*

In the family of the child developing a compressed structure, the child's impulses are not refined or modified as they usually are through socialization. The fact that the child has *any impulses at all*, particularly if these conflict with the will of the caregiver, is considered unacceptable (Lowen, 1971). Therefore, impulses do not exist merely to be modified, refined, and shaped. They are to be ignored and eliminated.

The child, to preserve his/her integrity of self against the benevolent or not-so-benevolent despotism of the caregiver, becomes locked deeply into a state of resistance. Later in life, long past the time when the caregiver no longer has power over them, people with a compressed structure sometime go to almost ridiculous lengths to avoid doing what is "good for them"—*even when what is resisted would be in their own best interests*. Because they were blocked from successfully completing the stage of development when their impulses needed to be freely expressed and limited appropriately by the caregiver, they were unable to move to the next stage in which they would learn to channel and sublimate their own impulses in the service of their own best interests. It is as if an automatic NO is embedded in the psyche of people with a compressed structure (Smith).

Digestion, assimilation, and elimination are central psychological themes in the universe of people with a compressed structure. The caregiver often expressed a need to control—sometimes even a morbid fascination with—everything that went into and out of the child. Following the theme "it's good for you," for example, there may be protracted battles over the child eating disliked foods or finishing all the food on the plate. "Having something shoved down one's throat" and "feeling forced to swallow something" are metaphors with which people with a compressed structure are usually familiar. They are forced to swallow not only food, but also the thoughts, feelings, and will of the caregiver (Perls, Hefferline & Goodman). These remain within the person as "undigested" or swallowed whole as introjections (see Chapter 3). When you are experiencing an introjection, you cannot distinguish your own will or desires from the caregiver's. The will of the person with a compressed structure is fused with that of the caregiver and can become fused with anyone with whom the person has an important relationship.

Struggling over food is a common event in bringing up a child. Not everyone who struggled over food has a compressed structure. However, for the person with a compressed structure, this struggle probably happened regularly, was about other issues besides eating food, and was done in the cause of imposing the will of the caregiver rather than in the spirit of caring about the child's well-being.

Along with a fascination with food going into the child's body, the caregiver may also need to control and observe what goes out, as with toilet habits (Lowen, 1971). The caregiver may have a compulsive need for cleanliness and view toilet functions—and all other functions of the lower half of the body—as "dirty." In the case of people with a compressed structure, parents, grandparents or other caregivers take excessive pride often in early toilet training. By early, we mean before the muscles of the pelvic floor and anal sphincter are developmentally capable and ready to exert the control needed to hold muscles in contraction. The child cannot always succeed, consequently early toilet training may initiate battles in which the parent wins and the child must capitulate, often resulting in considerable damage to the child's self-image. All children obviously must learn to control elimination functions, but premature timing and undue emphasis serve to break the will of the child, especially if humiliation tactics are used. Shaming and other such tactics cause a child to feel "dirty" and worthless. The child's feelings are often nonverbal, which makes them difficult to deal with in verbal therapy.

The child with a compressed structure may even feel that his parents "own" him. The caregiver's pressure on the child to produce certain actions or feelings tends to rob the child of the sense that he acts and feels by his own volition and that his actions or feelings "belong" to him. Instead, the child feels disconnected from those actions and feelings, and they then "belong" to the caregiver. Furthermore, the caregiver may be insensitive to the child's normal need for privacy and self-possession and may talk to friends or strangers about such issues as the child's toilet training, mistakes, and other potentially humiliating and embarrassing circumstances or crassly boast about the child's accomplishments. This childhood experience of being "owned" may lead people with compressed structures to feel enslaved or imprisoned in contemporary relationships of all kinds. The only way the child can preserve any autonomy and integrity is to refuse to cooperate.

The parent is by far more powerful, but the child also has strategies, tactics, and weapons. One way the child learns to have any control is by *holding in*, that is, retaining bodily functions on the physical level and feelings on the emotional level and resisting the caregiver's enormous pressure to "produce." Since outward, overt resistance is not feasible, the child will covertly *withhold*. Using withholding eventually becomes a defensive tactic against any perceived pressure, whether it is elimination, eating, or cooperating. The motto of people with a compressed structure becomes *"I won't."* Withholding also forms the matrix for the patterns that others find most irritating in dealing with people with a compressed structure: passive resistance and **passive aggression** (see the definition).

The aggression of children with a compressed structure must become passive in nature because if they were to express it freely, then they would be punished, even humiliated. Such punishment, humiliation, and subsequent guilt contribute to a severe lack of self-esteem and self-hatred. This self-hatred, along with a need for resistance, fuels the passive aggression. If a friend or therapist attempts to aid or help the person with this structure, a deep sense of mistrust stemming from their feeling worthless, as well as an expectation of retribution, foils the attempt.

Appearance

The type of armoring found with the compressed structure is sheath armor. The wall of the sheath psychologically provides protection from assaults from the outside world, and at the same time forms a barrier against expression of impulses arising from the interior world. The sheath may even effectively deaden the experience of the impulses themselves, thereby deadening feeling.

The armoring of the compressed structure tends to be thickened, dense, and numb. It has a rubbery quality to the touch. Skeletal and muscular surface definitions are obscured, giving an overall appearance of smoothness. For example, the scapulae may not be detectable on the surface of the back. The sheathing does not follow regular anatomical patterns, so it can be confusing at first to someone familiar with anatomy, such as a massage therapist. The holding patterns tend to form transverse rings or bands. These rings or bands are often found around the shoulder and pelvic girdles. There may be additional rings or bands and, if these are extensive enough, they sometimes form one great sheath.

The density of the tissue has a muffling effect on all sensation; thus, they may feel as if their body is encased in styrofoam or plastic and may long to feel both sensation and emotion. However, this longing to feel is usually not expressed outwardly. The tissue may also bulk up, giving the impression that the person is able to carry or withstand great loads of weight or responsibility.

The ring or band-like organization of the armoring acts to squeeze and hold them *and their impulses* in. This in turn creates a sensation of pressure building up. As an analogy, if a garden hose is squeezed hard, only a trickle of water can flow out. But behind the squeezed choke point, water is a building up at increasingly higher pressure. Similarly, the pressure of the energy dammed behind the armoring of the compressed structure creates a sensation of explosiveness in the individual, who has no means of releasing the pressure and gaining relief.

Most people with a compressed structure look as if they are being compressed, as if someone has put an enormous weight on top of their heads and their bodies

Passive Aggression

Dealing with emotional conflict or stress by indirectly and unassertively expressing aggression toward others is termed *passive aggression*. A passive aggressive person maintains a front of outward compliance or inability that masks hidden resistance, resentment, or anger. For example, acting inept or being forgetful can disguise anger and resistance. Passive aggression often happens in response to calls or suggestions for independent action or performance, or lack of satisfaction of dependent wishes (i.e., not getting what you want). An example of passive aggressive behavior is to agree to do something, but purposely (consciously or unconsciously) do it half-heartedly, incorrectly, or not at all. Another example is to lag behind on a hike or some other activity, which causes the other person(s) to slow down or fall behind, rather than ask for a break or opting out of the activity in the first place. The classic passive aggressive transference pattern in psychotherapy is to ask for help and then both to defy it and to suffer from it. For example, such a client seemingly complies with a therapeutic suggestion, but not very well, and then claims it was a poor recommendation and it failed.

From a defensive standpoint, the purpose of passive aggression is to preserve personal worth, needs, and convictions in a hidden way that causes less personal vulnerability. However, it often does so at someone else's expense and risks agitating others; that is, it involves overidealization of the self and devaluation of others. This sense of vulnerability is often psychologically based on a history and an expectation of being emotionally injured by a negligent and cruel caregiver whenever the individual expressed his needs or autonomy. Passive aggressive behavior is not exclusive to compressed character types. Some ways of dealing with people who exhibit passive aggressive behavior are to be cooperative rather than judgmental, angry, or controlling; be completely accepting of who they are; and not to expect or want anything from them.

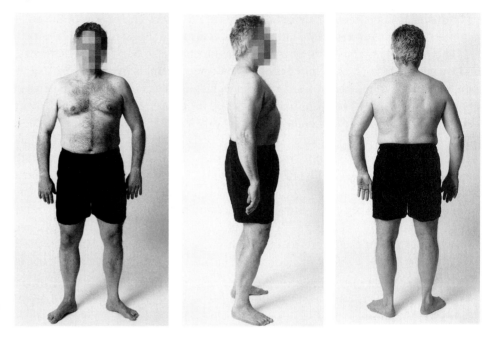

Figure 8.6
Male compressed structure. **Front view:** *Note thickened neck, barrel chest, banding at shoulder girdle, upward displacement of energy, banding at pelvic girdle causing an external rotation of the legs at the hips.* **Side view:** *Note forward displacement of the head, shelf-like appearance at junction of neck and shoulders, and anterior tilt of pelvis (which are moderate features in the individual in this photo).* **Back view:** *Note smoothness of sheath armor, holding in the back, tension in buttock area, and general appearance of being compressed.*

are being pressed down and crushed. The transverse banding that also squeezes the compressed structure is often visible in the form of an indention at the deltoids and the hips.

Many people with a compressed structure have barrel chests. Their chests are held in a permanent inflation without the relief of adequate expiration. Attempting to exhale fully is difficult. Even though they seem to be retaining a lot of air, the inflated position of the chest does not mean that they are able to use the air itself (Keleman). The chest rarely moves in respiration, with most of the movement occurring in the belly.

While the abdominal area moves in respiration, it is also tightly and deeply contracted (Lowen, 1971). At the surface, the belly may look almost swollen and distended. The belly itself is energetically isolated between the lid of a tight diaphragm and the bowl of a tight pelvic floor. They may experience substantial digestive and elimination problems.

The lower halves of people with a compressed structure may vary in appearance. Some men have an exaggerated lateral rotation of the legs, with the holding muscles making the buttocks look pinched, forming a "frog-leg" stance. The legs with this pattern are usually muscular with well-developed or overdeveloped calf muscles. Other men may have tightened buttocks with legs that are distinctly smaller in development than their chests (Figure 8.6). Women may have heavier lower halves with a specific kind of fatty tissue that is numbed and almost insulating in terms of sensation. The pelvis is often in a posterior tilt, which can appear to be a "tail between the legs" position (Lowen, 1971). The pelvis looks undercharged and is so (Figure 8.7).

The stance of people with a compressed structure often involves the feet being planted somewhat wide apart. This may involve the turnout discussed above or what is called the "Colossus stance" with the feet wide part and the knees straightened. The stance looks powerful, but is actually deceiving. A person with this stance can be pushed over quite easily. The feet and legs look well grounded, but are not well grounded at all. The person with a compressed structure is grounding through his or her will. Looking carefully at the ankles often reveals that the ankles seem pushed down or driven into the foot.

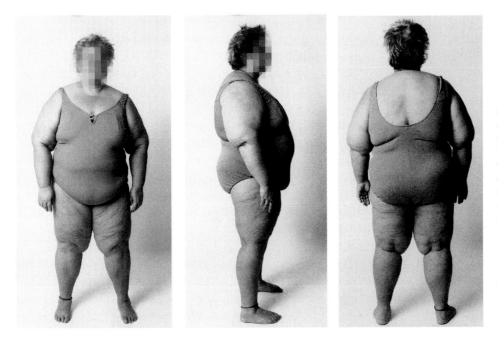

Figure 8.7
Female compressed structure.
Front view: *The female compressed type has a somewhat different appearance. Note the "Colossus" stance" (legs are externally rotated and feet placed far apart, giving an illusion of strength), although some other female compressed types may show a downward displacement of weight (pear-shaped).* **Side view:** *Note holding around hips, similar "shelf" at junction of neck and shoulders, posterior tilt of pelvis.* **Back view:** *Note sheathing in back, tightness caused by band around shoulder girdle, tension in buttock area.*

As strong as the stance of people with a compressed structure looks, such people do not feel "strong." The body is undercharged, particularly in the back. Although they may look physically stubborn and defiant, they cannot feel their back and lack the sense of "backbone" (Lowen, 1971).

The shoulders are often overdeveloped, with a holding pattern we call the "yoke," which is how people with a compressed structure experience it. The yoke consists of the shoulders being rounded forward so that the back of the body appears to be creeping into the front, with the arms medially rotated and held out in front of the body (often because of holding in the latissimus dorsi muscle), sometimes giving an "apelike" carriage.

The yoke pattern also forms a shelf-like structure at the top of the shoulders where the neck meets the torso. This also gives a feeling of weight on the back of the neck, making it difficult for people in the compressed structure to comfortably hold their head up or "stick their neck out" (Keleman). The neck is often thick and shortened and may appear like the neck of a turtle just coming out of its shell. The involvement of the sternocleidomastoid muscles in this positioning of the head and neck also connects to strong holding in the jaw. The jaw is often very tightly held and may sometimes give a stubborn expression. Holding is frequently found in the scalene muscles as well (Keleman). They may experience a lot of holding in the throat area and sometimes have a whiny voice as a result (Lowen, 1971).

Therapeutic Strategy

The dense sheath armoring of clients with a compressed structure is an important factor to deal with in massage. Soft or feathery touch can often, though not always, be highly irritating and frustrating to such clients. The numbing of the body often found in the compressed structure causes light touch to feel distant and like a tease, which is frustrating for such clients because they feel both the possibility of contact and deeper sensation in their body, but that it is also barely attainable. If the massage therapist does not understand this situation while working with clients with a

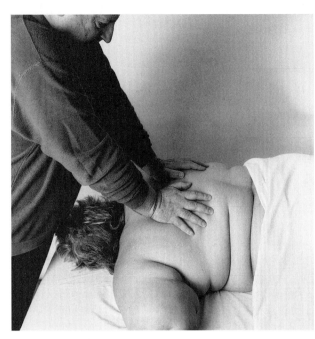

Figure 8.8
Technique of applying compression to back. *Using the entire palm or both palms and slowly applying weight to the dense sheathy tissue accomplishes it. Initially, this should be done only with the bands of holding in the back.*

compressed structure, then any angry and irritated responses from them to techniques that are usually relaxing may surprise the therapist.

A technique that works well with people with a compressed structure is what we call "taking over the holding." This technique involves holding, pressing, or supporting the client's body or body part in a way that duplicates the pressure created by the client's armoring and the containment and protection the armoring provides, so that the client does not have to hold, which facilitates a release of the holding pattern. With clients with a compressed structure, the massage therapist can take over the holding by applying heavy pressure to the dense rings around the body, particularly from the direction of the back. Using this technique, such clients no longer have to use their muscles to hold themselves and can deeply relax from the *inside out*. They *decompress* (Keleman). The relaxation can happen while applying pressure or when the pressure is released and the therapist moves away from the client. When a release takes place, the therapist will see a slow progressive expansion of breathing and signs of differentiation in the surface musculature ranging from subtle to dramatic. Another response from the client may be an active impulse to move and resist. While the client may spontaneously throw the therapist's hands off, the client is more likely to say something like, "I'd love to throw you off right now."

A form of taking over the holding is a technique called *compression* (different from the technique of the same name used in sports massage). Using the entire palm or both palms, the massage therapist slowly applies weight to the dense, sheathy tissue. The pressure needs to be applied broadly, rather than with point pressure, such as with finger or thumb tips. This is because pressure distributed along the circumferential banding found in this structure affects the entire band and releases it, whereas point pressure tends to be absorbed and have little effect. Initially, this should be done only on the bands of holding in the back. The front of the body can be approached in this way only when a deeply trusting relationship has formed between the massage therapist and the client. Because compression can evoke several types of responses—accommodation, resistance, struggling, or relaxation—going slowly and sensing the client's response is important. The pressure applied in compression needs to be sustained for a minimum of 5 minutes to be effective. Some clients like compression so much that they ask for it for much longer. However, massage therapists must also pay attention to their own bodies, since sustaining compression can be stressful and tiring (Figures 8.8, 8.9, 8.10).

Techniques such as taking over the holding and compression work because clients with compressed structures are *holding themselves in*. They are pressuring and squeezing themselves so that they do not let anything out, that is, to contain their impulses.

These techniques often stimulate a transference response that involves the issue of *accommodation*, manifesting usually on the bodily level. As previously mentioned, the lives of people with a compressed structure revolve around the accommodation of others. For example, when using the compression technique, during the first moments of applying heavy pressure, you might notice that the client can accommodate the pressure with very little discomfort. The client might even make remarks when this is pointed out, such as "I'm used to taking it" or "This feels familiar."

Upon applying more pressure, the therapist may notice progressive accommodation of the weight. At a certain point, the accommodation stops. This is a point at which the therapist should sustain steady pressure, but let the client know that at any time he or she is free to ask the therapist to lighten up, that is, reduce pressure. Asking undemandingly at each stage of applying pressure how it feels to the client also may be important. If such clients' histories are true to form, others have rarely inquired about how the client feels so that they can make things better or more comfortable. Instead, the situation usually is that others inquire in order to get the client to do something.

Clients who like compression sometimes ask us how they can get the same relief at home. Although nothing can replace the sustained pressure applied by the human hand, there are some alternatives. We have suggested that people put bags of kitty litter, sand, or bird shot on their backs, and they have reported that they do get some relief. Some types of athletic clothing have embedded weights, which also give some relief. They can also try having one or more people lie across their back, but they should not continue this if their response is not positive. The initiative to do this at home should come from the client, not as a homework assignment by the therapist.

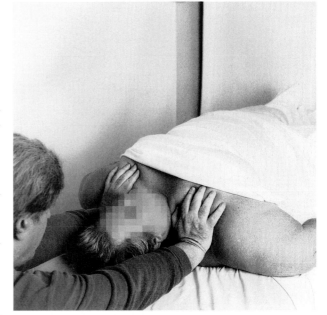

Figure 8.9
Technique of applying compression to shoulders.

Another form of massage that clients with compressed structures respond well to is deep tissue work, because the work is deep enough for them to begin to feel their body. As with compression, an adaptation that needs to be made when using deep tissue work with such clients is to use broad pressure, because direct specific pressure from the fingertips can be experienced as invasive or irritating because it does not release the banding pattern of tension. Wait until the sheath armoring has been loosened before trying direct pressure.

As we have seen, people with a compressed structure *learn to endure discomfort* until it goes away, rather than taking steps to get rid of the uncomfortable object or remove themselves from an unpleasant situation. They may not even know that they have the option of getting rid of what pains or irks them. This is why inquiry into the client's emotional state is so important when using the compression technique.

On the other hand, clients with a compressed structure may also benefit from energy work. Although this may seem to contradict the previous paragraph about deep tissue work, several energetic methods differ from the sort of light touch that may be frustrating to the client. At times, energetic methods can get underneath the armoring and undermine it. In other words, the work may stimulate or support the flow of vegetative energy on the endodermal level, which can erode the armoring "from below" by opening up deeper feeling.

Joints are another area to focus on with the work. Stretching the limbs and the neck and opening the joints can give clients with a compressed structure enormous relief (Keleman) (Figure 8.11). This effect happens because much of the compression in their structure affects the joints. Following this type of stretching, clients often report feeling longer and taller and experience their bodies the way they would feel without the

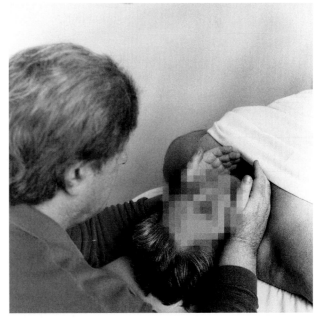

Figure 8.10
Technique of applying compression to masseters on jaw.

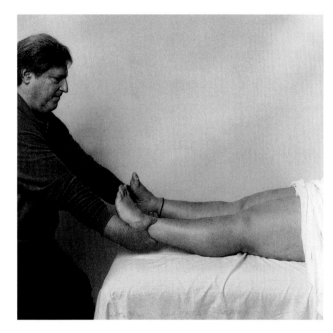

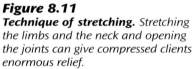

Figure 8.11
Technique of stretching. *Stretching the limbs and the neck and opening the joints can give compressed clients enormous relief.*

armoring. Another way of working with the joints is to apply pressure to each joint individually or the corresponding joints on each limb simultaneously. Pressure should not be applied directly to the knees, but can be applied directly above. This pressure can also give relief. Finally, simply holding joints for extended lengths of time with still (i.e., not moving) hands can also create an opening (Figure 8.12).

Because of the need for space that clients with a compressed structure have, not hovering over them is important. We have found that after using a technique, moving physically away from them to give them room to assimilate what has happened is effective. We often tell them that we are moving away, but we are still nearby. In this way, we are trying to counteract any early physical experience related to being invaded, hovered over, or hounded by the caregiver(s). Remembering that a primary conflict for clients with a compressed structure is relationship versus autonomy (i.e., love versus freedom), we want to let them know in a nonverbal way that they can be themselves, experience what they need to experience, and still be related to us.

The massage therapist must try to give up harboring any expectations or plans for the outcome of the session as well as a therapist can do so. Clients with a compressed structure tend to experience directive techniques, particularly verbal ones, as a demand. This triggers physical and emotional resistance, producing a counterproductive response. For example, many massage students learn to ask their clients to breathe, especially when encountering a place where tension is stored or to relax if they sense the client is tensing muscles. However, this well-meant suggestion backfires unexpectedly with clients with a compressed structure. Asking them to breathe is heard (usually unconsciously) as an order, which quickly takes them away from their own experience and plunges them into a dilemma of having to choose between complying with or defying the "order." Their attention then becomes dominated by what the therapist wants or thinks, taking them away from their inner awareness. This produces the *opposite* result of what is intended and reproduces their existential bind.

How can the massage therapist work with the dilemma of working to create a positive result, but not being able to direct the client toward the goal? Simply ignoring restricted breathing or constricted muscles is not a useful solution. An effective way to approach the dilemma is to frame suggestions as choices or experiments, because clients with a compressed structure need to make a choice or act on volition, rather than to act or follow a direction merely to please the therapist. Having choices can present to these clients an opportunity to exercise their will without initiating action, which would be more threatening. Experiments can open options for them as long as the massage therapist has no hidden expected outcome. For example, instead of telling the client to breathe, a massage therapist speaking in a more experimental frame might say, "See what happens if you deepen your breathing," or "See what happens if you hold your breath while I'm working." Then, the client can be asked what the result of the experiment was. Finding out ways of relaxing for themselves through experience, instead of being told how to do it, is more useful for clients in the compressed position. The *client* must be the one to reach the conclusion of the experiment or activity. We do not mean to suggest that the massage therapist cannot ask clients with a compressed structure to do movements required to release soft tissue, for example, to move the leg while working on the psoas muscle. This simply needs to be done in the right way.

The type of statements to avoid are indirect, open-ended suggestions, especially about *feeling*, and truisms or platitudes. Such statements induce a stuck feeling in clients with a compressed structure. They are inwardly trying to achieve the attitudes or actions suggested by the statements and simultaneously resisting and resenting them, while also feeling humiliated by the expectations implied in the statements and shameful of their resistance *all at the same time*. This reveals why the best intentioned therapist can end up with a client who makes little progress, seems bogged down, and makes the therapist feel ineffective.

Because of the tendency of people with a compressed structure to accommodate, asking too much of them in terms of shifting appointments or other changes in logistics may be easy—often too easy—for the massage therapist. Such clients try to make themselves amenable, and the massage therapist may think it is easy for them to comply. Therefore, to ask sincerely whether a change is inconvenient is very important. Otherwise, clients with a compressed structure tend to accommodate until they reach a point at which they become angry. Unfortunately, this anger is often expressed inappropriately, through sulking, withdrawal, leaving, and occasionally exploding (only if they cash in enough brown stamps, as Richard did in the case study).

Another phenomenon that occurs in the massage therapy relationship with clients with compressed structures is that they attempt to establish a friendly relationship by doing favors, that is, becoming a "go-fer" or "do-fer." This is not a conscious attempt to manipulate the therapist, but a "people-pleasing" way to relate to another person . . . on the surface, at least. Their expectation is that they will be valued because of what they can do for the other person. The favors or services they offer are often quite useful and they do not ask for anything in return, which makes it easy for the therapist to accept the favors. However, at some point after these favors accumulate, such clients become resentful, but do not express their feelings. The therapist must resist the temptation to accept these favors and not participate in what is essentially collusion with the client's pattern.

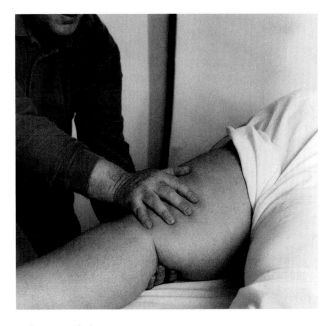

Figure 8.12
Technique of energy work at joints. Energy work with the joints is done by simply holding them for extended lengths of time with still hands.

Vanessa and Alison

Vanessa told her client, Alison, that she was moving her massage practice to a new office. Alison said, "Do you have your movers already? I know some great guys. They're the best. And they'll do it cheap. They owe me."

"Well, I don't have anyone yet," said Vanessa, "But I really can't ask you to do that."

"At the prices these guys charge, you can't ask me *not* to do that," Alison insisted, "Let me do this for you. It's nothing."

Vanessa, with some hesitation, said, "Well, I guess this would be alright. It's a referral, after all."

"Great, " said Alison, "I'll make the call. Don't worry about it. After all, you'll be the one paying."

A few months later, Vanessa, making conversation, said brightly to Alison, "Well, it's that time of year again. Gotta go home and calculate what I owe Uncle Sam!"

"Do you have a good accountant?" asked Alison.

Vanessa and Alison

"My accountant is okay," said Vanessa, "She hasn't saved me a fortune, but I guess she's alright."

"You have to meet my accountant," Alison responded, "She's saved me tons of money, and she also cleared up a misunderstanding I had with the IRS. I'll call her and see if she has room to see you."

"I don't know," demurred Vanessa.

"Oh c'mon. She'll save you oodles of money. What harm can that do?" asked Alison.

"Well, okay," said Vanessa.

Alison arranged for Vanessa to meet her accountant. Vanessa liked the accountant and she did, indeed, save her a lot of money. A little while later, Vanessa was ordering some new window treatments for her office. She had the swatches set up in the waiting room so she could look at them between sessions.

"Hmmm," said Alison, as she walked through the waiting room to the treatment room, "Swatches. Looking to change your curtains? I have a friend and I have a discount with her. A big one. She's a professional decorator. I'll let you use it. I'll arrange it."

"No, I can't take it," replied Vanessa.

"Sure, you can," said Alison, "I'll never use it."

"No, I really can't," said Vanessa, "Now, let's start your massage and pay attention to you."

A few days later an envelope arrived in the mail. It was from Alison. In it was the certificate for the discount. Vanessa decided that since Alison wasn't using it, it couldn't do any harm for her to use it.

Vanessa found that it became slightly easier each time to accept favors from Alison. She also found that she was beginning to think subconsciously of Alison as an easy opportunity for getting help when she needed it. Even though she had never solicited help from this client, she unwittingly placed herself, with the unconscious aid of her client, in the position to use her. This reaffirmed Alison's perception of herself that she is only good enough to be of service to others.

Next we will discuss the rigid character structure, which has several substructures. Because this is a comparatively longer discussion, we have placed it a separate chapter.

REFERENCES

Berne, E. (1994). *Games people play*. New York: Random House.

Brown, M. (1990). *The healing touch*. Mendocino, CA: LifeRhythm Press.

Johnson, S.M. (1985). *Characterological transformation: The hard work miracle*. New York: W.W. Norton.

Keleman, S. (1985). *Emotional anatomy*. Berkeley: Center Press.

Knapp, B.L. (1995). *Manna and mystery: a jungian approach to Hebrew myth and legend*. Wilmette, IL: Chiron.

Kurtz, R. & Prestera, H. (1976). *The body reveals*. New York: Harper & Row.

Lowen, A. (1967). *The betrayal of the body.* New York: Macmillan.

Lowen, A. (1971). *The language of the body.* New York: Collier Books.

Lowen, A. (1975). *Bioenergetics.* New York: Penguin Books.

Lowen, A. (1980). *Fear of life.* New York: Macmillan.

Montagu, A. (1986). *Touching.* New York: Harper & Row.

Perls, F., Hefferline, R. & Goodman, P. (1951). *Gestalt therapy.* New York: Dell.

Robbins, R. (1990). *Rhythmic integration.* Barrytown, NY: Pulse.

Rosenberg, J. L. & Rand, M. (1985). *Body, self, and soul-sustaining integration.* Atlanta: Humanics.

Shapiro, D. (1965). *Neurotic styles.* New York: Basic Books.

Shapiro, D. (1989). *Psychotherapy of the neurotic character.* New York: Basic Books.

Shapiro, D. (2000). *Dynamics of character.* New York: Basic Books.

Smith, E. (1985). *The body in psychotherapy.* Jefferson, NC: Macfarland & Company.

9

Armoring: The Rigid Character Structures

THE RIGID STRUCTURES

The primary traits of the *rigid* structure are to hold back on impulses to open and reach out emotionally, a high degree of control over behavior, and a good contact with reality that is used defensively against pleasure and letting go. The rigidity, which is like steel, also serves as a defense against giving in. While growing up, people with a rigid structure experienced frustration in striving for gratification. Connection and approval were gained through means other than simply reaching out for love. Indeed, such reaching out was often discouraged in various ways. Generally speaking, the rigid structure is overcharged, overgrounded, and overbounded (Lowen, 1971). However, this is not so with all of the rigid substructures, as explained later in this section. The holding patterns, which vary among the substructures, are held up, held back, or held out.

The discussion of the rigid structures varies from those of the other character structures in Chapter 8 because of the greater complexity introduced by the presence of several rigid substructures. We first discuss the common psychological dynamic threads that run through all. Then we discuss each substructure in greater detail.

General Psychological Dynamics

The structure that massage therapists are most likely to encounter in their practice is the rigid structure. It is the most prevalent structure, perhaps in part because the characteristics of the rigid structure are strongly supported and valued by our society (and most Western societies). Simply put, rigid patterns in the body allow the individual to suppress or repress feeling to achieve goals or maintain control. Achievement and control are thus valued over satisfaction and feeling. In other words, this structure is the embodiment of chronic "delayed gratification." The catch is that gratification may never happen because even after accomplishing a goal, the individual in the rigid position continues to need to maintain control or sets new goals to pursue, thereby continually prolonging the postponement.

Function over feeling is the common hallmark of all rigid structures and is the key to understanding why the term "rigid" is used. These highly functional people may appear to gain gratification from the material goods and status symbols that our society offers, as well as from their pursuit of activities that provide a high level of sensory experience. However, a persistent lack of *true* satisfaction and pleasure dwells under the surface. People with a rigid structure do not give in to their feelings, especially if this would deter them from reaching a goal. Their inability to give in to or surrender to their feelings keeps them from experiencing true satisfaction and pleasure.

The goals that people with a rigid structure pursue may exist in the external, material world. For example, the goal may be making a good salary, achieving social status, gaining power, or becoming an athletic champion. Alternatively, the goal may be internal and psychological, such as never letting oneself slip from a certain standard of polite behavior or be vulnerable in a relationship.

Feeling is threatening to people with a rigid structure, not only because of the fear that it will cause poorer performance, but also because of the belief that feeling is not acceptable and that it is shameful and a sign of failure. Comments we frequently hear from clients in the rigid position are, "If I lie down or rest, I'll never want to get up again," or "If I start crying, I'll never stop." Giving up effort and giving in to feeling is regarded as a failure to be avoided at all cost. Rigidity keeps them going despite any need or desire to stop. Their rigidity also keeps them from losing enough control to feel.

The rigid structure is designed to override emotional and physical pain, and discomfort coming from any source, to focus the entire being on the goal. Goal-driven performance requires focus, which is an intentional narrowing of information to accomplish a goal. On the other hand, feeling tends to diffuse focus and brings in more information. People with a rigid structure believe that considering broader information interferes with their performance, and therefore is neither productive nor useful. Extreme political movements, like totalitarian parties, are an extreme example of how a "rigid" ideology places ideas above feelings. All human feeling considerations are despised and disposed of in order to achieve their goals.

Will is a central component in rigidity. However, people with a rigid structure may or may not recognize that they are willful. If the will is directed toward the service of others, then it is likely that they will not recognize it as willfulness, but instead as "having good values," "knowing what to do," "doing the right thing," "getting the job done," or "doing what must be done." People interacting with an individual with a rigid structure are much more likely to perceive the overload of will, sometimes experiencing such a person as uncompassionate, heartless, pushy, competitive, unbending, superior, dominating, or insensitive. But the people with a rigid structure themselves rarely admit to having these qualities. *Their will must reign over feeling.*

People with a rigid structure may express their drive to perform in a variety of ways. These different performance modes are expressed in the body in different energetic and muscular holding patterns, accompanied by somewhat different psychological defense structures. Therefore, a variation of substructures within the rigid character category can be observed. Generally, the performance modes are

Table 9.1. *Summary of Character Structure Qualities*

Qualities	Disembodied Structure	Collapsed Structure	Compressed Structure	Rigid Structure (in General)
Charge	Overcharged	Undercharged	Undercharged	Overcharged
Grounding	Undergrounded	Undergrounded	Overgrounded	Overgrounded
Bounding	Underbounded	Underbounded	Underbounded	Overbounded
Armor	Knotty armor at joints and neck, holding in diaphragm	Flaccid, some knotty armor at joints, may have holding in upper back as compensation	Sheath armor, particularly at shoulder and pelvic girdles	Knotty armor, with holding in the upper and lower back; may have mesh armor
Holding	Held together	Held down, holding on	Held in	Held up and/or held back
Primary wound	Hostility or coldness, rejection	Deprivation	Crushed, invaded	Rejection, or seduction and rejection
Internal conflict	Not allowed to exist	Not allowed to need	Not allowed to be autonomous **and** loved, love vs freedom	Not allowed to feel, not allowed to love
Motto	I don't exist	I can't	I won't	I will
Compromise	I'll live without feeling and contact the world through my ideas	I'll live without reaching out and contact the world by giving and waiting	I'll live without asserting my independence and contact the world through submissiveness	I'll live without love and contact the world by making myself successful and/or attractive

based on control, achievement, being entertaining, and romanticizing or sexualizing relationships. These are referred to as rigid substructures or subtypes.

Having discussed some psychological characteristics that all rigid structures have in common, we now discuss these four rigid substructures: controlled rigid, achieving rigid, entertaining rigid, and romantic rigid.

THE CONTROLLED RIGID STRUCTURE

Psychological Dynamics

The hallmark of the *controlled* rigid structure (we refer to each substructure as a structure throughout the rest of this chapter) is using rigidity to control behavior according to an embedded code of personal conduct that regards certain forms of behaviors as "virtuous" and others as "bad." The bad behaviors and expressions are repressed by the rigidity. The controlling type of rigidity may be deeply involved with the organization of objects, time, other persons' behavior, eating, cleanliness, and so on, resembling to varying degrees (but not identical with) the traits of obses-

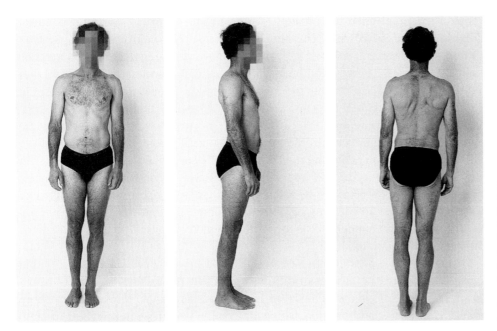

Figure 9.1
*Controlled behavior rigid structure. **Front view:** Note appearance of being slightly held in and held up. **Side view:** Note slight shelf at the shoulders, "turtle shell" in upper back, and splitting between the front and back halves. **Back view:** Note "rods" in lower back. There's a slight amount of sheath armoring in the upper back.*

sive-compulsive personality disorder. The deepest motivating belief of people with a controlled rigid structure is that if they can organize either themselves or the world perfectly, they will be able to feel secure (Shapiro, 1965). As a result, perfection is their goal, buttressed by an unconscious belief that they can attain perfection. This structure is overcharged, overgrounded, and overbounded (Figure 9.1).

People with a controlled rigid structure value predictability and fear spontaneity, so they keep as much of their life as they can under control. Spontaneous behavior is a problem because it cannot be controlled very well and "something can slip." Whatever "slips" or leaks out may be somehow incorrect, and people with this structure greatly value being correct. Thus, they try to maintain a smooth, even, almost monotonous rhythm in their lives, which is reflected in the energetic rhythm of their bodies. The rhythm incorporates and absorbs anything that is sudden, surprising, or spontaneous. When feeling threatens to break out—or break in—the armoring pattern quickly acts to cut it off and return things to "normal" somewhat like a self-sealing tire that immediately and rapidly responds to seal off any leaks.

The arcade game with toy moles randomly popping up out of holes that the player has to bash back into the hole with a club (often called *Whack-a-Mole*) serves as a metaphor for how people with a controlled rigid structure keep anxiety at bay. The moles represent internal impulses or anything unpredictable or disorderly in the external world, and the holes represent the unconscious, their origin. Whacking the moles represents the characteristic behavior that attempts to control impulses and spontaneous events. From the therapeutic point of view, the ultimate triumph for a person with a controlled rigid structure would be not to notice a mole pop up, but if seeing a mole, to say, "The heck with it . . . I think I'll take a break for a while."

The controlling behavior generated by this structure tends to focus on an area that is central to the person's life and attempts to make it orderly and clean. For example, if the person is drawn to aesthetics, then the person's emphasis is on beauty, grace, and order, with a fear of ugliness, awkwardness, messiness, and tawdriness. If the person is drawn to religion, then his or her world is ordered around staying morally clean, with a fear of moral disorder, sexual dirtiness, and chaos.

People with a controlled rigid structure appear to be absorbed by manners, social ritual, and social correctness. This characteristic may also manifest as an obsession with physical cleanliness of self and surroundings, which regards dirt and mess as constant enemies. The dirt and mess are symbolic of a profound discomfort with interior feelings and the organic nature of humanness. People with this structure in a sense are scared stiff of the messy, sticky, mushy nature of their internal feelings and spontaneous existence.

Money can also be a central focus of people with a controlled rigid structure. Unlike people with an achieving rigid structure (discussed in the next section) who may have a need to make a lot of money, people with a controlled rigid structure may concentrate on counting it, saving it, and going to extraordinary lengths to make a good deal, clip coupons, or otherwise control its flow. Whatever the central focus of the control happens to be, it overtakes much of the self, life, and sometimes the lives of those around them.

Encountering a person with a controlled rigid structure often leaves one with a sense of emotional dryness or aridity. However, this differs from a sense of heartlessness. The excessive emphasis on functioning and doing leaves little energy available for feeling and emotion, which flattens the person's emotional expression. They are often judgmental both of themselves and others. People with a controlled rigid structure may intentionally or inadvertently give others the feeling that others are messy, ugly, dirty, clumsy, ill mannered, bad with money, stupid, or immoral. Children raised by a parent with a controlled rigid structure tend to feel oppressed by the parent's need for perfection and lack of emotional contact.

Etiology

People with a controlled rigid structure are brought up by parents that emphasize the *propriety* of the child's behavior. Such parents focus excessively on rules and principles and expect the child to behave according to these rules "to the letter of the law." To do this, the child develops a high level of self-control, which is why this structure is referred to as controlled rigid. People with this structure hold back their impulses to a degree that is found in no other structure (Lowen, 1971). In this structure, *function* completely defeats feeling.

The parents are so focused on behavior that they fail to connect with the child emotionally. As a result, the child learns that the parents are pleased by the ability to be controlled, but do not value attempts to connect emotionally.

The parents also have a high level of anxiety about order and fear being overwhelmed by the inner world of instincts, impulses, and the body. They transmit these anxieties and fears to the child, but also that these can be vanquished by the adequate application of will and volition; that is, if you apply your will, you can order reality in such a way that everything will be secure. Willpower and control provide security because they bottle up the threatening and messy inner impulses and desires that roil within.

Security is highly prized within the family system. Striving for security can manifest as seeking physical safety, financial security, social correctness, aesthetic perfection, cleanliness, or religious or moral purity.

The parents punish any loss of control, lack of restraint, and spontaneous exploration and experimentation. Punishment can take the form of actual penalties, but their disapproval is more painful and inhibiting for the child. What makes disapproval in the case of this structure particularly potent is that the disapproval is absolute and makes the child feel inherently bad, dirty, and inferior and strive to be good, clean, and superior.

What is present with this type of rigid structure that is not with the others is *pressure*. While people with a controlled rigid structure also have the attributes of blocking feeling as the others do, they are under pressure to control their behavior and impulses. The parents believe that without intense observation and pressure, the child will fall prey to inner impulses, such as being lazy, unpurposeful, self-indulgent, sexual, and generally *giving into pleasure*. The parental pressure not only applies to behavior, but also to appearances. Therefore, people with this structure must also appear perfectly controlled under all circumstances. The pressure accounts for why the controlled rigid structure forms some sheath armor in the upper back, in contrast to the other rigid structures.

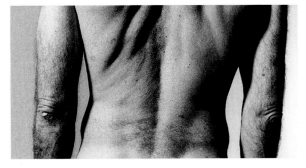

Figure 9.2.
"Rods" in back of controlled behavior rigid structure. Thickening of the muscles on either side of the spine forms the impression of rods holding up the rest of the upper back. As a result, these "rods" are supporting the upright body, rather than the legs.

Appearance

The controlled rigid structure is primarily what we term a "held-up" structure. Such people are most concerned with preventing falling and failing. The held-up aspect can be seen primarily in the long extensor muscles of the posterior half of the body (Keleman). Energetically, the back of the body is charged, whereas the front of the body seems dry, vacant, or absent. When looking at the posterior side one can see a thickening of the erector spinae from the lumbodorsal hinge downward to the pelvis. The thickening of these muscles on either side of the spine give the impression of rods holding up the rest of the upper back. As a result, these "rods" in the back, rather than the legs, are supporting the upright body (Figure 9.2). If we look at a person with this structure from the side, we can see that this is indeed what this formation is doing. These "rods" brace the body and keep it from falling down, collapsing, or otherwise giving in (Keleman). The pelvis often has a slight anterior tilt.

The head is slightly displaced anteriorly, which results in the appearance of a shelf-like formation at the base of the neck. We call this the Atlas formation—not having anything to do with the first vertebra—because this is the place where this structure is figuratively holding up the world as the mythical figure Atlas did. If a weight is actually placed on the shoulders of a person with the Atlas formation, you can see that their body seems to accommodate to the weight with little effort. They bear up to practically any burden, whether it is actual weight or *emotional* weight, without appearing to be actually pressured or burdened.

The "shelf" in the upper back tends, in part, to form a turtle-like shell. This means that the shoulders are curled forward and the chest is narrowed in the front. The tissue in the upper back tends to be thicker than what is usually found with knotty armoring, since it has some qualities of sheath armoring and is what allows this person to bear so much physical weight or emotional burdens without feeling it (Figure 9.3). In contrast to the compressed structure, whose primary armor pattern is the sheath pattern, the controlled rigid structure does not tend to appear as dense or compressed. Although both structures were programmed to bear excessive amounts of responsibility as children, the will of the controlled rigid structure was *encouraged*, even to excess, rather than crushed. As a result, the rigid pattern is

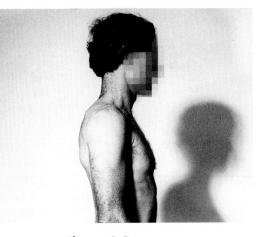

Figure 9.3
"Turtle shell" of upper back. The "shelf" in the upper back tends, in part, to form a turtle-like shell of the entire upper back. This means that the shoulders are curled forward and the chest is narrowed in the front. The tissue in the upper back tends to be thicker than knots. It has some qualities of sheath armoring and is what allows this person to bear so much physical or emotional weight or burdens without feeling it.

predominant, whereas there is some sheath armoring also in the upper back area owing to the emphasis on duty.

Energetically, this structure has a controlled, even, almost monotonous rhythm. This physical rhythm allows the person to stay mentally and emotionally tightly organized. Interruption of this rhythm causes the person to feel off balance.

Therapeutic Strategy

The strategy for massage for a client with a controlled rigid structure should include breaking up the system of knots along the posterior half, especially along the back. Some compression may be useful for any sheath armor that may be present in the upper back, although this is much less developed compared with the compressed structure. The back half should be substantially softened before doing deeper work on the chest and abdominal areas.

Softening the thick, ropy "rods" formed mostly by the erector spinae muscles that start around the diaphragmatic line and extend down into the lumbar region is particularly important. Since these rods act as a "brace" in the lower back, softening them is intended to enliven and open more connection to the sacrum and legs. Hopefully, this allows the client to begin to experience the pelvis and legs as support, rather than simply using the rods in the back.

After some progress has been made, it may be interesting to try some nonrhythmic tapotement (tapping). As previously mentioned, the controlled rigid structure tends to establish a very monotonous energetic rhythm in their bodies and lives that stifles spontaneity. Some nonrhythmic work that the client cannot "track" or predict can help disorganize this internal rhythm. Shaking the limbs, hands, and feet can also break up this rhythm. This is especially effective if the entire limb, particularly from where it is attached to the torso, is shaken. For instance, grasp the shoulder and wrist of the client, either both at the same time or separately, and shake nonrhythmically though a pulling motion or a push-pull motion. This begins to loosen up the upper back in a way that the armoring cannot anticipate. Experimenting with other kinds of nonrhythmic shaking movements such as the therapist putting the hands on the tops of the client's shoulders and gently pushing in a start-stop rhythm (push-push-push-stop-push-push-stop, and so on.) may also be helpful. Using the technique *Japanese Trepidation* (which involves picking up limbs, arhythmically shaking or swaying them, then periodically dropping them), if it is familiar to you, is also effective. If you are introducing a new technique into the massage, inquiring about how the client is experiencing the movement is helpful.

The massage therapist may notice the client making small constant, rhythmic movements, such as light finger drumming or toe crunching. This kind of movement is unconsciously ritualistic and designed to keep the client feeling "safe" (the discussion on compulsions in Chapter 10 gives further explanation). The massage therapist can suggest that the client experiment with feeling the movement more consciously, with feeling what is happening when it occurs, and noticing how he or she feels when stopping it.

Any behavior by the client that lacks decorum—bad jokes, silly behavior, contemptuous remarks, or tangential talking—during the massage may be considered an emotional release for someone with this structure. Behavior like this may seem insignificant in contrast to crying, screaming, or writhing in pain, but for someone who is encased in rigid ideas about behavior and being under control, such "improper" behavior can be a profound emotional release and highly therapeutic.

THE ACHIEVING RIGID STRUCTURE

Psychological Dynamics

A second type of rigid structure is overly concerned with *achievement*, driven to delay gratification to achieve a goal, that is, to be productive and competitive and to accumulate material goods or accomplishments as evidence of one's success and rectitude (Johnson). The body of a person with an achieving rigid structure may include a held-up pattern, but the entire body is more energized than that of the controlled rigid structure. We have had some clients with this structure report that they feel as if they are still standing up when they are lying down, which is due to their highly charged position of being "upright." This structure is likely to have the held-back pattern in combination with being held up. The holding back corresponds to the delay of gratification. This structure is also overcharged, overgrounded, and overbounded.

Because this structure values achievement above all else, anything that deters from this goal is to be avoided and is threatening. In psychological terms, people with an achievement-oriented rigid structure fear feeling and defend against feeling by hardening the body against their feelings. They may come across as hard, judgmental, in command, and righteous (Keleman). However, some people with this structure also can be affable, extroverted, and relate well with others as long as they feel they are in control. However, when they are challenged or diverted from their purpose, or asked to deepen a relationship, the hardness may appear. Vulnerability is very threatening and is avoided at all costs.

People in an achieving rigid structure are often more comfortable being aggressive than are people in other structures. The aggression enables them to get things done, "hit the ground running," and sustain energy over an extended period of time to achieve the goal (Keleman). Indeed, they are usually highly functional individuals. The aggressive and assertive energy enables them to be competitive both with others and with themselves. When taken to an extreme, they can become hostile and belligerent, and "must" win at everything no matter what (Smith).

People with an achieving rigid structure do come for massage, but often to maintain the body rather than to explore, deepen, or change personal experience. It is as if they want to maintain a well-oiled machine and the massage therapist is seen as a technician or even a mechanic. Although this is a reasonable use for massage, people with an achieving rigid structure must, because of their pattern, see it as the only reason. Ironically, this particular structure of rigidity rejects any good feeling or pleasure that does not come from their own actions.

People living within the achieving rigid structure can work for the pleasure of a Ferrari, a sum of money, a large house, career advancement, or sex, but these pleasures are *symbolic*, rather than *embodied*. The satisfaction gained lies more in *obtaining* them and what they may represent, rather than *experiencing* them directly. For example, a person with an achieving rigid structure may gain great ego satisfaction and affirmation from being seen in a Ferrari, rather than experience joy and fun driving the car and enjoying its unique capabilities. The achievements may also provide an escape from anxiety and pain, rather than deep satisfaction. So although they may even appear hedonistic, people with this structure are actually afraid of and resistant to actual pleasure and relaxation.

Pride and shame drive the achieving rigid structure (Smith). They also seek pride through achievement and acquisition. The right car, right house, right spouse, and right family are pivotal to self-esteem. Anything less than the best is often a source of shame.

The driven quality of the person with an achieving rigid structure is connected to an overdeveloped ability to focus mentally, or "overfocus." They need to maintain this overfocused mental activity because it responds to an overly highly charged energy system in the body. The overfocus acts as a micromanager of the overcharge. If the energy does not have somewhere to go, it feeds anxiety. Without the overfocused activity, the driven energy would torment the person with this structure. If their armoring breaks down, this is indeed what happens, and then the discomfort and anxiety caused by the driven energy may cause them to seek therapy.

Consequently, people with an achieving rigid structure have a great investment in maintaining an overfocus—or as we might say in our terms, being over-grounded—at all costs and resist experiences that undermine this overfocus. For example, the idea of just "going with the flow" or "zoning out" might sound good to a massage therapist, but would be treated as highly threatening by a client with an achieving rigid structure. The idea of having a massage just to relax would have no appeal to such a client, which might seem confounding to a massage therapist who does not have this type of structure.

The phenomenon of the mental critic is crucial to understanding the rigid structure in general, but especially the achieving rigid structure. This is because of a strongly developed, sometimes even absolute, sense of what is right and wrong. The picture of what is *ideally* right and wrong is then used as an internalized template for criticizing themselves, others, and the world. People with an achieving rigid structure see this critical part of themselves as positive and carrying a high standard. They often also experience it, however, as extremely painful and debilitating because they can never satisfy this internal critic. The harshness of their internal critic then becomes the basis for similar treatment of others. We like to describe this internal mental critic as being a "perpetual motion misery machine." All it does is make the person miserable, never letting up. If the person comes close to satisfying a demand of the internal critic, then it raises the demand, diminishes the person's attempt, or switches to something else to criticize. The critic is never satisfied.

An additional factor is that the achieving rigid structure is overcharged, which fuels the drive to keep going and to achieve the goals set down by the critic. Analogously, the critic is the driver, the charge is the horse, and the body is the cart. Although people with an achieving rigid structure seem in control, they are actually *not* in control at all. *The critic and the high charge control the person.* Although they may seem decisive, they are not able to make choices for their lives outside the critic's tight strictures. The energy system fuels the capacity of the critic to impose unbending, impossible ideals and harsh judgments. The charge becomes *part of the survival mechanism* and therefore, *is not easily surrendered.* Massage therapy potentially presents an ambivalent situation for the achieving rigid structure because massage tends to reduce the overcharge and threatens the internal critic. The critic needs the energy supplied by the overcharged system to attempt to accomplish the goals imposed by the critic. If people with an achieving rigid structure are not perpetually striving for the goal, then there is no security for them. This explains the paradox presented by the achieving rigid structure: "*I want to relax, but I don't want to relax.*"

Emotional release can happen with someone with this structure, but it may be rare. The entire achieving rigid structure is defended against letting down and giving in. Having feelings may be experienced as "losing control" and therefore embarrassing and shameful, and may make people with this structure feel far too vulnerable (Keleman). Emotional release is most likely to happen with clients with an achieving rigid structure when life has dealt them a blow that they cannot solve by taking action or hardening up, such as a divorce or breakup, a death, the loss of a job, an accident, or a life-threatening or disabling disease.

Etiology

The achieving rigid structure develops during two different periods. The first is between 4 and 7 years old as the child begins to be related to the father as well as the mother. Other important events during this time are that socialization begins and children begin their schooling. The children must begin to increasingly shift their energies from play into goal-oriented activities. The parents emphasize achieving those goals and doing them well.

The predominant value in the family of origin is *function over feeling*. This may be explicitly stated through nostrums such as, "big boys don't cry," "don't be such a baby," "get over it," "keep your chin up," "straighten up and fly right," or it may be demonstrated through example by the parents (Keleman). In the family, certain behaviors related to achievement are rewarded, whereas other behaviors related to feeling and emotional expression are ignored or even punished. For example, expressions bidding for attention or requests for nonproductive toys or outings are ignored or discouraged. The emphasis on productivity differs in quality from what is seen with the compressed structure. The achieving rigid structure's productivity has a greater emphasis on idealism and attaining goals, in that the person must accomplish a certain status in life by accumulating money, honors, material "trophies," or fame or infamy, and that he or she does so with a driven quality.

The roots of this overgrounded overfocus comes from anxiety within the parents. The parents have the very legitimate goal of equipping the child to be successful. However, anxiety also is transmitted (usually nonverbally and unconsciously) to the child through emotion and through overdirecting the child. An example is the parents who schedule their child into "teaching and learning" situations from the time of early childhood. The child goes from lesson to lesson all day long with no time available to just "be" or do nothing. Relaxation or "unproductive play" is not valued. The body of the child loses the memory of the "doing-nothing" experience (if the child ever did have such an experience). Doing nothing becomes "bad" or "worthless."

The second period occurs in adolescence as the normal hormonal changes give an extra boost to the ability to be aggressive and assertive. The parents, while legitimately attempting to focus the teenager, may create a child who is actually very outward oriented, consumed with attaining approval through achievement. The child may feel that the parent's love is contingent on performance related to accomplishment (Smith).

As with early childhood, these adolescents may be overworked and overscheduled, for example, trying to develop an impressive list of achievements to get into the best schools and colleges. The adolescent must learn to bear the enormous pressure of the school's and parents' expectations for him or her to succeed. The adolescent wants to make the parents, school, and the community proud (Smith). Failure or even a less than stellar performance can cause anxiety and shame. He or she is striving to be "good enough," which may actually be a striving to be perfect (Smith). The young person may compensate for the shame by trying harder, working more, and rising above the shame. Shame and self-criticism, however, become fixed in the psyche of the adolescent at both conscious and unconscious levels.

Appearance

The rigid structure is overcharged. There is a fairly even charge throughout the body, except for a slightly higher charge in the top half and the back half of the body. This high level of charge "feeds" a high level of tension in the body. Despite the tension, people with achieving rigid structure learn often to adapt to the tension and become well coordinated in their movements. After all, the rigid structure that is driven for performance also is motivated to appear to be very functional. Consequently, people with this structure often appear to be a "together person," very functional, and not burdened with many problems.

The musculature in people with this type of rigid structure carries sufficient tone to be functional in the world. People in this structure have an awareness of the distinction between themselves and others that is centered in the body. At times, however, the armor pattern leads people with an achieving rigid structure to be overbounded.

The armoring found in people with an achieving rigid structure is knotty. The knots in the back of the neck in particular form patterns that keep the person perpetually upright, that is, alert, functional, and withheld emotionally. Metaphorically, the knots in the neck work to keep the head on top, which is symbolic of the premium placed on maintaining rationality above all else.

Knots form in two areas of the back in particular. The knots affect the shoulder girdle, which has the effect of holding back the arms and hands. This is related to the holding-back pattern referred to earlier (Keleman). It holds back or blocks expression, particularly aggressive movements such as reaching out, hitting, grasping, pushing, and pulling. The holding back pattern also diminishes breathing, since the muscles in the back affect the movement of the chest. The holding-back pattern also is expressed through a distinctive contraction of the muscles around the scapulae, such as the trapezius, and rhomboid.

The other area where knots appear involves the held-up pattern (Keleman). This occurs in the paraspinal muscles, particularly in the lower thoracic and lumbar regions, as described in the previous section. The knots in this pattern occur in the form of bunching, rather than small hard knots. They can take on a rod-like form and appearance. These rods act to hold the person up constantly without letup. In this held-up pattern, the rod-like holding helps brace the body and takes the place of well-grounded legs and feet in terms of balance. Although the person at first glance may appear well grounded in the lower body, a closer examination shows that this is an illusion. Because the rods in the back absorb the stress that the legs and feet should be absorbing, the person is really grounding him- or herself through the will. The person in the achieving rigid structure is actually overgrounded rather than well grounded (Figure 9.4).

As with the controlled rigid structure, the rods are part of a system of support in the back that are designed to tolerate pressure. Again, the held-up armoring forms a system of knots in which the individual is able literally to bear up under high pressure without buckling or noticeably showing any distress.

The chest with both the held-up and held-back patterns is tight, and respiration is less than what it could be. Although there is no difficulty inhaling, complete exhalation and the "letting go" that accompanies it do not take place. With the held-back pattern, some charge in the chest is present, but less than in the upper back. In contrast, the chests of those with the held-up pattern have a significantly lower charge as if the chest is dried out and starved of aliveness.

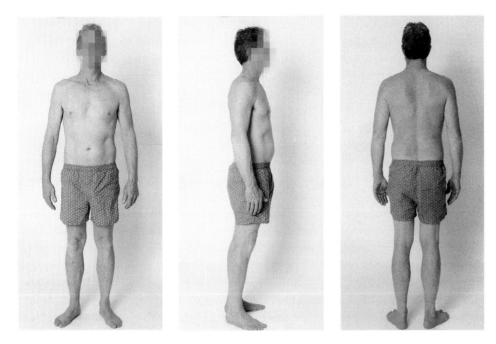

Figure 9.4
Achieving rigid structure. Front view: Note the uniform appearance of the body, and general tension. *Side view:* Body is tensed, prepared to act, and very upright (i.e., rigid). *Back view:* Note the held-back system of knots.

People in both patterns may have significant holding in the jaw and chin. Very often they have a determined-looking chin and jaw and, at times, a stiff upper lip. "Chin up," "taking it on the chin," and other expressions of determined attitude often seem to apply to the person with this structure (Johnson).

Therapeutic Strategy

The strategy for massage with a client with an achieving rigid structure should include dissolving the system of knots along the posterior half, especially along the back. The held-back and held-up areas should benefit from deeper work. The back half should be substantially softened before doing deeper work on the chest and abdominal areas. Teaching the client to let go through breathing while receiving deep tissue work can be very productive. The client should receive strong support for any deep relaxation or release of emotion, which may help to quiet the internal critic.

People with an achieving rigid structure may have one or both patterns of holding. In working with the knots, seeing what function the pattern of knots is performing is important. Working randomly can be effective from a purely physical point of view; however, from a holistic view it is not as effective as working with the pattern as a whole. If worked with "in pieces" the pattern can keep asserting itself, which then leads to less change and the client is less likely to become aware of the purpose that the tension is serving. This greater awareness can be very helpful to the client and can enhance the process.

Since *performance* is the key value for people with an achieving rigid structure, they prefer to see massage as enhancing or maintaining performance, thereby helping them to keep going. In fact, they may use it to help them maintain an extremely stressful schedule, rather than reducing stress by changing their schedule. Since performance is the highest goal, they must reject anything that interferes with performance. If massage appears to interfere with performance, they will eliminate it, too. For example, despite the benefits of massage, if they find that the massage appointment no longer fits their schedule, it is entirely possible that they will drop the massage rather than change the schedule. Or, on a smaller scale, they might say they cannot make it, ask you to change their time, and if you cannot do so, they may say they can do it.

In the list of priorities of a person with an achieving rigid structure, the job or the goal comes first. The massage therapist should not be surprised that massage may take a back seat. Often, when people with this structure are going through a life-changing event, the need for performance decreases, and during that time they are able to use massage at a deeper level. They are more emotionally open and therefore more able to take in the nurturing aspects of massage. However, the massage therapist should be aware that any changes that happen during this period could lead to a backlash later when the crisis is over.

Because you are not in the role of psychotherapist with the client, you are not in a position to intervene by working on the problem with them. However, this information is hoped to help you understand what is happening. Sometimes during this period of openness, clients with an achieving rigid structure may come up with all kinds of insights about themselves that is stimulated by the work on their body. They may be able to continue this flow of awareness, or the armoring may reconfigure and return the person to previous patterns. Depending on your relationship with them, you may be able to remind them of how much more alive or better they felt when they were working with their body at more than a maintenance level. However, the draw of performance is very strong, and although they may be able to acknowledge the correctness of what you are saying, they may continue to stay in a maintenance mode.

An example of how a massage therapist might encounter the mental critic of a person with an achieving rigid structure is what occurs during or after a session that seems to the massage therapist to be effective because a degree of release or relaxation took place. Instead of the expected positive response, clients with an achieving rigid structure have a reaction ranging from disinterest to disdain. If and when the client lashes out critically, it is frequently an externalization of his or her own critic. If you, as a massage therapist, have ever been stung in this way, the experience can give you an understanding and appreciation of the sort of pain that this person lives with in his or her own reality. It hurts to be constantly bashed and not be able to make it abate.

Despite the threatening aspects of massage, it can also be safe. Understanding the struggles of people with an achieving rigid structure to accept the nonstriving, nonachieving, simply "being," qualities of massage is important. They may feel safer with being able to rationalize the massage session as something that will improve them in some way and that meets some kind of goal. For example, they may frequently need to ask for "progress reports" from the massage therapist, as in the following case.

Rex

The attachment of the achieving rigid structure to rationality and the fear of pleasure may create surprising interactions for the massage therapist. Hiroshi had a standing appointment for several years with Rex, a client with an achieving rigid structure. Rex went to massage therapy to maintain his health and support his racquetball game. One day, however, during a massage, Rex burst into tears on the table. Rex did not talk about it during the session and left without saying anything.

Just before the next session, Rex canceled his session with Hiroshi. "Something has come up in business," Rex explained to Hiroshi. After several more cancellations, Rex informed Hiroshi that his schedule had become too busy for massage and he would not be able to come any more. Hiroshi was very surprised, thinking Rex' last session had been such a good one. "Why would Rex quit after such a good session?" Hiroshi wondered to himself.

Rex, as would likely be the case with a client with an achieving rigid structure, did not understand why he canceled and then quit. Somehow, in such a situation, rigid clients can explain to themselves in their own mind why massage is no longer important, essential, or a priority. You, as the massage therapist, are baffled. You may think you have done something wrong, despite feeling that you have done good work. You do not understand, after many massage sessions, why this individual who seemed to like your work so well no longer values the work. Although it may be that you cannot regain your client, knowing why the client has left may be important to you.

Whenever someone acts out of character, a reactionary or rebound effect often happens later. As illustrated by the example of Rex, expressing such open emotionality for this structure is out of character and actually quite threatening. Their defenses are constructed to keep such emotional outbursts under control. To cry on the table violates their emotional rules and leads to psychological inner recrimination later. What may seem to the therapist to be a positive event, for the client is an awful experience. To avoid being in such a situation again, the client may terminate massage therapy. This keeps the client in a safer position. Without any understanding of the situation, clients are unaware of their "real" reasons for terminating massage. They really believe they do not have the time, or whatever the excuse may be.

THE ENTERTAINING RIGID STRUCTURE

Psychological Dynamics

Like people with an achieving rigid structure, people with an *entertaining* rigid structure also have a performance-oriented pattern, but perform by being entertaining, personable, funny, artistic, dramatic, pleasing, outgoing, charismatic, or scintillating. They have "star power."

Along with being overcharged, the entertaining rigid structure is also undergrounded and underbounded. The undergrounded aspect is frequently part of the charm people with this structure have. The lack of grounding accompanies a strong relationship to fantasy and creativity that they can incorporate into their performing behavior. Such people also may seem spontaneous and unpredictable. However, the same undergrounding may lead them not to be able to depend on themselves because they can never "land on the ground" or sustain energy without "jumping around." Therefore, their undergrounding may make it difficult to make and keep commitments both to self and others, leading them to be perceived by others as flighty and "lightweight."

The underbounded aspect can also be charming, but disastrous. The lack of boundaries can also foster more fantasy and creativity, since people with an entertaining rigid structure do not have tightly formed mental constructs. People with this structure tend to think and perceive in an impressionistic fashion, which can be highly useful (Shapiro, 1965). However, being underbounded may make it exceedingly difficult for them to concentrate (Shapiro, 1965), because they often cannot think in more structured, factual, and logical ways. This is not an issue of intelligence, but of psychological defense.

The underboundedness of people with an entertaining rigid structure can also be highly confusing interpersonally. Such people tend to quickly relate to others in an emotional way. They "jump in with both feet." They seem to open up to the other person quickly and often to get the other person to open as well. The ordinary social boundaries and the time it takes to get to know someone seem to shrink around them. Just as quickly though, they can pull away from a seemingly close relationship.

Although their high charge, excitation, and underboundedness attract others, what might not be immediately evident is that the same qualities also keep people from getting too close emotionally to people with an entertaining rigid structure. They withdraw if someone wants to get too close. However, they do not retract their energy, as one would experience with people with a disembodied structure, but instead "disappear" by *shifting their attention*. They move away from a specific person, rather than withdraw into themselves, suddenly avoiding contact. For example, they may not return phone calls, may break dates, or visibly shift their attention to another person.

Such developments can be terribly confusing to the person on the other side of such a social transaction. The ability of people with an entertaining rigid structure to focus their highly charged attention onto the other person is also attractive. This can lead the other person to believe that the person with this structure wants to be closer, as if feeling pulled closer by their energy. The message seems to be "come here." If the other person follows the message and attempts to get closer, they may find the person with an entertaining rigid structure shifting away, that is, disappearing. Then the message seems to be "go away," and they feel pushed away. This pull-push or turn on-turn off pattern causes a lot of grief. The confusion is compounded because people with this structure tend to bring the kind of intensity present in romantic, sexual relationships and encounters to nearly all kinds of relationships.

The *coup de grace* in the social interaction happens when people with an entertaining rigid structure deny that they extended any kind of invitation or opening to become closer. This denial makes the person on the other end feel bad, perhaps foolish, or as if they imagined something. If the person with this structure were to say, "I got scared, so I needed some distance," the interaction would seem more understandable. However, the person tends to act as if nothing was going on, which is perplexing. He or she is more likely to say, "What are you talking about?"

The pull-push dynamic may lead the other party in the transaction to feel he or she has been "seduced." In this case, seduction can be emotional, sexual, or both. A hallmark of seduction is that something is offered, but then not really delivered, which differs from a change of mind or heart taking place in a relationship. The person who is seducing feels no need to care or offer an explanation about why his or her feelings have changed. The person may even deny offering a closer relationship in the first place.

The seduction is not based on a conscious intent to deceive the other person, but stems from deep confusion about feelings and expressing feelings. People with an entertaining rigid structure experience having to pull attention and love toward themselves by being entertaining, attractive, and charming. In other words, they have to seduce love toward themselves rather than expressing what they may be feeling, such as, "I want to get to know you better," "I like you," or "I'm interested in you." Because they cannot be direct, they must attract the other person toward them *without becoming vulnerable themselves.* Imagine what it would be like if you had to use magnetism instead of asking or reaching out directly to get emotional contact.

Seduction is ultimately about *power.* The ability to cause another person to be attracted to them becomes an act of power. While the common, popular view of seduction may be that it is about sex, *seduction is about the power of making another person do what you want them to do or feel what you want them to feel.* In the case of people with an entertaining rigid structure, they want the other person to be attracted to them, and they use whatever means they have at their disposal to do so. Because the attraction feels like love and power, it fills their emotional void within. The syndrome of seduction is like being addicted to emotional junk food. It feels good and is temporarily filling, but is not emotionally nutritious in the sense that it *satisfies a felt need,* often for intimacy. The person who is the seducer ultimately comes away emotionally hungry, dissatisfied, and needing another round.

People with an entertaining rigid structure appear to have ready access to their feelings and can be quite emotional. However, they may be completely cut off from deeper feelings. This paradoxical relationship to emotions can create difficulties for both the client and massage therapist. Remembering that the emotions that the client may be expressing are real is important. However, *these very real emotions serve as a defense against experiencing more threatening feelings. In essence, the defensive strategy of this structure is to use more superficial, less well-formed emotions as a way to preempt the emergence of more threatening, deeper feelings.* It is also important to understand that these defensive emotions may not appear or be experienced as superficial. (The term superficial is used here to refer to the defensive layering of emotions in the entertaining rigid structure.) Simply put, *the emotions are real, but they are defensive* (Shapiro, 1965). Therefore, the holding pattern is *held out* because they are keeping feelings at a surface level.

The defensive, undergrounded emotions prevent people with an entertaining rigid structure from truly knowing how they feel, despite their appearing to be extremely aware. Their emotions seem to be unanchored, fluid, and mercurial. The lack of contact with core feelings often leads them to feel a lack of identity or an unstable identity (Shapiro, 1965). This can often be seen in people with this structure as they "try-on" different personas through different clothing, enthusiasms, and fads.

The hyperexpressiveness sometimes combines with physical hyperflexibility in people with entertaining rigid structures, which can make them seem to embody perfectly the goals of some therapies to be loose and in touch with emotions. Indeed, at first glance, they may seem to have very little tension. However, their *inner* experience is very different. They constantly *feel* very tense, and no matter how much they stretch, they cannot rid themselves of the tension. It is as if they are caught in a flexible onion bag or string bag in which they can stretch almost infinitely, but never quite break through.

The person with an entertaining rigid structure must maintain a high charge of energy to avoid what is underneath all the excitement—a layer of deadness and depression. The "dead layer" feels numbed and paralyzed to them, the antithesis of all the excitement at the surface. When they begin to contact this layer, they begin to experience intense boredom, which they fear. Part of the intensity of the fear is due to the belief that this layer is "all there is" to them. They have no idea that there may be another source of energy deep inside them that is neither overly charged nor deadened. If given the choice between the boring dead layer and the excited hyperexpressive layer, they choose excitement. This explains how the high level of excitement within them is a defense against the dead layer. For people with an entertaining rigid structure, to be deadened *is* deadly.

Because people with an entertaining rigid structure fear a lower charge, they also fear and avoid rest and relaxation. Any activity, including work, socializing, creative pursuits, romance, family life, sports, play, *and massage therapy*, might be an occasion for being driven to be productive (Shapiro, 2000). As a result, one often sees people with this structure going and going to the point of exhaustion, and then collapsing. They do not get tired, but *exhaust* themselves. This is the only acceptable way they can rest because their collapse appears to be compelled, rather than by choice. This exhausted collapse may also take the form of illness.

The entertaining rigid structure also is a form of energy management. People with this structure often experience moderate to high amounts of anxiety (Lowen, 1971). They may unconsciously manage the anxiety by finding a new and more interesting activity, such as switching jobs or career, finding a new relationship, a new creative outlet, a new spiritual path, and so on. Switching objects of attention lowers anxiety and also prevents contact with deeper, more threatening feelings. The saying, "A rolling stone gathers no moss," fits them well.

Etiology

One of the origins of the need to maintain a high charge comes from the person's role within the family. Love, approval, and attention came to them through the capacity to excite, stimulate, and entertain family members. As a result, people with an entertaining rigid structure may believe (usually unconsciously) that their ability to be charming or talented is their only way to get love. If they are not "on," then they may begin to anticipate and fear a loss of love and approval. This happens anytime that their high energy begins to diminish. They associate a lowering of energy with a diminishment of their capacity to perform, which in turn is associated with a loss of ability to get the psychoemotional "goodies." Therefore, not being able to perform *and* having a lower level of charge are threatening.

People with an entertaining rigid structure are brought up in environments in which the parents are uncomfortable with expressing feelings. This is not to say that the parents do not care, but they do not *express* feelings like affection, warmth, and caring or feel comfortable with expressing such feelings (Keleman). The experience within the family is not one of intimacy and true interchange of feeling. To contend with the situation, the child may learn to draw out the parents by being cute, entertaining, or charming. Although being charming is something most children do naturally to some extent, the difference in the case of people with an entertaining rigid structure is that this becomes the *primary* mode of relating.

Furthermore, the entertaining rigid structure pattern is reinforced as the parents respond primarily to the child's charm, rather than to their own feelings. Therefore, such children effectively learn that they will not get the reaction they crave *without* using that behavior. At the same time, these children are also developing or have developed a discomfort with intimacy that is similar to that of their parents. As a result, people with an entertaining rigid structure as adults act out this pattern in which they are energized or emotionally fed by being able to cause another person to be attracted to them, but they become anxious if the person becomes too close or expresses "real" feeling. Love is what they are really craving, and they think they are getting it, but are not. In other words, *they have mistaken the energy of attraction for love.*

People with this structure also have other confused emotions, including sexuality. Since feelings in general are repressed within the family, sexuality is not well accepted either, especially when the child reaches adolescence. If the parents are uncomfortable with expressions of affection and sexuality, they cannot teach their child healthy attitudes regarding touch, affection, love, and sexuality. When feelings are not well understood or appreciated, being confused or engulfed by another kind of feeling becomes easier. For example, differentiating pure sexual attraction from feelings such as love, caring, delight, enjoyment, appreciation, and many others becomes difficult, and one feeling can be confused for the other. Fear of one particular feeling leads eventually to the pushing down of *all* feelings, including those that would have allowed healthy closeness and nonsexual intimacy. Parental emotional confusion leaves them without a means to share loving feelings and a means for the child to learn them. Instead, the parents unwittingly teach emotional confusion to the child (Lowen, 1971).

If sensual touching and sexual touching become confused, then touching in general becomes unacceptable. In turn, the child ends up not knowing how to deal with sexual energy and has difficulty differentiating between having a feeling and acting on the feeling, that is, differentiating *feelings versus actions*. The person becomes vulnerable to accepting or giving sexual advances because he or she may have misinterpreted such behaviors to be the love and confirmation that he or she lacked at home.

A further complication is that any attraction that the parents feel toward the child becomes tinged with forbidden sexuality. If the parents cannot handle this, they respond by cutting off their feelings even more. The message the child learns is that his or her sexuality caused him/her to be rejected; that is, it is the child's fault. Once the child's own sexuality becomes a threat, then he or she must defend against these feelings and disown them.

Appearance

The entertaining rigid structure is distinguished by mesh armoring, which we introduced in Chapter 7. Mesh armoring is constituted by a high charge at the surface of the body that is so high that it may feel "buzzy" to the touch. That is, with some training and practice, one can sense a highly modulated sensation or vibration when touching mesh armoring. Mesh armoring also is characterized by excessive heat on the surface of the skin.

The high charge of excitement associated with mesh armoring serves two purposes. It distracts mesh-armored people away from the deadness, sadness, and depression that they might feel underneath in response to not really connecting emotionally within their family of origin. It also sustains the excitement and attractiveness to others that has become their only way to feel emotionally alive (and block the deadness). They fear losing this high charge, but this is *exactly* what must happen for them to relax and feel themselves (i.e., be in contact with their core) more deeply.

Visually, clients with this structure tend to have a fairly well-proportioned physical structure, as most rigid types have. They also tend to have a system of knots, but the characteristic mesh predominates. Mesh armor cannot be seen, but only felt through touch. They may seem restless or frenetic, constantly on the move, speak rapidly and in a staccato manner, or they may use an enormous amount of range and flexibility of subject matter when speaking. They are likely to be physically flexible, even hyperflexible, as well.

Therapeutic Strategy

Just as society rewards rigid people who achieve, so are the people with an entertaining rigid structure rewarded by society for their performing. The massage therapist needs to be aware of the ability of a client with this structure to charm. This "energetic sleight of hand" may divert or deflect the massage therapist's attention away from serious physical problems or patterns. For example, they may have the massage therapist rolling on the floor with laughter about all the stressful misadventures that they have encountered. This keeps the massage therapist from questioning how the stressful behavior contributed to the condition of their body.

The diversion from what is taking place on a deeper level to the more superficial aspects is, in a way, acting out the energetic situation of clients with an entertaining rigid structure. Just as they prefer to stay at the surface of their bodies, they need to stay at the surface of their lives and how they live (Shapiro, 1965). This is not to say that people with this structure seem superficial or trivial. To the contrary, they may share rather profound experiences and insights. However, the distinction is that while they are authentic, they are not connected to their core. *The diversion from core connection is the problem* for people with this structure. The importance of this realization to the therapist is that it may be hard to create real change if the diversion consistently throws the therapist off, and the therapist does not realize that stress and anxiety may be lurking underneath the surface.

This situation has a potential for countertransference. The client may be living in a way that the massage therapist wishes she could, making things "look easy," thus keeping the massage therapist from seeing the stress involved in maintaining this structure and its living style.

Because of their hyperawareness, clients with an entertaining rigid structure may give the therapist voluminous feedback about many different parts of their body, and descriptions of their bodily sensations can be relatively detailed. This may cause the therapist to be drawn to work on many different areas seemingly all at once. In a sense, when working with a client with this structure, the therapist can be drawn into "chasing" the tension all over the body. Supplied with a much richer stream of feedback than usual, the therapist can become very engaged in the hunt, which stimulates the client's hyperawareness or vigilance even more. The chase can then become even more exciting for both the client and therapist.

The key to deep relaxation, however, is *not* to chase the tension, but to use sustained touch, or what we term *still-handed touch*, by which the therapist places the hands on one area of the client's body and, without moving the hands, sustains the touch for several minutes. The therapist uses the entire palmar surface of the hand in this structured touch (Figure 9.5). The stillness of the hands enables the client to feel supported without having to "watch" or to produce or perform anything for anyone else. The still-handed touch also discharges the high energy charge in that part of the body. Movement of the hands would reinforce the hypervigilant state because the client tends to be constantly aware of where the massage therapist's hands are going while simultaneously internally second-guessing the expectations of the therapist. The client—and often the therapist—is not aware that this is what is happening. As a result, they unconsciously and unwittingly collude to maintain a heightened state of vigilance (within the client) and what appears to be awareness ends up masking the defensive quality of the hypervigilance. This phenomenon is significant because it blocks a therapeutic pathway to affect a core aspect of the armoring, which is the tendency for feelings to remain superficial. An analogy would be an airplane that constantly circles the airport, but never lands.

Discharging the energy with a technique like still-handed touch allows such clients to feel themselves at a deeper and more diffuse level. A diffuse level means in this context a mode of awareness that is not sharply focused, which allows one to experience internally images, insights, sensations, and memories that a sharp focus excludes. Such clients deeply need to make this kind of contact with themselves.

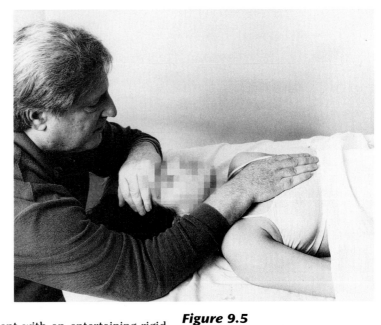

Figure 9.5
Technique of still-handed touch as applied to entertaining rigid type.
Still-handed touch involves placing the hands on one area of the client's body and, without moving the hands, sustaining the touch for several minutes. The therapist uses the entire palmar surface of the hand in this type of touch. (Standard draping procedures were not used in this photo so that the placement of the therapist's hands would be visible.)

A useful place to use still-handed touch on a client with an entertaining rigid structure is on the scapulae, with the client in either a supine or prone position (this was depicted in Figure 6.3). The high charge of energy in the upper back maintains the client's overly active mind and body. As this area becomes less charged, the client is more able to experience his or her body and psyche in a way that the high charge had been screening. Another area on which to use still-handed touch is the forehead. In this case, adding some pressure to the still-handed touch helps the client let go of the incessant mental chatter and commentary going on in the mind. The pressure should not be painful, but done to the point at which it feels good to the client. The pressure should be applied slowly with an open, full hand. Sometimes, the therapist can also use still-handed touch on the belly, if this is not too threatening to the client, while touching the forehead. The mind often interferes with gut feelings and intuitions, so this touching on the belly helps create more open awareness within the head and allows fuller feeling in the body as a whole (Figure 9.6).

The client may sometimes resist still-handed touch, which will manifest in feelings of restlessness and boredom. If the therapist can sustain the touch long enough, the client passes through this phase into a deeper state of relaxation. The feeling of wanting the therapist to "do something" is a feeling that the client constantly has regarding him- or herself. Activity and survival are unconsciously synonymous for people with this structure. For this precise reason, the client may initially tend to feel uncomfortable with the still-handed touch. If simply sustaining the touch for a longer time does not work, then this may indicate the client is still too defended. In this case, the therapist can go back to a more active way of working and try still-handed touch again later.

Still-handed touch, which we also term *nurturing touch*, could conceivably be used for an entire hour, but is usually used in the beginning portion of a session for 5 or 10 minutes. Although still-handed touch may appear similar to certain subtle energy work techniques, it is not. Still-handed touch is not used to move energy in the body. It provides a sense of security that diminishes the hypervigilant high charge. This allows the client to feel and experience the deeper flow of endodermal energy that is already present within, but unfelt. Generally, massage often becomes more effective after the high charge is drawn down. Techniques to soften any tense area can then be used more effectively.

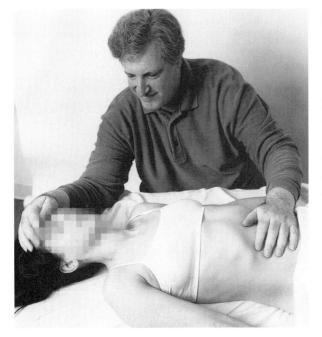

Figure 9.6
Technique of still-handed touch on belly and forehead. The therapist can also use still-handed touch on the belly while touching the forehead. The mind often interferes with gut feelings and intuitions, so this touching on the belly helps create a more open space for a different kind of awareness. (Standard draping procedures were not used in this photo so that the placement of the therapist's hands would be visible.)

THE ROMANTIC RIGID STRUCTURE

Psychological Dynamics

People with a *romantic* rigid structure also have the characteristics of being achieving and entertaining, but the structure's main defense involves sexuality. In comparison, although people with an entertaining rigid structure are unconsciously seductive, *people with a romantic rigid structure are consciously and deliberately seductive.* Also, the focus of the entertaining rigid structure is primarily on attraction, but the romantic rigid structure's focus is specifically on romantic and erotic attraction. For people with this structure, sex and romance are very important—sometimes the most important—aspects of their lives. Imagine what it was like at some point in your life to be preoccupied with romance and sex, despite whether there was any actual sexual activity involved. For most people who do not have this structure, this preoccupation was much greater at some times than others. However, for people with a romantic rigid structure, this preoccupation is almost constant.

This is evident in their seeing the world through romantic and sexual fantasy lenses, which is built into their thought process (Shapiro, 1965). The entire sexualized romantic fantasy is about giving into impulse, losing boundaries, and merging with the other person in a fantasized way. This also reveals why people with a romantic rigid structure have a held-back pattern. They feel tremendous conflict between holding back and giving in. The fantasy aspect of the romantic feelings keeps feelings at the surface. This is the *held-out* aspect of the romantic rigid.

The central motivating principle for people with a romantic rigid structure is whether or not they are attractive in a sexual and romantic way. While everyone to some extent "reads" signals from other people, the people with this structure almost always read signals about sex and romance rather than other signals. For them, the world is divided distinctly into two groups: those who are desirable and those who are not. This means that the person who is considered desirable witnesses a different form of behavior from them than the person who is considered undesirable. Their seductiveness may be directed intensely at the desired person, or set simply like a net, waiting for anyone desirable to fall into it. In this sense, they may present somewhat different "faces" to the therapist, depending on whether or not they are attracted.

We would like to clearly distinguish potential clients with a romantic rigid structure from people who believe that massage is a form of prostitution and therefore seek out massage solely for sexual gratification. People with a romantic rigid structure *do not* go for massage with an intention to seduce the massage therapist. However, since their self-image depends on their sexual attractiveness, they may be seductive toward the therapist. The difference tends to be that the person with a romantic rigid structure is not relating to the therapist as a sex object, but rather as someone with whom they want to be "involved."

People with a romantic rigid structure *are* seeking relationship, but they can do so only within romanticized or sexualized contexts. Even sexual conquests are a form of relationship for them, though not a healthy one. Relationships for them can take all kinds of forms. However, they do not sustain these relationships. The romantic rigid structure shares with the entertaining rigid a tendency to and a fear of boredom. They do not realize that the boredom they fear lies within themselves and not within the other person, nor is it the other person's responsibility. Like people with an entertaining rigid structure, people with a romantic rigid structure must maintain a high charge within themselves, but must do so through romance and sexuality. Continuous relationships provide the charge they need to stave off boredom. If people with a romantic rigid structure are engaged in a pattern of sexual conquest, they may need to make many short conquests to stave off deadness and depression (Lowen, 1975).

If people with a romantic rigid structure have a more romantic bent, they may take a longer time to seduce someone who is seemingly unavailable, only to drop them shortly after the other person has fallen for them (Johnson). A more pernicious form of this sort of conquest is a triangulation in which the person with a romantic rigid structure seeks to win a romantic target away from someone else. This form of romantic "game" repeats the early situation of their childhood in which they attempted to win the parent of the opposite gender away from the parent of the same gender. The object of the game is to be more sexually powerful, and the twist is that the more the "loser" feels (e.g., hurt, angry, betrayed), the more valuable the person with a romantic rigid structure feels.

People with a romantic rigid structure believe they are seeking fulfillment, but they are actually seeking gratification. The gratification does not satisfy a deeper and more unconscious hunger for a genuine connection with themselves and with another person. Essentially, they do not really know how to connect with another person in an intimate way. Sex and romance substitute for intimacy with both self and others.

One final issue concerning people with this structure merits discussion because of its gravity. The sexualizing of all relationships may, in this case, be a cry to pay attention to severe emotional wounding, and *possibly* sexual abuse. Often, people who have been abused feel that sex is the only way they can get or express love, because through their abuse they have been taught that this is an appropriate way to get love and affection. Another effect of sexual abuse can be that the abused child's sexuality is awakened prematurely and can lead to a need to repeat this kind of contact. Note that *not all individuals who have been sexually abused act out sexually*. Such abuse does, however, lead the person to view the world through a sexual lens. In some cases, this may stem from sexual fears that trigger avoidance of intimate contact, and in others it may stem from being confirmed as lovable and attractive and stimulates seeking contact. Note also that *only some people with a romantic rigid structure have been sexually abused*. However, sexual confusion has certainly existed in their environment.

Etiology

People who have developed a romantic rigid structure have not been able to complete a matrix of development occurring within two distinct periods in the maturing process. The first period occurs between ages 3 and 7, during which the child begins to relate to the wider world and socialization is begun through school (Lowen, 1980). The second period is puberty, when the hormonal surge causes the child to relate more to others in a romantic and sexual way. Whether the child lives in a traditional family in which there is a mother and father present, or in other types of families, such as single parent/same gender, family, a blended family with a stepparent, or a family with two parents of the same gender, the child goes through a process driven by both the psyche and biology to establish a relationship with a caregiver of the opposite gender.

The attempt to establish a close relationship may be accompanied by the rejection of and competition with the caregiver of the same gender. Who has not known some 4-year-old boy who has declared that he will "marry Mommy" when he grows up or a 6-year-old who is "Daddy's little girl?" This early period may be seen as a normal practice period for romantic relationships that develop later. In healthy families, the parents understand this period and make it safe for the child to experience it. They do not take advantage of the child's naïve adoration of the opposite gender caregiver or the rivalry between themselves to play out their differences with their life partner (Lowen, 1980). The naïve romance of the child for the parent disappears at about 7 years and reappears just before puberty in another form (Lowen, 1980).

In the adolescent incarnation, there is occasionally less emphasis on the connection to the parent of the opposite gender and more on the conflict with the parent of the same gender. During this time, the child seeks to have his or her masculinity or femininity accepted and affirmed by the caregiver of the opposite gender. In the case of a girl, this would mean that while a father notices his daughter's sexual development, he stays present to her and does not withdraw out of fear. In a healthy family, he creates a protective environment to help her ground her own feminine attributes and also to help her face and understand the world of men. An example of this would be a father who tells his daughter how very pretty she is and also how to take care of herself around unwanted advances from men *without* making her fearful of men in general. In the case of a boy, the mother may affirm his developing masculinity by supporting his growing independence and decision-making capabilities within the context of firm limits and boundaries. She welcomes his relationships with girls and supports this by her own letting go of being the "main woman" in his life.

In the family of a person with a romantic rigid structure, an inordinate emphasis—positive *or* negative—is made on sexuality and sometimes on gender roles. Depending on the upbringing and character structure of the caregivers, the emphasis on sexuality and gender can begin at birth and extend throughout the development of the child (Cornell and Ludwig). Excessive, intrusive verbal emphasis can be placed on the child's primary and secondary sex characteristics through jokes and remarks or, more repressively, make sure the child knows that those parts of the body are "bad" or "dirty" (Lowen, 1980).

Sometimes, a child becomes a favorite of the parent of the opposite gender, while the spouse is denigrated or unappreciated. In effect, this makes the child a "substitute spouse," who fills the emotional needs of the parent and becomes the recipient of that parent's special affection. Even though no overt sexual abuse may occur, the relationship often carries a romantic charge.

The parent of the opposite gender might become scared by the sexual development of the child and emotionally and physically withdraw. As a result, the parent may no longer hug the child closely or walk with his or her arm around the child. When the parent withdraws out of fear, it is done often with no explanation. The child ends up feeling very rejected and blames him- or herself for wanting and needing the parent's love. The child may feel rejected for wanting any sort of relationship. However, the adolescent child still needs relationship and may turn to romantic and sexual liaisons with peers in an excessive and dependent fashion.

Another scenario is that the parent of the opposite gender may be emotionally or physically absent. As with the withdrawing parent, as such children move into puberty, they discover that their sexuality may be a way to gain the affection that has been missing or withdrawn by the parent of the opposite gender. Finally, cases of abuse in which actual sexual contact has taken place may lead to this structure forming.

Appearance

The armoring pattern of the romantic rigid structure is knotty with some mesh armor mixed in sometimes. People with this structure are more likely to be held back, rather than held up. A high charge in the upper back and a strong contraction between the scapulae are found often. Like most rigid structures, the romantic rigid structure is overcharged. As the charge of the person in the entertaining rigid structure manifests in performing, the romantic rigid structure's charge manifests in being overtly or covertly seductive in a romantic and sexual way (Lowen, 1971). In other words, the charge is related to and directed at romance and sexuality.

People with a romantic rigid structure are also undergrounded. The feet of people with this structure do not appear to be on the ground. Their primary orientation is to be in a romantic or sexual relationship and like to be "walking on air." Although this structure is considered to be overcharged, the feet and legs are undercharged. The direction of energy flow in the body appears to be upward. In addition, the pelvis is "cocked back" in an anterior tilt—like a pistol that has not fired. This holding pattern supports the entire body being overcharged.

Underbounding is also found in people with a romantic rigid structure. Again, *relationship* is a primary desire, so they maintain low boundaries in order to connect easily. The chest may be slightly deflated and appear to be undernourished. Even if the muscles have been built up with weight training, the undernourishment can be identified through the lowered energy in the chest. Despite the undernourishment, the chest is hard, guarding their heart and their softer feelings (Lowen, 1971). This combination of underboundedness and hardness in the chest creates a conflict about closeness for people with a romantic rigid structure as they constantly seek love and relationship, but cannot feel it once it is available.

An energetic break is often found around the diaphragm, leaving the impression of a split between the upper and lower halves of the body. The neck is held stiffly, with a large amount of tension at the occipital ridge, creating another energetic break (Lowen, 1971). The holding at the base of the skull also connects with holding in the scalenes and the jaw. This body pattern is often expressed psychologically as the person being unable to bring his or her head, heart, and pelvis together.

A notable holding pattern that occurs in the romantic rigid structure is a mask-like pattern similar to the mask worn by the film and television character Zorro; that is, it is a band that covers the eyes from mid-forehead to mid-nose. This holding pattern can manifest as headaches, particularly at the temples and the forehead, and also as a sensation of dissociation. People with a romantic rigid structure display a range of emotional states through their eyes, ranging from dullness, deadness, and absence when they are more dissociated, to high intensity and seductiveness when they are trying to connect with someone as a romantic partner (Lowen, 1971).

Women with a romantic rigid structure have distinctive movement patterns associated with flirtation (Lowen, 1971). They appear restless and sometimes cannot sit still, but the movement pattern often has some sort of twisting involved. One can often see women with this structure sitting so that the upper body twists one way and the lower body in the opposite direction. A stance one can see frequently is with the hip cocked in one direction and the hand on the opposite hip, with the weight on the leg on the side of the cocked hip. Women with this structure often find it difficult to stand with their weight evenly distributed on both feet. They often feel uncomfortable standing on both feet and end up shifting their weight between their feet several times while standing.

Therapeutic Strategy

People with a romantic rigid structure may manifest sexualizing behavior in the setting of massage therapy in two ways. One is that they may be directly and overtly sexually seductive. Direct sexual seduction may consist of inappropriately touching the therapist, sexualized language, inappropriate sexually suggestive movement and sounds, or attempts to direct the therapist to make touch sexually stimulating. This differs from being involuntarily aroused, such as having an erection that is unintended. Someone who is involuntarily aroused is not likely to try to intensify and extend the arousal or to take it as a prompt to become more sexually aggressive.

The other manifestation is that they act out the seductiveness *in the relationship*, rather than on the table. This response is more likely from clients with a rigid romantic structure. Rather than seeking immediate sexual gratification during the session, they attempt to seduce the therapist into a romantic relationship or at least the possibility of one. Their pattern does not always include an intent to engage in sexual activity. In some cases, the pattern involves mainly the seduction, but it also includes a fear of actual sexual activity. The emphasis is often to get the other person seduced, rather than to have sex with them. To make the distinction clearer, the following is an example of how a dialogue might be in each case.

Dialogues with a Client with a Romantic Rigid Structure

This dialogue involves a client who is simply attracted to the therapist. This is Jennifer's third session with her therapist, Sam.

Jennifer arrives for sessions dressed in her business clothing. As with nearly everyone who is in a state of undress in the presence of someone of the opposite gender, she has been modest about dressing and undressing and maintaining the draping. Until this point, Jennifer has not asked Sam any personal questions, nor has she made any personal comments about him. Jennifer is lying on the table while Sam is working on her feet.

Jennifer: Do most massage therapists hang their diplomas on the wall? My last massage therapist didn't, but you do.

Sam: I think it's important to display your credentials. It's something that I think is professional.

Jennifer: Have you always practiced here in town?

Sam: No, I moved here from Florida about 5 years ago.

Jennifer: Did you move here by yourself?

Sam: Yeah, during a semester break from massage school I visited some friends here and thought this might be a good place to start a practice.

Jennifer: Your office is in such a great neighborhood. I don't have to go very far to get here. Do you live near here?

Dialogues with a Client with a Romantic Rigid Structure

Sam: Uh-huh, about 5 or 10 minutes from here. I don't like to commute much and you're right, this is a nice area.

Jennifer: Oh, are you in one of those townhouses by the park?

Sam: Yup, I really like it there.

Jennifer: They're kind of expensive for one person. Do you have a family or do you have roommates?

Sam: Roommates.

Jennifer: Do you use the park much?

Sam: I use the tennis courts a lot. They're really well maintained.

Jennifer: Oh, really? I play tennis, too. I thought you might, I saw your racket in the closet in the waiting room.

Sam: That's right. Sometimes I play after work.

Jennifer: I play after work, too, usually around 7. Maybe we could play sometime?

Sam: I'd like to, but I've found that as a massage therapist it's important to not see clients socially. I mean, if I'm working with someone, I don't do things with them outside of the office. Do you understand what I mean?

Jennifer: Sort of . . . I'm not sure.

Sam: What don't you understand?

Jennifer: Well, it's just tennis.

Sam: First, if I offended you or put you off, I didn't mean to do that. It's just that the massage therapy relationship is special. I'm working with your body, but I'm also paying attention to the connections between your mind and your feelings and your body. That means I need to focus on *your* needs and create a safe space for you to experience them. Even if you just feel more relaxed in your shoulders after the massage, I still need to make that safe space for you in case you need it. That focus doesn't change when we walk out this door. That's why I don't socialize with clients.

Jennifer: Well, what's mixing me up is it seems you're saying we can't even be friendly with each other, like if I see you on the street I have to ignore you?

Sam: No, I'm not saying that. I am saying that making social arrangements, like playing tennis, having lunch, or going to the movies changes the focus of the relationship. Then you begin to think about me and my life and my needs, just like you would any other acquaintance, even if it's casual. That can pull away from your concentration on your own experience when we do massage. If I see you on the street, I'll be glad to see you. And it's okay for us to be friendly with each other. I want all my clients to feel comfortable and feel welcome. It's just that I have a professional obligation to my clients to keep my professional life and my social life separate.

Jennifer: Well, I don't quite understand it, but I trust you and it seems okay.

Sam: I'm glad you trust me and we can always talk more about this if you need to.

In this sample dialogue, Jennifer is simply attracted to her massage therapist. She is not sexualizing the situation and is reasonably open to an explanation of the situation. In this case, being sensitive to the possibility of the client feeling shamed or rejected is important. However, with a sexualizing client, a somewhat different approach is called for.

Dialogues with a Client with a Romantic Rigid Structure

The next dialogue takes place during the third session, with Warren as the sexualizing client and Lucy as the therapist.

Warren: That's a great blouse you're wearing. Is it new?

Lucy: No, it's just a polo shirt, the same kind I wear all the time to the office. Nothing special.

Warren: Well, it really looks different . . . wonderful. Maybe it's you. Have you been working out?

Lucy: Well, I've been working out for several years, so I haven't been doing anything special lately that would make me look all that different.

Warren: Well, I gotta tell you that you do look good, but I'll bet you hear that all the time.

Lucy: Thanks, but not really.

Warren: Well, then you've been neglected. Sounds like Mr. Lucy can't see what he's got.

Lucy: Well there really isn't a Mr. Lucy.

Warren: I can't believe it. Someone like you? No boyfriend?

Lucy: Uh-uh.

Warren: Hard to believe! Oh, be sure not to forget to work on my left shoulder too. I pulled it out swing dancing.

Lucy: Hmm, swing dancing! That's pretty 'in' these days. It's even getting play on MTV. I can sure see how you could pull something though. There are a lot of throws involved.

Warren: Yeah. I love it though. I like dance styles where I can touch my partner. I bet you're a great slow dancer. You have a wonderful touch.

Lucy: Right and I have two left feet.

Warren: I'll bet I could teach you in one night how to get those feet going together.

Lucy: I don't think so. This has been going on since I was a kid. I'm hopeless.

Warren: I'll bet you aren't. Someone as in touch with her body as you are probably just *believes* she can't. You need a good leader.

Lucy: Maybe. Is that sore there?

Warren: Mmm. Ummm. Yes. But such nice hands. They make me feel better. You know, you have a great grip. I'll bet it would feel great to have you hold onto me while I spin you around the floor.

Lucy: Don 't be so sure.

Warren: Oh, come on. Let's give it a try. I know you'd love it. I know you'd loooove dancing with me. You know every inch of my body. Of course, you'd be able to follow my lead perfectly.

Lucy: Warren, I don't think so. I don't see any of my clients socially. I can't.

Warren: Oh, come on Lucy. It's just a little dancing. Besides, aren't I an exception? I won't bite you.

Lucy: I know that. But whether or not we would have a good time isn't the point. I don't see any of my clients socially because when I work with people I feel I have an obligation to have my focus on their needs. If I get involved socially with someone, it obviously can't be like that.

Dialogues with a Client with a Romantic Rigid Structure

Warren: Dancing with me would be focusing on my needs. Come on, Lucy, what harm can a little dancing do? After all, rules are made to be broken . . . especially when you and I could have such a good time together.

Lucy: I'm sure we would have a good time. But that's not the point either.

Warren: So what *is* the point? Don't you like me? If we like each other, why is it wrong to have some fun?

Lucy: I like you, but in the way a therapist has a positive regard for a client. As I said, my policy is I do not get involved socially with any of my clients. I realize this might not be making much sense to you right now, but my not socializing with any of my clients creates a kind of environment in which they're free to experience what they need to during their massage without worrying about how it might affect me or the therapeutic relationship. The focus of the massage is entirely on you and your needs and you don't have to think about my needs or taking care of me like you would in a friendship . . . and especially a dating relationship.

Warren: But what do you mean I'm free to experience? You just told me I'm not allowed to like you! Isn't liking you part of my experience?

Lucy: Of course you're allowed to like me. It also means not following through on it socially . . . like dating or going dancing.

Warren: Mmm . . . well, okay, I don't completely get it, but I guess that's the way you feel.

Lucy: Yes, it is. Thanks. We can always talk more about this if you need to. Now, back to your shoulder!

Letting this kind of client know that your boundary applies to everyone, has no exceptions, and is absolutely inviolable is very important. If the massage therapist does not close the door completely, the defenses of clients with a romantic rigid structure will compel them to squeeze through that door one way or another. Closing this door firmly may be difficult if the therapist also has an attraction to this client. However, *it is absolutely essential that the therapist clearly closes the door*. Not doing so prolongs the client's fantasy of winning the massage therapist over into a romantic or sexual relationship, and the client will continue flirtatious or seductive behavior. On top of this, not closing the door may be interpreted as a seductive signal to keep trying. As a result, the client cannot focus on relaxing, which is the work at hand. By eliminating this defensive route, the massage therapist can allow something else to happen for that client.

This may be an uncomfortable interaction for the massage therapist, as well as the client. In an effort to "save" or protect the client's feelings, the therapist may have a tendency to leave the door open for a possible future social interaction. For example, the therapist may be reluctant to appear to be rejecting, so he or she will avoid establishing a clear boundary. Such interactions are fertile ground for countertransference issues (discussed in Chapter 3). Uncomfortable feelings are not a sign of weakness nor is making clear boundaries a sign of toughness; however, these kinds of reactions *can* be signs there are issues that the therapist needs to examine.

Another way to leave the door open is to make statements that can be construed as indefinite enough to be indirectly inviting further probing, as if the therapist is saying, "I cannot say yes, but I would like to if only you can get me to overcome my ethics." For example, "We can have feelings, but we cannot follow through on them," implies that the massage therapist does have feelings for the client, but is forbidden to act on them. This may be true, but the client with this structure interprets this as meaning that the right person could break down the therapist's barrier. Of course, this client believes that he or she *is* that person. In addition, the forbidden quality of the interaction can make it all the more attractive and may spur the client to even greater efforts.

Another pattern expressed by people with romantic rigid structures is more directly concerned with getting sexual contact, than with establishing a relationship with the therapist. This kind of sexualizing begins very early, most likely even in the first session. This type of client with a romantic rigid structure experiences almost all bodily sensations as sexual feelings. They are prone to interpret and experience most touch as sexual. A very important characteristic is that their sexualizing of touch and bodily sensation is unconscious, meaning that in most cases they do not have a premeditated goal of getting sexual contact from the massage.

This behavior manifests as genitally centered excitement, which may lead to various outcomes. To be clear, this refers to a person who has a spontaneous erection or another similar physical response triggered by *psychological* factors and *not* to responses triggered by physiological and physical factors. One outcome is that the person may be uncomfortable with the physical response and try to endure it while it is happening. The other is the person may experience the excitement as an inducement to seek sexual contact or just greater excitation. However, it is not planned.

In either case, the therapist's approach can be the same. The approach is to *encourage these clients to experience the sensations of the massage throughout their entire body or in other parts of their body so that they do not focus the sensations on and in the genitals.* Moving away from the torso, to the periphery of the body—hands, feet, and head—and encouraging the client to allow feeling these other parts of the body can be effective. If a nonverbal approach is not effective, then the therapist may say directly to the client that focusing on sexual sensations is at cross purposes with massage therapy because sexualizing the treatment requires excitation rather than relaxation. In addition, the therapist cannot allow the behavior because it is clearly against legal and professional codes. If the client persists, then gently but firmly stopping the session is necessary. The client's armoring is probably too strong in this situation for the client to be able to stop his of her behavior.

In working with any clients with a romantic rigid structure, recognizing weak spots in their own boundaries is important for the therapist. In some cases, this may take the form of being vulnerable to flattery or seductiveness by an attractive client. It may involve going a little farther than the therapist would like in order not to hurt the client's feelings or not to appear uptight. It also may manifest as being easily overwhelmed by seductive or sexually aggressive behavior and not being able to say no, despite the fact that the therapist is not actually attracted to the client. On the other hand, the seductive or sexualizing behavior may be so threatening or repulsive to the therapist that the therapist may react too harshly, and instead of creating a firm boundary, reject the client emotionally. For example, the therapist may perceive the client as a violator to be summarily tossed out, which prevents the therapist from being able to take a therapeutic stance with a client with a romantic rigid structure. In this case, an example of a therapeutic stance would be to use the interventions mentioned above that are intended to allow the client to experience sensation in a different, noncharacteristic way.

Table 9.2. *Summary of Rigid Character Substructure Qualities*

Qualities	Controlled Rigid	Achieving Rigid	Entertaining Rigid	Romantic Rigid
Charge	Overcharged	Overcharged	Overcharged	Overcharged
Grounding	Overgrounded	Overgrounded	Undergrounded	Undergrounded
Bounding	Overbounded	Overbounded	Underbounded	Underbounded
Armor	Knotty	Knotty	Mesh, some knotty	Mesh and knotty
Holding	Held up	Held up & held back	Held out	Held back and held out

Even if the therapeutic intervention is not effective and the therapist must end the session, there is still a therapeutically sound way of doing so. For example, "I need to end this session because it appears that you are unable or unwilling to hold your sexual sensations back and it looks as if you want to expand them into something more, which is not acceptable and not part of this work. This is an absolute boundary and if you agree to recognize that, we can talk about your feelings if you choose. If not, this session will end immediately." Please note that it is optional for the therapist whether to offer to discuss the client's feelings. If the therapist does not have the skills or does not feel sufficiently emotionally centered to do so, not doing so is best. Respecting the limitations of your training and skills, along with your emotional preparedness, is *always* important. A client with this structure in most cases ultimately needs to work with a skilled psychotherapist or counselor to resolve his or her character issues.

Massage with a client with a romantic rigid structure otherwise can be very similar to the work with the other rigid structures. One more point needs to be emphasized. The undergrounding in people with a romantic rigid structure is a very important element in keeping them in fantasy. Therefore, working to bring tangible sensation and feeling into the lower legs and feet is important. Again, experiencing bodily sensations throughout their body, rather than only localized in parts, especially erogenous areas, is also very important for clients with a romantic rigid structure.

REFERENCES

Cornell, W. & Ludwig, M. (2002). *The body as a retreat from relateness: Exploring autistic and hysterical defenses.* Presentation, United States Association for Body Psychotherapy Third National Conference.

Johnson, S.M. (1985). *Characterological transformation: The hard work miracle.* New York: W.W. Norton.

Keleman, S. (1985). *Emotional anatomy.* Berkeley: Center Press.

Kurtz, R. & Prestera, H. (1976). *The body reveals.* New York: Harper & Row.

Lowen, A. (1975). *Bioenergetics.* New York: Penguin Books.

Lowen, A. (1980). *Fear of life.* New York: Macmillan.

Lowen, A. (1971). *The language of the body.* New York: Collier Books.

Robbins, R. (1990). *Rhythmic integration.* Barrytown, NY: Pulse.

Rosenberg, J. L. & Rand, M. (1985). *Body, self, and soul-sustaining integration.* Atlanta: Humanics.

Shapiro, D. (1965). *Neurotic styles.* New York: Basic Books.

Shapiro, D. (1989). *Psychotherapy of the neurotic character.* New York: Basic Books.

Shapiro, D. (2000). *Dynamics of character.* New York: Basic Books.

Smith, E. (1985). *The body in psychotherapy.* Jefferson, NC: Macfarland & Company.

Understanding Mental Health Conditions and Disorders

10

Chapter

Psychological and psychiatric conditions and disorders are widespread in society, perhaps more than most people think. One in 10 Americans—some sources say even more—experience some disability from a diagnosable mental illness, which implies that a massage therapist *inevitably* encounters one or more such clients. Therefore, massage therapists need to be familiar with conditions that should be treated primarily by a mental health professional. For this reason, we present here basic information about the more commonly occurring conditions that a massage therapist may encounter and that potentially should involve a referral to a mental health professional.

The main purpose of this chapter is to help you become more familiar with major psychological and psychiatric disorders so that you will be able to:

▶ Recognize and have a basic understanding of the terms and conditions reviewed
▶ Have a sense of problems that may be outside the scope of practice of massage therapy
▶ Be aware of psychological conditions that need to be referred to mental health professionals
▶ Be conversant about these conditions and disorders, at least on a basic level, with other professionals, especially mental health professionals
▶ Have a sense of how massage can safely and effectively be used with clients who present these problems, usually in their less serious forms
▶ Respond knowledgeably and confidently when a client mentions these conditions
▶ Use this information to avoid projection or inappropriate subjective conclusions when facing various psychological characteristics in clients
▶ Read and learn more about these problems on your own

Box 10.1

WHAT IS THE DSM?

The DSM-IV is the *Diagnostic and Statistical Manual*, which is published by the American Psychiatric Association and is the psychiatric profession's official guide for defining emotional and mental illnesses or conditions. The *DSM* influences the other mental health professions, including decisions made concerning systematic research, drug trials, and insurance coverage. The *DSM* played a key role in the 1970s when psychiatrists moved their field from Freudian insight and analysis toward a classification similar to other medical specialties, linking mental illness to brain disorders, and thereby more closely aligning with the medical model. Although the medical model—and the *DSM*—include some use of talk therapy and other psychotherapeutic techniques for treatment, the main direction of modern psychiatric research and practice has been drugs that affect brain chemistry.

In a sense, this chapter presents a brief mental health primer for the massage therapist. However, our purpose is not to teach diagnosis, but to impart sensitivity to mental health conditions. In other words, this information is not given to assist you in making a diagnosis or in "figuring out" what is wrong with a client, but to understand what it means and what is involved when a client or a health care professional gives you mental health information and to have a sharper idea of when and why to refer a client for a mental health related reason.

All psychiatric symptoms can be produced or mimicked by a medical disorder, so keep in mind this prescription: "*Think medical unless proven otherwise.*" For this reason, referring a client to his or her primary care provider is often the first action to take when you believe you are confronting a psychiatric symptom. An example of the importance to "think medical" is the classification of *organic disorders*, all of which are conditions stemming from physical causes, such as acute organic brain syndrome (delirium state), chronic organic brain syndrome (dementia), and psychiatric disorders secondary to brain dysfunction.

The most significant and relevant disorders have been included. The psychiatric diagnostic nomenclature is extensive, so not all disorders and terms have been included here. Also, the most relevant information about each disorder that we believe will be useful to a massage therapist has been included, whereas of necessity other information is not. You can always see the *DSM-IV* (Box 10.1), *Merck Manual*, or other resources for more information. Sources have variations concerning terms and systems of categorization, so you may find such variations in this chapter also.

GENERALIZED ANXIETY DISORDER

Generalized anxiety disorder involves experiencing constant, exaggerated worrisome thoughts and tension about everyday routine life events and activities for at least 6 months. A person with generalized anxiety disorder typically anticipates the worst, even if there is little reason to expect it would happen. It is commonly accompanied by physical symptoms, such as fatigue, trembling, muscle tension, headache, sweating, or nausea. As with the other anxiety disorders, the symptoms substantially surpass "normal" worries in intensity, duration, and unrealistic basis to such an extent that the person is debilitated by the anxiety.

Generalized anxiety disorder, sometimes called "free-floating anxiety," affects 2.8% to 5% of the U.S. adult population and is twice as common in women as in men. Also, up to 60% of people affected have a history of at least one other mental disorder (NIMH, 2001; Nathan et al.). Generalized anxiety disorder, panic disorder, obsessive-compulsive disorder, post-traumatic stress disorder, and phobias all are classified as *anxiety disorders*.

The effect of massage therapy to reduce anxiety is clearly beneficial for generalized anxiety disorder.

PHOBIAS

The essential feature of a *phobia*, as described in the *DSM-IV* (p. 405), is a persistent fear or anxiety response that is "excessive or unreasonable that is cued by the presence or anticipation of a specific object or situation . . . .Most often, the phobic stimulus is avoided, although it is sometimes endured with dread. The avoidance, fear, or anxious anticipation of encountering phobic stimulus interferes significantly with the person's daily routine, occupational functioning, or social life, and/or the person may be markedly distressed about having the phobia." Phobias usually first appear during childhood or adolescence and tend to persist into adulthood. The psychoanalytic literature and twin studies show a connection between phobias and separation traumas in childhood. Although the term phobia has entered popular usage when referring to forms of discomfort or emotional "hang-ups," a phobia in clinical terminology involves a much more intense level of feeling than simple fear or discomfort. The fear is usually intense enough to be virtually paralyzing. Phobias affect about 11% to 13% of adult Americans sometime during their lives and are twice as common in women as in men (NIMH, 1996; Nathan et al.).

Phobic fear can be prompted by anticipated harm from or losing control upon exposure to: animals or insects; elements of the natural environment (e.g., storms, heights, or water); bodily functions such as bleeding, infection, or injury; specific situations (e.g., public transportation, tunnels, bridges, elevators, escalators, flying, driving, or being in open or enclosed places); situations that may lead to vomiting, choking, or contracting an illness; "space phobias" (which involve fear of falling down if away from walls or other means of support); and children's fears of loud sounds and costumed characters (e.g., fear of clowns, called *cloutrophobia*).

Phobias are divided generally into two categories: social phobia and specific phobia. People with a *social phobia* have an overwhelming and disabling fear of scrutiny, embarrassment, or humiliation in social situations. People with a *specific phobia* experience extreme, disabling, and irrational fear of something that poses little or no actual danger. Some authorities consider a third category of phobia to be *agoraphobia*, which is the fear of being alone in any place or situation from which the person believes that escape is impossible or difficult.

People with phobias end up in treatment when their phobias interfere with normal living patterns, for example, when the fear of insects or being outside or in open spaces causes the person to remain shut up in a meticulously controlled environment. The form of treatment that has shown the most success treating phobias is a form of behavior therapy known as *systematic desensitization* (involving repeated exposure to the dreaded situations, while practicing specific cognitive-behavioral techniques to become less sensitive to them), which is provided primarily by a psychiatrist or psychologist.

Although massage therapy may not be used for direct treatment of phobia, the effect of massage to reduce anxiety is beneficial for people with a phobia. Massage may also be effective in teaching relaxation to a client with a phobia.

PANIC DISORDER

The essential feature of *panic disorder* is: "Recurrent, unexpected panic attacks followed by at least one month of persistent concern about having another panic attack, worry about the possible implications or consequences of the panic attack, or a significant behavioral change related to the attacks. Panic disorders do not include any situations caused by the direct physiological effects of a drug of abuse or medication or general medical condition (e.g., hypothyroidism) or situations that can be better accounted for by another mental condition" (DSM-IV, p. 394). However, panic disorder can be accompanied by other disorders, such as depression. Panic attacks, the hallmark of panic disorder, are believed to occur when the brain's normal mechanism for reacting to a threat—the "fight or flight" response—becomes inappropriately aroused. Females are affected two times more frequently than males. In the United States, 1.7% to 3.5% of the adult population will have panic disorder at some time in their lives (NIMH, 1996; Nathan et al.).

Panic attacks are distinct, often sudden, periods of intense fear or discomfort that can have no noticeable stimulus or triggering event and that reach a peak within 10 minutes. They often occur while a person is engaged in some ordinary activity like driving a car or walking to the store. People who have had panic attacks describe the fear as intense, and they often have an urgent desire to flee from what they perceive as the source of the attack. Panic attacks also involve physical symptoms, such as greatly increased heart rate, rapid breathing, trembling, dizziness, nausea, feelings of choking, and cold or hot sweats. Psychological symptoms may involve feelings of unreality or being detached from oneself, fear of losing control or going crazy, or fear of dying. Initial panic attacks may occur when people are under considerable stress, for example, from overwork or the loss of a family member or close friend. Attacks may also follow surgery, a serious accident, illness, or childbirth. Excessive consumption of caffeine or use of cocaine or other stimulant drugs or medicines, such as the stimulants used in treating asthma, can also trigger panic attacks.

The anxiety that is characteristic of panic attacks differs from generalized anxiety by its intermittent, almost paroxysmal, nature and its typically greater severity. A panic attack is spontaneous, and, in contrast to phobic reactions, is not associated with a situational trigger; that is, it occurs "out of the blue." The frequency and severity of panic attacks can vary widely. Individuals with panic disorder harbor typical worries about the consequences of the panic attacks, often leading to avoidance behavior related to activities believed to provoke another attack. For example, the person becomes afraid of being in any place or situation in which escape might be difficult or help unavailable in the event of a panic attack. Anxiety about another attack, and the avoidance it causes, can lead to disability. If the panic attacks are unpredictable, then the person is further debilitated by feeling the possibility of another panic attack striking at any time and by always being on guard. Several other conditions are found to coexist with panic disorder, such as phobias, depression, obsessive-compulsive disorder, substance abuse, irritable bowel syndrome, and mitral valve prolapse.

People with panic disorders often need to be treated by a mental health professional. Also, a number of books are now available that describe non-drug alternatives for treating panic disorder.

Massage therapy is not used for direct treatment of panic disorder, but the effect of massage to reduce general anxiety and counter some of the possible physical reactions is beneficial for people with panic disorder. Although it is very rare, it is possible that someone could have a panic attack during a massage or in a massage therapist's office. Sometimes, slowing breathing rate and use of grounding techniques help. Having the client breathe into a paper bag can help control hyperventilation (by increasing the carbon dioxide level) and resultant symptoms of tetany (cramped fingers, toes, and lips; tingling sensations; light-headedness). However, sometimes "stopping" a panic attack is not possible, so do not feel discouraged if you are unable to stop an attack or determine why it happened. Sometimes, this may not be a good idea anyway.

Also, trying to figure out why the panic attack happened while the person is having a panic attack is not very useful and may even make it worse. If you find yourself with someone who is having a panic attack, the best thing to do is to remain grounded yourself and protect the person from harm. When the panic attack ends—do not worry, it *will* end—you can offer support and comfort. After an attack, clients often need to talk over what happened, why it happened, and how others have treated them because of their attacks (Box 10.2).

Be aware that helping a client successfully deal with a panic attack can create a situation in which transference can develop. A client may begin to look to you as his or her source of a safe, secure place and person. This can be perfectly fine if the client is receiving other help. However, if the client is not or has been in psychotherapy before with limited success, he or she may transfer the need for psychotherapy or simply support to the massage therapist and to the use of massage as an outlet.

OBSESSIVE-COMPULSIVE DISORDER

The disorders grouped under *obsessive-compulsive disorder* (OCD) have three varieties: obsession, compulsion, and obsessive-compulsive. OCD affects 2.3% of the adult population, meaning that it is more common than schizophrenia, bipolar disorder, or panic disorder (NIMH, 1999).

Box 10.2

COPING WITH A CLIENT IN PANIC

In the event that your client experiences a panic attack, these suggested strategies (directed toward the person experiencing the panic attack) may help:

► Although your feelings and symptoms are very frightening, they are not dangerous or harmful.
► What you are experiencing is just an exaggeration of normal bodily reactions to stress.
► Try not to fight the feelings or try to make them go away. The more you are willing to face them, the less intense they will become. Try to slow your breathing.
► Try not to think about what *might* happen, which will add to the panic. For example, you could say, "Instead of asking 'what if,' tell yourself, 'so what!' Think about how good you will feel when you succeed this time."
► Let's both stay in the present, and notice what is happening in the here and now. Focus on mundane bodily awarenesses. Focus on feeling your feet on the ground (or table) or back or front side on the table (or chair).
► Rate your fear level from 0 to 10 and watch it go up and down, noticing that it does not stay at a very high level for more than a few seconds.
► When you realize that you are thinking about the fear, instead focus on and carry out a simple and manageable task such as counting backward from 100 by threes or by snapping a rubber band on the wrist.
► "When the fear comes, expect and accept it. Wait and give it time to pass without running away from it or adding to it. B r e a t h e!"
► Have you had medication prescribed for panic attack? Do you have any medication with you?

(Adapted from National Institute of Mental Health. Understanding Panic Disorder. Publication No. 95-3509. Bethesda, MD: NIMH, 1995.)

Obsession

An *obsession* involves an intrusive fixation on a thought, image, person, event, or condition and causes distress or anxiety. Clinically speaking, obsessions are: "Persistent ideas, thoughts, impulses, or images that are experienced as intrusive and inappropriate and that cause marked anxiety or distress. Such thoughts, impulses, or images are not simply excessive worries about real-life problems. The person attempts to ignore or suppress such thoughts, impulses, or images, or to neutralize them with some other thought or action. (DSM-IV, p. 418)." The sort of excessive worry associated with generalized anxiety is distinguished from obsessions by the fact that excessive worrying involves concerns about real life circumstances, whereas obsessions do not. For example, an excessive concern that one may lose money in the stock market would constitute a worry, not an obsession. In contrast, the content of obsessions does not typically involve real life problems, and the affected person experiences the obsessions as inappropriate (e.g., the intrusive distressing idea that "God" is "dog" spelled backward). Common obsessions include contamination, safety, doubting one's memory or perception, concerns with symmetry, scrupulosity (need to do the right thing, fear of committing a transgression), and sexual/aggressive thoughts.

Compulsion

A c*ompulsion* is a fixation involving an action and is usually repetitive. Compulsions are, clinically speaking, "Repetitive behaviors or mental acts that the person feels driven to perform in response to an obsession or according to rules that must be applied rigidly. The behaviors or mental acts are aimed at preventing or reducing distress or preventing some dreaded event or situation, . . . [but] either are not connected in a realistic way with what they are designed to neutralize or prevent or are clearly excessive (DSM-IV, p. 418)." Typical repetitive behaviors are hand washing, cleaning objects, putting things in order, checking, hoarding, and asking for assurances, whereas examples of repetitive mental acts are praying, counting, list making, and repeating words mentally.

At one time, all obsessions were considered mental events, and all compulsions were thought of as behavioral events. However, now compulsions can be considered mental or behavioral. For example, a mental ritual, such as counting numbers repeatedly, serves the same purpose as a behavioral ritual by reducing the anxiety associated with an obsession.

Obsessive-Compulsive

Obsessive-compulsive disorder involves both conditions being present. The person with an obsession usually attempts to ignore or suppress such thoughts or impulses or to neutralize them with some other thought or action, that is, a compulsion. The individual feels driven to perform the compulsion to reduce the distress that accompanies an obsession or to prevent some dreaded event or situation. For example, people with obsessions about being contaminated may reduce their mental distress by washing their hands until their skin is raw, people distressed by obsessions about having left a door unlocked may be driven to check the lock every few minutes, or people distressed by unwanted blasphemous thoughts may find relief in counting to 10 backward and forward 100 times for each thought. OCD, as well as simple obsessions and compulsions, all are essentially security operations in that they are intended to prevent harm and assure physical or psychological safety, rather than provide satisfaction or pleasure. They are also time-consuming, disabling, or extremely personally unpleasant.

The simple presence of obsessions and compulsions does not always constitute OCD. The clinical features of OCD are: "Recurrent obsessions or compulsions that are severe enough to take more than one hour a day or significantly interfere with the person's daily life (*DSM-IV*, p. 419)." People with OCD often have varying degrees of insight. Sometimes, they recognize that their obsessions and compulsions are unrealistic (this knowledge is called *intact insight*), but other times they are unsure of their fears or believe in their validity. OCD sufferers tend to hide their disorder rather than seek help, often learning how to work around their characteristic rituals, which accounts largely for why it takes an average of 17 years from the time this disorder begins until a person obtains treatment (Nathan et al.). For most individuals, the symptoms are chronic and long-lasting, although they may become less severe from time to time.

OCD is now considered to be primarily a brain disorder and may have genetic origins, rather than being primarily the result of life experiences. The search for causes now focuses on the interaction of neurobiological factors and environmental influences, as well as cognitive processes. Researchers have found that an afflicted person's brain may not register or recognize that a certain action has been completed, so the action is repeated. For example, checking behavior—repeatedly checking to see if a light is switched off or a door is closed—is one form of OCD. When the person switches off the light, the brain does not "know" that the action of flicking the light switch has been made and completed, so the action has to be repeated.

Some coexisting disorders are depression, eating disorders, substance abuse, one of the personality disorders, attention-deficit hyperactivity disorder, or another of the anxiety disorders (OCD is categorized as one of these). Medication and systematic desensitization are often used as treatments.

Other disorders included in the obsessive-compulsive spectrum are body dysmorphic disorder (distorted body image, also considered a somatoform disorder by some), trichotillomania (hair pulling), Tourette's syndrome, and neurotic excoriation (skin picking or scratching).

OCD differs from the popular use of the term as a synonym for worrying or being neat and should not be confused with what is described as being "compulsive." People may be so described because they hold themselves to a high standard of performance and are perfectionistic and very organized in their activities. When such traits are more a part of a person's character, rather than having a neurobiological basis, this may be considered *obsessive-compulsive personality disorder*. These traits differ from the life-wrecking obsessions and rituals of the person with OCD. The symptoms related to OCD are much more intense and debilitating and interfere with normal life.

POST-TRAUMATIC STRESS DISORDER

Post-traumatic stress disorder (PTSD) is the "development of characteristic symptoms following exposure to an extreme traumatic stressor . . . The characteristic symptoms include: persistent re-experiencing of the traumatic event, persistent avoidance of stimuli associated with the trauma and numbing of general responsiveness, and persistent symptoms of increased arousal . . . [causing] significant distress or impairment in social, occupational, or other important areas of functioning (DSM-IV, p. 424)." About 3.6% of U.S. adults have PTSD during the course of a given year and 15% at some time during their lifetime, although PTSD can occur in people of any age. More than twice as many women as men experience PTSD after exposure to trauma. The high frequency level of PTSD, in the opinion of many researchers, reflects the high level of interpersonal violence in American society. About 30% of the people who have spent time in war zones and 31% of women who have been raped develop PTSD (NIMH, 2001; Nathan et al.).

PTSD can be started by a variety of events. *Personally experienced traumatic events* that lead to PTSD include combat, violent personal assault (sexual assault, physical attack, robbery), sexual or physical abuse (Widom), being kidnapped, being taken hostage, terrorist attack, torture, incarceration as a prisoner of war or in a concentration camp, natural or manmade disasters, severe automobile accidents, or diagnosis with a life-threatening illness. *Witnessed events* that happen to others that lead to PTSD include observing the serious injury or unnatural death of another person or unexpectedly seeing a dead body or body parts. *Events experienced by others that are learned about later* that lead to PTSD include violent personal assault, serious accident, or serious injury experienced by a family member or close friend, or learning that one's child has a life threatening illness. The problem may be especially severe or long-lasting if the stressor is of human design. The person's response involves intense fear, helplessness, or horror.

Many people with PTSD repeatedly re-experience the ordeal as flashback episodes, memories, nightmares, or frightening thoughts, especially when they are exposed to events or objects reminiscent of the trauma. Anniversaries of the event can also trigger symptoms. Other anxieties may appear, such as sleep disturbances, hypervigilance, exaggerated startle response, feelings of doom, depression, anxiety, and irritability or outbursts of anger. Feelings of intense guilt are also common (Davidson). Most people with PTSD try to avoid any reminders or thoughts of the ordeal. Avoidances may include amnesia or cutting off from the external world by "psychic numbing" or "emotional anesthesia" (Feeny et al.). Physical symptoms, such as headaches, gastrointestinal complaints, immune system problems, dizziness, chest pain, or discomfort in other parts of the body, are common. Although anyone may experience one of these symptoms for a brief period, PTSD symptoms are present for more than 1 month. Depression, alcohol or other substance abuse, or other anxiety disorders (PTSD is an anxiety disorder) frequently co-occur with PTSD.

Symptoms of post-traumatic stress may appear during a massage and lead the client into considering treatment. Fragmentary "body memories" are the most likely symptoms that may appear during massage. Working in conjunction with a psychotherapist at this point is important for even an experienced massage therapist. Massage therapy can be an effective approach to the problem of numbing and dissociation if it facilitates the person's ability to tolerate being in their body. One study of children with severe PTSD symptoms who received massage had lower levels of anxiety and depression and improved relaxation (Field et al. 1996). Because of the great controversy involving "recovered memories," or "false memories," massage therapists can put themselves in a legally risky situation by attempting to elicit further memories without the aid of a therapist trained in PTSD treatment. Although body memories may be a symptom of PTSD, they are not necessarily always PTSD symptoms.

ATTENTION-DEFICIT HYPERACTIVITY DISORDER

Attention-deficit hyperactivity disorder (ADHD) is characterized by (1) *inattentive behavior*, such as failure to pay close attention to details and making careless mistakes, difficulty in sustaining attention in work or play, not seeming to listen when spoken to directly, not following through on instructions and failing to complete tasks, difficulty organizing activities and often losing things, disliking engagement in tasks that require sustained mental effort, and being generally forgetful and easily distracted; (2) *hyperactivity*, such as fidgeting and squirming, an inability to remain seated, inappropriate running and climbing, difficulty being quiet, acting as if driven by a motor, and excessive talking; and (3) *impulsive behavior*, such as difficulty curbing immediate reactions or thinking before acting, for example, blurting out answers to questions before they have been completed, difficulty awaiting one's turn, and interrupting or intruding. ADHD affects 3% to 5% of all children, perhaps as many as 2 to 5 million American children. About 3% to 4% of elementary school-aged boys and 1% to 2% of same-age girls are affected (NIHM 1996; Nathan et al.).

ADHD has replaced the former classifications of attention-deficit disorder (ADD) and hyperactivity disorder (HD). Instead, ADHD now has two subtypes: primarily inattentive or primarily hyperactive.

People with ADHD do not have distinct physical signs that can be seen in tests. The signs can be identified only by looking for the characteristic behaviors of inattention, hyperactivity, and impulsiveness, which vary from person to person. To be considered ADHD, these behaviors must be excessive, long-term, and pervasive; occur more often than in other people the same age; and be a continual problem rather than a response to a temporary situation. Onset is in childhood. The fact that many medical and other psychiatric conditions such as a learning disability, epilepsy, and middle ear infections also cause inattention further complicates the picture.

There is little argument among researchers that ADHD is a disorder of the brain with multiple causes, but these have yet to be pinpointed. Implicated in the development of ADHD are genetic irregularities, low glucose metabolism in the brain, frontal cortex structural abnormalities, neurotransmitter aberrations, and prenatal exposure to alcohol and nicotine, along with other pre- and immediate postnatal risk factors. Compounding the difficulty in identifying the causes is evidence that the causes combine differently in different individuals. Experts generally agree now that ADHD is *not* caused by too much television, food allergies, too much sugar, poor home life, or poor schools, although there is some emerging support for gluten sensitivity as a cause. However, parenting styles and environmental factors do play a role in the development of aggressive and antisocial behaviors that sometimes accompany ADHD.

These symptoms may be similar to the kind of things many people go through as children, but ADHD symptoms are more extreme, cause problems in more than one area of a person's life, and tend not to change much as the person becomes an adult. Until recently, adults were not thought to have ADHD. However, it is now believed that half the children with ADHD continue to have symptoms through adulthood, although the symptoms tend to change with the passage of time as hyperactivity and impulsiveness diminish, but not inattentiveness. The recent recognition of adult ADHD means that many people may finally be correctly diagnosed and helped.

People with ADHD often have low self-esteem because they have experienced numerous failures in school or in the workplace, often despite a normal or high level of intelligence. Massage therapy as an adjunctive treatment can help people with ADHD in several ways. Benefits include a calming effect and reconnecting the person with his or her body in a way that significantly increases the person's ability to directly experience and organize physical sensations. The increased sensory awareness allows such a person to focus better and be less distractible and more organized in a cognitive sense. For example, if you are more focused in your body, you are more focused on picking up a pen or some other specific task. As is generally true, massage therapy also benefits self-esteem when unconditional positive regard is communicated through the touch of the therapist. One study on the effect of massage on adolescents with ADHD confirmed such positive effects and showed decreased inattentiveness and hyperactivity with massage (Field et al., 1998).

Box 10.3

CHARACTERISTICS OF ADDICTION

Addiction is characterized by:

Loss of *control*: The user cannot predict what will happen when using the substance or cannot control how much he or she will use. An overwhelming urge to keep on using occurs (called "priming," which is believed to involve the neurotransmitters beta-endorphins and dopamine), sometimes only occasionally. For example, one day the person may stop after one drink or one line of cocaine, and the next day he or she may not be able to control such use at all.

Compulsive need: Compulsion, in contrast to craving, is an unconscious drive. The user also spends a great deal of time thinking about (technically, an obsession) the substance or the experience. Compulsion to use substances or engage in certain behaviors means it becomes such a high priority—even the most important activity in the person's life—that it crowds out or endangers other previously important priorities.

Continued use despite negative *consequences*: The person's use or behavior continues despite problems caused by that use or behavior. Family becomes concerned and relationships become strained, or there may be a change in friends and a growing tendency to isolate. Problems develop at the workplace, such as too much time missed from work or conflicts with coworkers, leading to complaints, grievances, or disciplinary action. The person engages in behaviors that contradict his or her values or sense of right and wrong. This causes feelings of anxiety, guilt, and anger, which can lead to symptoms that mimic mood disorders, manic depression, personality disorders, and even some types of psychosis. Physical and personal safety is jeopardized by increased risk of accident, being beaten up, robbery, and sexual assault. Legal consequences can include impaired driving charges, license suspensions, possession charges, assault, disorderly conduct, or professional and ethical disciplinary charges (Hyman 2001).

ADDICTION AND SUBSTANCE ABUSE

Addiction and substance abuse are included here because they are, as a group, among the most common of all mental health problems and occur across all segments of the population. In the United States, approximately 6% of the population abuse illegal drugs, 12% abuse alcohol, 25% are addicted to nicotine, and, conservatively, 10% are addicted to prescription medications (NIMH, 2001).

Considerable controversy swirls about over what constitutes addiction to and abuse of substances like alcohol and drugs. *Addiction* is the *compulsive* need to engage in and the inability to *control* certain behaviors despite their destructive *consequences* (Hyman, 2001). Note that addictive behavior is not determined by how much or how often a substance is used (Box 10.3). Substances involved in addiction include alcohol, depressants (sedatives), stimulants (amphetamines), cocaine, hallucinogens (LSD), inhalants (glue), opiates (heroin, morphine, opium), steroids, caffeine, and nicotine, as well as legal (prescription) drugs. The concept of addiction has been expanded more recently to include in addition to substances a variety of behaviors, including compulsive gambling, eating disorders, sex addiction, and even excessive work or exercise. Although some contention exists over whether such behaviors can be considered addictions when physical or chemical addiction is absent, some researchers have found the behaviors themselves also can lead to physiological changes.

Excessive, compulsive substance use that develops into a persistent pattern of destructive behavior leading to clinically significant social, occupational, or health impairment that interferes with normal activities is called *substance abuse* (Nathan et al.). The difference between addiction and substance abuse evokes one of the areas of debate, which centers on the question of dependence. Behavior leading to actual physiological dependence is called *substance dependence*. At one time, increased tolerance and withdrawal symptoms upon stopping were considered necessary signs of addiction (see the definition). Essentially, abuse (the psychological/behavior element) plus dependence (the physical element) equaled addiction. However, experts on the subject no longer agree about whether tolerance and withdrawal should be included as signs of addiction. It is now better understood that although tolerance and withdrawal are often present to varying degrees, they are not necessarily present in people with substance dependence. For example, the binge alcoholic is still alcohol dependent a month after his or her last binge; or, early in the course of addiction to alcohol and cocaine physical dependence is not present, yet a clear diagnosis of dependence or addiction may be made. In other words, although physical addiction always has a psychological element, not all psychological dependence is accompanied by physical dependence (Szamraj; Pursch).

The notion of whether substance abuse or addiction is voluntary or involuntary is at the core of the debates. Spinning off from this question are polarized arguments, such as disease versus bad behavior, treatment versus punishment, or reducing demand by prevention and treatment versus restricting availability. Models of causation emphasizing morality or individual conscious choice, biological or disease vulnerability, behavioral learning patterns, or cultural-environmental concerns all have held sway at various times. The biopsychosocial model seems to be leading at the present, which views substance abuse as a complex interaction of all of the other models. The clear and unambiguous message from volumes of scientific research is that substance abuse and addiction are complex, dynamic processes, with voluntary and involuntary components to every stage. Research on effective treatment indicates treating the whole person works best.

People who have low self-esteem have a higher rate of addiction and abuse. They abuse substances or behaviors to enhance or create pleasure or to decrease constant emotional pain in their lives as a way of "self-medicating" their insecurities and bad feelings about themselves. The better a person feels about him- or herself, the less likely he or she is to use or abuse. *The benefits of massage intersect with the addict's or abuser's psychological needs to produce pleasure or avoid pain.*

Alcoholism

Because *alcoholism* is such a widespread problem, we look at it in more detail as an example of a substance abuse problem (see the definition). The cause of alcoholism is not certain, but strong evidence exists for genetic, psychosocial and environmental origins. Given the inherited risk, a variety of psychological and environmental factors (e.g., depression, broken home, alcohol misuse by other family members) appear to influence the expression of that risk in the individual. Once begun, alcoholism typically progresses over 10 to 20 years. Because the progression is gradual, however, determining exactly when a person becomes an alcoholic is difficult. Currently, estimates of the number who abuse alcohol or are alcoholic range from about 17 to 34 million in the United States (NIMH, 2001).

Although one may assume alcoholism is noticeable, this is not always the case, and alcoholism may not be evident to a massage therapist. Indeed, in the early stages, few outward signs of a problem are evident. The person may function normally most of the time, but a few personality changes may appear, along with the inability to handle stress and increased conflict with family members. Although these changes do not necessarily indicate an alcohol problem, additional signs are present to others before the person accepts them. One way a massage therapist may become aware of alcoholism is if alcohol consumption or drinking behavior comes up while taking a history before beginning working with a client. A massage therapist may also take in information on a client's drinking habits through conversation or observing behavior over time (Box 10.4).

People do not need to have all four of the signs stated in Box 10.4 to be considered an alcoholic. Those who have significant problems controlling their drinking and functioning in social situations because of alcohol may be considered alco-

Tolerance and Withdrawal

Tolerance is the need for significant increased amounts of a substance or behavior to achieve the desired effects (e.g., in drug abuse, getting high), or causes significant diminished effects with continued use of the same amount of a substance or behavior.

Withdrawal is the suffering of uncomfortable and sometimes harmful symptoms after a reduction or cessation in the intake of a substance or expression of a behavior over a prolonged period. Classic symptoms may include sweating, hand or body tremors, nausea, vomiting, agitation, insomnia, anxiety, hallucinations, illusions, or seizures.

Alcoholism

The National Council on Alcoholism and Drug Dependence defines *alcoholism* as a primary, chronic disease with genetic, psychosocial, and environmental factors influencing its development and manifestations. The disease is often progressive and fatal. It is characterized by continuous or periodic: impaired control over drinking, preoccupation with alcohol, use of alcohol despite adverse consequences, and distortions in thinking, most notably denial.

Box 10.4

SIGNS OF ALCOHOLISM

A variety of lists of the signs of alcoholism exist. These signs fall into four areas:

▶ Recognition by the individual of alcohol excess or the need to "control" drinking. For example, alcoholics may intend to have two or three drinks, but before they know it, they are on their tenth.
▶ Negative effects on others, such as continued use of alcohol despite social, family, and work problems.
▶ Adverse consequences, such as anxiety, depressed mood, drunk driving arrests, dyspepsia and gastritis, elevated liver enzyme levels, hepatitis or cirrhosis, recurrent minor injuries, seizures and delirium tremens, sleep disturbance, and victim or perpetrator of violence.
▶ Evidence of alcohol tolerance, actual chemical dependence, or the need to manage a withdrawal syndrome. Withdrawal symptoms include anxiety, agitation, increased blood pressure, and, in extreme cases, seizures. These symptoms may persist for several days (NIAAA).

holics without the physical signs, tolerance, and withdrawal. The most prevalent and pervasive symptom exhibited overall is that of *denial*. The alcoholic person believes that no problem exists. They attribute chronic drinking and other related problems to other causes (NIAAA; NIMH, 2001).

Some other symptoms of alcoholism are:

▶ Making excuses to drink
▶ Feeling annoyed when criticized about drinking
▶ Keeping and hiding alcohol in unlikely places
▶ Drinking first thing in the morning to avoid a hangover
▶ Showing aggressive behavior while drinking
▶ Solitary drinking
▶ Missing work
▶ Losing interest in social activities
▶ Neglecting physical appearance
▶ Impaired memory, forgetting what happened during drinking episodes
▶ Difficulty with thinking clearly, confusion
▶ Irritability
▶ Redness and enlarged capillaries in the face (red eyes, puffy face) (NIAAA; NIMH, 2001).

Some authorities distinguish between alcoholism and alcohol abuse. The latter is a less severe problem. Unlike alcoholics, alcohol abusers do not develop physical withdrawal or compulsive alcohol use. However, like alcoholics, their drinking has negative health, economic, and social effects.

In the past, alcoholism carried a tremendous public and social stigma. This was a barrier to many people who were fearful of employment, family, or social retribution. Today, this stigma has diminished greatly owing to the increased awareness that alcoholism is a disease rather than a choice or lifestyle, which has made treatment more accessible.

Understanding your own attitudes regarding alcohol consumption is important for the massage therapist. If you are a teetotaler, you might conclude that any regular alcohol consumption constitutes alcoholism. A massage therapist who has not dealt with alcoholism with a close relative or friend or has not had the problem him- or herself, might miss signs that someone's drinking has gone over a line into alcoholism and requires treatment. We suggest that you read the above signs and symptoms and notice what your response is concerning yourself and those close to you.

It is not necessary to stop doing massage if you discover a client is alcoholic, but suggesting treatment if the person is bringing up or acting out any psychological phenomena with you as a massage therapist is important. If a client comes for a session "under the influence," not only treatment can be suggested, but the client also should be informed that being under the influence is not an acceptable condition for receiving and giving massage. One of the situations you may encounter if you do suggest a referral for alcoholism is that the client may not act on it. If the client refuses such treatment and continues to introduce psychological issues into the massage therapy session that require the intervention of another health professional, then this may be a time when the massage therapist may consider terminating with the client. The massage therapist is not in a position to forcefully direct clients to follow suggestions regarding any and all aspects of health; that is, massage therapists are not the "health police," but they can make decisions when the client's behavior may undermine the effects of the massage. The example given of alcoholism can be extrapolated to some degree to other addiction and substance abuse problems.

EATING DISORDERS

Anorexia and bulimia are the two major eating disorders. The incidence of eating disorders is highly gender dependent. Females are much more likely than males to develop an eating disorder. An estimated 85% to 95% of people with anorexia or bulimia are female. Estimates of the number of people who suffer eating disorders during their lifetime have a wider range than those for other disorders, which is about 1% to 4%. However, the rates of bulimia are thought to be almost 10 times that for anorexia. Eating disorders frequently occur with other disorders such as depression, substance abuse, and anxiety disorders (NIMH, 2001; Nathan et al.).

Anorexia

According to the *DSM-IV* (p. 539), the essential features of *anorexia* are: "The person refuses to maintain a normal body weight, is intensely afraid of gaining weight, has a significant distortion in the perception of the size or shape of the body and is characterized by dieting, fasting, and excessive exercise" (Box 10.5). One of the characteristic dynamics of anorexia is the extreme need to *control* something—anything—such as the body, believed to stem from a feeling of powerlessness and being controlled by others, such as an overly harsh parent (Nathan et al.). In a quest to gain control of bodily needs, the person may also overuse laxatives and exercise excessively. A person with anorexia usually has *body image disturbance*, which means that the person perceives (not just believes) his or her body is substantially different from what it really is. From time to time, we may have seen photos in magazines or special reports on television that show the extreme condition of starvation in which people with anorexia live. What another person views as an emaciated body is perceived by someone with anorexia as closer to the "perfect" body. Other predisposing factors are low self-esteem and a fear of maturing.

Although its causes are not completely understood, it is believed anorexia, as well as

Box 10.5

SIGNS OF ANOREXIA

Signs of anorexia include:

► **Resistance to maintaining body weight at or above a minimally normal weight for age and height**

► **Intense fear of gaining weight or becoming fat, even though person is actually underweight**

► **Disturbance or distortion in the way in which the person's body weight or shape is perceived or experienced; undue influence of body weight or shape on self-evaluation; or denial of the seriousness of the current low body weight**

► **Infrequent or absent menstrual periods (in females who have reached puberty)**

(Adapted from National Institute of Mental Health. Eating Disorders. Publication No. 01-4901. Bethesda, MD: NIMH, 2001.)

bulimia, has roots in family history and can also be culturally induced. The fashion industry, with its emphasis on extremely thin preadolescent and adolescent bodies as models, has helped create a surge in such problems. In addition, particular athletic pursuits such as gymnastics and ballet demand body compositions for participants and generate body images for others that are not compatible with health for the majority of people. The course and outcome of anorexia vary. Some individuals fully recover after a single episode, some have a fluctuating pattern of weight gain and relapse, and others experience a deteriorating course of illness over many years.

Massage therapists may encounter anorexia in two different kinds of situations. In one situation, the person with anorexia may not yet be in any kind of treatment. This is a difficult situation because the person's physical health is likely to be declining at regular intervals. When someone is losing large amounts of weight over time, the reasons may be stemming from physical illness or an eating disorder, so finding out the cause for the weight loss rather than making assumptions about it is important. However, in many cases, when someone has an eating disorder that has not been "officially" diagnosed, they may not be able to respond to your questioning by giving you the exact cause.

Sometimes, people suffering from anorexia may be proud of a weight loss that looks excessive to someone else. Recognizing that they have an eating disorder can be the first step in their treatment, so someone with anorexia who has not had treatment should not be expected to tell you that he or she has anorexia. The massage therapist has to use a best sense of judgment when dealing with the question of whether to say something about it or suggest seeking eating disorder treatment, keeping in mind that anorexia can threaten both health and life (e.g., it can cause an imbalance of electrolytes needed for normal functioning of the nervous system, serious heart conditions, and kidney failure), with mortality rates of 10% to 15% (Nathan et al.). It is also a tenacious disorder, and the person who has it may be so resistant to hearing what the therapist or anyone else says that this may break the relationship.

In the other situation, the person with anorexia may be in treatment. Here, massage therapy may be very effective, although not a panacea. Anorexia is a condition in which concern about body image and control of the body can dominate the person's entire life, including all body sensation. In other words, feeling bad, fatigued, sick, and weak are a small cost to pay for the "perfect" body. There is a loss of healthy sensation in the body. In addition, the kinesthetic sense of body size or proportion is distorted or weak. Massage therapy can begin to let the person feel his or her body size from the "inside out." One study showed that a group of women with anorexia who received massage showed decreased anxiety, stress, and body image disturbance levels (Hart et al.).

Massage therapy can also be threatening for exactly the same reasons. When touching or working at any level with the body, the massage therapist is disturbing this radical control. When the control mechanism is weakened, then the person is more likely to experience feelings that may be unpleasant and difficult to handle. That is, the anorectic pattern is blocking or "defending" them from being in touch with these problems. If such material comes up during massage sessions, encouraging the client to bring this to sessions with the primary psychotherapist with whom he or she is working toward recovery from anorexia can be important.

Bulimia

Features of *bulimia* are "Binge eating and purging, which may include vomiting and the misuse of laxatives, diuretics, or enemas" (*DSM-IV*, p. 539), (Box 10.6). Bulimia is a condition in which a person tries to maintain a body image through following binge eating (eating an excessive amount of food within a discrete period of time accompanied by a sense of lack of control over eating) with purging what they have eaten. Bulimia also often involves body image distortion and a lack of self-worth as paramount issues. Bulimia can be a hidden condition because a person with bulimia may appear to have a normal weight. Another reason it is hidden is that they often perform the behaviors in secrecy, feeling disgusted and ashamed when they binge, yet relieved once they purge. The therapist may never know about this condition unless the client admits it or leaves clues. The kind of clues could be traces of vomit in your restroom or the client mentioning the use of laxatives.

Bulimia is a serious eating disorder and can be health and life threatening. For example, the digestive acids in the purged vomitus can damage the soft tissue leading from the mouth to the stomach, as well as the teeth. Sometimes, ipecac is used to induce vomiting, which is dangerous because ipecac is also a muscle poison that can accumulate in the body and damage vital organs such as the heart.

As with anorexia, the person with bulimia may be highly resistant to seeing her (bulimia usually affects females) behavior as a problem. Even if the therapist is able to refer the client to resources, the client may be unable or unwilling to use them. This is because the person with bulimia is highly invested in the bulimic behavior. Whether or not the person with bulimia accepts other professional help, massage therapy can continue, and it may have a positive effect on body image problems that accompany bulimia. One study on the effects of massage on bulimia showed lower levels of anxiety and depression for massaged subjects (Field et al., 1998). After a professional referral, the massage therapist may need to work very hard at letting go of being invested in the client changing the behavior.

Other Eating-Related Problems

Not all people with eating-related problems are underweight. A person coming into massage therapy who is obese is probably already painfully aware of the condition. Because body acceptance is one of the building blocks of healing in obesity, the massage therapist should avoid raising the issue of the client's weight. The client may come to massage to experience the body in a different way, not to be reminded of how he or she appears. If a client raises the issue, this may be an opportunity for a dialogue to begin.

Understanding their attitudes toward weight is essential for massage therapists. A therapist's negative attitudes toward overweight people can stand in the way of the self-acceptance that a client may need to develop to deal with the problem. For some people, self-acceptance is a precursor to losing weight. There clearly are many possible causes of obesity—many of which are not psychological—and no simple, single explanation in most cases. If there were, the solution would be easier.

Box 10.6

SIGNS OF BULIMIA

Signs of bulimia include:

▶ Recurrent episodes of binge eating, characterized by eating an excessive amount of food within a discrete period of time and by a sense of lack of control over eating during the episode
▶ Recurrent inappropriate compensatory behavior to prevent weight gain, such as self-induced vomiting or misuse of laxatives, diuretics, enemas, or other medications (purging); fasting; or excessive exercise
▶ Both binge eating and inappropriate compensatory behaviors occurring, on average, at least twice a week for 3 months
▶ Undue influence of body shape and weight on self-evaluation

(Adapted from National Institute of Mental Health. Eating Disorders. Publication No. 01-4901. Bethesda, MD: NIMH, 2001.)

SOMATOFORM DISORDER

Somatoform disorder (also spelled *somatiform*) involves physical symptoms that appear to be or are presented as a general medical condition; however, the physical symptoms or their severity and duration cannot be explained by a general medical condition, other mental disorder, or substance. The symptoms do cause distress and are not under the person's conscious control (Kroenke et al.; Merck). Somatoform disorders can be notoriously difficult to diagnose and constitute a specialty for which mental health practitioners can take extra certification. Reliable statistics on the occurrence of somatoform disorder are hard to come by because of the nature of the disorder (if you thought you were physically ill, you probably wouldn't go to a psychiatrist or psychotherapist!), but the frequency could be one of the highest of all psychiatric disorders.

The following are types of somatoform disorders. *Somatization disorder* is characterized by multiple somatic complaints that cannot be explained adequately based on physical examination. To make a body-oriented analogy, somatization could be looked at as a form of body-focused generalized dissociation. *Hypochondriasis* is characterized by unexplained physical symptoms related to fear of a specific medical condition or developing a serious disease, which often persist despite medical evaluation. People with hypochondriasis focus on the feared disease, in contrast to people with somatization disorder, who focus on symptoms. Hypochondriasis could be looked at as a form of body-focused panic. *Conversion disorder* is characterized by a loss or disturbance of a bodily function that does not conform to current concepts of the central or peripheral nervous system. Examples, although rare, are blindness, deafness, or paralysis, which cannot be accounted for by any physical cause. Conversion could be looked at as a form of body-focused dissociation (i.e., more extreme than somatization). *Somatoform pain* is a disorder characterized by persistent pain that is distressing, disabling, or both. The person's description of the pain exceeds what would be expected and is often felt in more than one place. *Body dysmorphic disorder* involves a disturbing preoccupation with an imagined physical defect or characteristic. Body dysmorphic disorder can accompany eating disorders, depression, and delusions. Some authorities include it as an OCD, whereas others state that it can accompany OCD. Body dysmorphic disorder even can be looked at as a form of body-focused OCD. Somatoform disorders do not include psychosomatic disorders and malingering (Kroenke et al.; Merck).

A causal explanation of somatoform disorders is that the body is expressing emotional conflicts that are translated unconsciously into physical problems or complaints. Considering that the number one complaint is some type of physical symptom and the bodymind has a central involvement in its psychodynamics, it is possible that a massage therapist may encounter a client with a somatoform disorder. People with a somatoform disorder are known to "shop around" and try different health care practitioners, especially when they do not want to accept what they have been told, so contacting a previous practitioner, if possible, may yield helpful information.

Massage clients with a somatoform disorder may benefit from anxiety reduction, increased body awareness, reconnection with the body, and increased tolerance for discomfort and bodily feelings and sensations. Improving grounding should also be beneficial. The massage therapist who is working with a client with a somatoform disorder should avoid being drawn into the client's transference issues with any of the client's therapists or health care providers. For example, the client may complain about another professional because he or she is dissatisfied with being told "it's in your head." In this case, the massage therapist should avoid colluding with the client, which could reinforce the pattern, yet should remain supportive. Also, avoid saying to the client that nothing is wrong, since acceptance by the therapist of the client's somatic symptoms as being real is important.

In terms of countertransference, as a body-oriented practitioner you may be tempted to try to "cure" the symptoms that have proved so elusive for probably many other health care providers. Such a countertransference can damage your objectivity as a practitioner.

MOOD DISORDERS

Mood disorders can be divided into two categories: depressive disorders and bipolar disorder (see the definition).

Depressive Disorders

Depressive disorders, also called *unipolar disorders*, are characterized by feelings of sadness or emptiness and diminished interest or pleasure in activities. Other signs and symptoms are identified in Box 10.7 These symptoms must be present for at least 2 weeks to be considered a depressive mood disorder. Women experience depression two times more often than men. Men, however, tend to express depression through being irritable, angry, and discouraged, rather than feeling hopeless and helpless (Blehar and Oren). Just as significant is that up to 15% of people with major depression die by suicide. In any given 1-year period, 9.5% of the population, or about 18.8 million American adults, suffer from a depressive illness, making depression the most prevalent mental disorder (NIMH, 2000; Nathan et al.).

Because *depression* affects so many people, some further discussion is warranted. We all have felt sad and depressed—"blue"—at some time in our lives, usually in response to a disappointment or loss. This kind of depression, called *acute situational depression*, does not last and is not considered a psychopathological condition. However, when a person does not recover as quickly and also suffers some loss of function, then this type of depression is called *major depression or clinical depression*. Major depression involves a combination of symptoms (see Box 10.7) that interfere with the ability to work, study, sleep, eat, and enjoy once pleasurable activities. Such a disabling episode may happen only once, but more commonly occurs several times in a life-

Mood

Mood usually signifies a longer-term emotional tone than does *affect* (displayed emotion). Mood may also be taken to mean a more internal and less observable state than affect.

Box 10.7

SYMPTOMS OF DEPRESSION AND MANIA

Signs of Depression

► Persistent sad, anxious, or "empty" mood
► Feelings of hopelessness, pessimism
► Feelings of guilt, worthlessness, helplessness
► Loss of interest or pleasure in hobbies and activities that were once enjoyed, including sex
► Decreased energy, fatigue, being "slowed down"
► Difficulty concentrating, remembering, and making decisions
► Insomnia, early morning awakening, or oversleeping
► Appetite and/or weight loss or overeating and weight gain
► Thoughts of death or suicide; suicide attempts
► Restlessness, irritability
► Persistent physical symptoms that do not respond to treatment, such as headaches, digestive disorders, and chronic pain

Signs of Mania

► Abnormal or excessive elation
► Unusual irritability
► Decreased need for sleep
► Grandiose notions
► Increased talking
► Racing thoughts
► Increased sexual desire
► Markedly increased energy
► Poor judgment
► Inappropriate social behavior

(Adapted from National Institute of Mental Health. Depression. Publication No. 00-3561. Bethesda, MD: NIMH, 2000.)

times. A less severe type of depression, *dysthymia*, involves long-term, chronic symptoms that do not disable, but keep one from functioning well or from feeling good.

Other forms of depression are *seasonal affective disorder (SAD)*; *postpartum depression*, which happens after childbirth; and *premenstrual syndrome* (PMS, or *late luteal phase dysphoric disorder*), which happens before menstruation. SAD is a pattern of major depressive episodes that come and go with changes in seasons. The most recognized form of SAD, "winter depression," is characterized by recurrent episodes of depression, excessive sleep, increased appetite with carbohydrate craving, and weight gain that begin in the autumn and continue through the winter (Saeed and Bruce).

In the not-too-distant past, experiencing depression was often regarded as a character flaw, and people were expected to "snap out of it." However, now a better understanding exists that many cases of depression have biochemical origins, so the old attitudes about it being a flaw that should be controlled by will power were unfair.

In a biochemically based depression, even excellent psychological work may not be enough. The client should be in the care of a psychiatrist, psychopharmacologist, or primary care physician to prescribe and monitor treatment. Medication is used to treat the biochemical causes and to control the symptoms so that the person can cope and be more receptive to psychotherapy. Medication for depression has undergone significant advancement in the last decade and continues to be a focus of research. Some medications prescribed for depression (depending on the type of depression) are Prozac, Zoloft, Paxil, Luvox, Effexor, Nardil, Parnate, Pamelor, Anafranil, Celexa, Remeron, Serzone, Wellbutrin, Tegretol, Depakote, Lamictal, Neurontin, and Lithium (Duralith, Eskalith, Lithobid). If a client mentions that he or she is taking one of these drugs during taking a history, for example, then this information could prompt you to think about the possibility of depression in the client and direct your inquiries and work accordingly. In more difficult cases of depression, a "cocktail," or a combination of several of these drugs, may be prescribed. More controversial treatments for depression are acupuncture, herbal therapy (primarily St. John's wort), and electroconvulsive therapy (electroshock or ECT).

Massage therapy can be an effective adjunctive therapy for nonpsychotic depression, but cannot serve as the primary therapy. Massage therapy may help the depressed client to feel more energized and less lethargic. One study showed that massage therapy lowered levels of depression and anxiety (Field et al., 1992), whereas another study showed similar effects for depressed adolescent mothers (Field et al., 1996). The touch contact provided by massage may also help create a greater sense of grounding and bounding, which should positively affect both depression and mania. Touch may also help the client to feel less isolated. If the person has a psychological history of emotional deprivation, the touch and energy provided by massage can be healthful.

Bipolar Disorder

The second form of mood disorders is *bipolar disorder*. Bipolar disorder is characterized by one or more depressive episodes accompanied by or alternating with manic episodes (manic symptoms are listed in Box 10.7). A *manic episode* is defined in the DSM-IV (p. 328) as a, "distinct period of persistently elevated, expansive, or irritable mood, lasting at least four days. [A manic episode is characterized by] inflated self esteem or grandiosity, decreased need for sleep, more talkative than usual, distractibility, flight of ideas, subjective experience of racing thoughts, increase in goal directed activity, or excessive involvement in pleasurable high risk activities (e.g., unrestrained buying sprees, sexual indiscretions, or foolish business investments)."

Bipolar disorder tends to cycle or swing between depressive and manic poles (hence *bi*polar, rather than one end or pole, which is *uni*polar). The individual may be exuberant and elated, become overactive, feel all-powerful, and feel an almost invincible state of well-being for a certain amount of time and then begin to plunge into a dark depression in which he or she becomes lethargic or almost inert (Figure 10.1). Bipolar disorder typically develops in late adolescence or early adulthood. However, some people have their first symptoms during childhood, and some develop them late in life. More than 2 million American adults, or about 1% of the population age 18 and older in any given year, have bipolar disorder (NIMH, 2000). At least 25% of people in the depressed phase of bipolar disorder attempt suicide, and up to 50% are suicidal when they begin treatment. Less than one third of people with bipolar disorder ever receive treatment, which is the *lowest* percentage of any mental health disorder (Nathan et al.).

Several variations of the bipolar theme are identified. The classic form of the illness, which involves recurrent episodes of mania and depression, is called *bipolar I disorder*. A mild to moderate level of mania is called *hypomania*. Hypomania may feel good to the person and may even be credited with fostering enhanced functioning and productivity, so the person may deny that anything is wrong. Without proper treatment, however, hypomania can become severe mania in some people or can switch into depression. *Cyclothymia* is marked by manic and depressive states; yet neither is of sufficient intensity or duration to be considered bipolar disorder or major depressive disorder. When milder episodes of hypomania alternate with depression, this form of the illness is called *bipolar II disorder*. Finally, some people have mania only.

The sort of depression experienced in unipolar depression and the depression experienced in bipolar disorder have some differences. For example, unipolar depression is usually associated with a later age at onset (36 years) than bipolar disorder (28 years); people with unipolar depression tend to have insomnia and agitation, whereas people with bipolar disorder typically sleep more than usual and are lethargic; and more blood relatives of people with bipolar disorder have mood disorders than do the relatives of those with unipolar depression.

Researchers have many theories, but do not yet understand exactly what causes the cyclical nature of the bipolar disorder or how it works. They do know that the cycles can be wide and slow or very rapid, which is called *rapid cycling depression* (defined as more than four major mood cycles per year). At one time, manic depression was automatically considered a form of psychosis. This is because the person may enter into a depressed or manic phase that is so intense or extreme that he or she loses touch with reality. For example, as a person moves toward the peak of a manic phase, the feelings of power and greatness may escalate until he or she comes to believe that he/she is a famous historical figure, such as Napoleon, a U.S. president, or Jesus.

A typical problem that arises is that as the person builds a feeling of invincibility and super well-being owing to the mania, he or she stops taking medication, believing that it is no longer necessary. Without the medication, the mania escalates unabatedly.

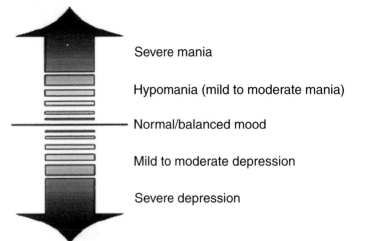

Severe mania

Hypomania (mild to moderate mania)

Normal/balanced mood

Mild to moderate depression

Severe depression

Figure 10.1
The bipolar spectrum. *The various mood states in bipolar disorder can be organized in a spectrum or progressive range. At one end is severe depression, then moderate depression, and then mild low mood, which many people call "the blues" when it is short-lived, but termed dysthymia when it is chronic. Next is normal or balanced mood, then hypomania (mild to moderate mania), and severe mania at the other end of the spectrum. (With permission from Bipolar Disorder, National Institute of Mental Health (NIMH) Publication No. 01-3679. Bethesda, Maryland, 2001.)*

As with depressive disorder, massage therapy can be an effective adjunctive therapy for nonpsychotic forms of bipolar disorder and mania, but it cannot serve as the primary therapy. Massage can be used for the depressive phases of bipolar disorder, as stated in the section on depressive disorder. Providing grounding and bounding through touch is also helpful. For manic phases, *for some people* massage therapy can provide a calming affect. For others, massage can either stimulate the mania or have no effect. Because there is no way to predict how a person with mania will respond to massage, you need to closely monitor the person's responses.

PSYCHOSIS

Psychosis is commonly thought of as "madness" or "crazy" behavior. It is clinically defined as a severe mental condition characterized by a loss of contact with common reality and by impaired thinking, perception, or judgment. It can be defined conceptually as a loss of *ego boundaries* (a sense of self and the ability to differentiate between oneself and the rest of the world) or gross impairment in *reality testing* (differentiating between reality and nonreality). Symptoms present in people with psychosis include delusions (false, strongly held beliefs not influenced by logical reasoning or explained by a person's usual cultural concepts), hallucinations (hearing, seeing, or otherwise sensing the presence of things not actually there), disorganized speech, and grossly disorganized or *catatonic behavior*. Catatonic behavior is physical immobility or stupor or purposeless excessive activity; an apparent motiveless resistance to all instructions or maintenance of a rigid posture against attempts to being moved; mutism; repetitive odd movements; or senseless repetition of a word, phrase, or movements of another person.

Psychosis can manifest as a brief episode lasting a day to a month. This is called a *psychotic break* or *episodic psychosis* and may occur once in a person's life or many times. It can also manifest as a longer-term disorder, *chronic psychosis*. Current research suggests that genetics, certain illnesses, or injuries cause chronic psychosis. However, substance abuse or extreme stress can also cause brief psychosis.

Subclassifications of psychosis can be roughly divided into schizophrenic spectrum disorders and psychotic affective spectrum disorders. *Schizophrenic spectrum disorders* (sometimes termed *thought disorders*) consist of various forms of *schizophrenia*, a chronic, severe, and disabling brain disease, typified by delusions, hallucinations, disorganized speech, and grossly disorganized or catatonic behavior and what are called *negative symptoms*—apathy, a flattening of emotional expressiveness, poverty of speech, social isolation, and socially deviant behavior. These symptoms may leave people with the disorder fearful and withdrawn. Their speech and behavior can be so disorganized that they may be incomprehensible or frightening to others. Schizophrenia is *not* "split personality," such as a Dr. Jekyll-Mr. Hyde switch in character. Approximately 1% of the population develops schizophrenia during their lifetime; more than 2 million Americans suffer from the illness in a given year (NIMH, 1999). Although schizophrenia affects men and women equal frequently, it tends to appear earlier in men, usually in the late teens or early 20s, whereas women are generally affected in their 20s to early 30s. Contrary to popular perceptions that schizophrenia follows an inevitable downhill slide into total dysfunction, about half of those afflicted improve or recover. However, 10% die by suicide (Nathan et al.).

Psychotic affective spectrum disorders (sometimes termed *mood disorders*) involve elevation or depression of a person's emotional state. Most mood disorders are *not* forms of psychosis and are considered psychotic only when general psychotic symptoms such as hallucinations, delusions, disorganized speech, and other grossly disorganized behaviors appear, that is, when psychosis is primary. The psychotic affective spectrum disorders are *major depression with psychotic features*, and *bipolar depression* or *mania with psychotic features*. The term *schizoaffective disorder* may be used to distinguish a schizophrenic disorder in which a mood disorder is independently present.

Although the cause of psychosis and schizophrenia is not fully known, current thinking is that it is a brain disease caused by a chemical defect or a physical abnormality of the brain or both. A person under treatment for psychosis is very likely taking certain antipsychotic medications. The following medications *may* indicate that the client is being treated for psychosis: Haldol, Stelazine, Thorazine, Prolixin, Navane, Moban, Risperdal, Zyprexa, Seroquel, Clozaril, Serentil, Trilifon, Mellaril, Geodon, or Loxitane.

Although psychosis is generally considered a contraindication for massage, if a massage therapist does proceed with a psychotic client, it is extremely important that the massage therapist works closely with the client's psychiatrist or psychotherapist *and* have training in working with psychopathological conditions. However, most massage therapists are not trained or experienced in working with people with psychosis, and you are strongly cautioned not do so unless you have such training and experience. For some psychotic individuals, receiving touch can be very disturbing, disorienting, or fragmenting. For others, it can be nurturing or supporting.

SEXUAL OR PHYSICAL ABUSE

Abuse is a highly charged topic about which much has been written. Symptoms of *sexual* or *physical abuse* may arise during massage (Box 10.8). It is sometimes the first place that someone begins remembering abuse. This is because massage deals directly with the body.

Box 10.8

SYMPTOMS OF ABUSE

The symptoms of abuse are extensive in number and nature. As lengthy as this list is, it does not include every symptom denoted in the literature. Because there can be many other causes for many of these symptoms, not making any assumptions about abuse simply because a person's symptom appears on this list is *essential*. Problems stemming from sexual or physical abuse can include:

- ▶ Absence of memories for a period of childhood
- ▶ Disinterest or excessive interest in sexual feeling or activities
- ▶ Inability to differentiate or combine sex, affection, and intimacy
- ▶ Various sexual dysfunctions
- ▶ Fear of dating or close relationships
- ▶ Feelings of shame
- ▶ Feeling as if something is inherently wrong or defective with oneself
- ▶ Low self-esteem
- ▶ Body image distortions
- ▶ Dissociative experiences (disconnection between mind and body, not being in one's body)
- ▶ Emotional "numbing"
- ▶ Depression
- ▶ Eating disorders
- ▶ Anxiety disorders
- ▶ Variety of self-destructive behaviors (alcohol abuse, drug abuse, self-mutilation, etc.)
- ▶ Inability to say no to others
- ▶ Difficulty nurturing self
- ▶ Not trusting own perceptions and feelings
- ▶ Physical symptoms with no medical cause
- ▶ Feeling betrayed and repulsed by own body
- ▶ Withdrawing or flinching from touch
- ▶ Difficulty with trusting self/others with intimacy
- ▶ Self-imposed isolation or excessive neediness
- ▶ Toleration of abusive patterns
- ▶ Issues with boundaries, control, and abandonment, along with symptoms of post-traumatic stress disorder, such as flashbacks, hypervigilance, agitation, and severe trouble sleeping

However, simply because the massage therapist's work was able to bring such material into consciousness or out into the open, it does not necessarily follow that the massage therapist alone is also able to help the client work through the issues involved with the abuse. As more is learned about working with abused people, it becomes clearer that it is a very complex situation to deal with therapeutically and calls for well-trained expertise. If a recovered memory was bad enough to be buried out of consciousness for many years, which is a complicated psychological defense, the solution to dealing with the abuse and all its psychological ramifications is a delicate and complex matter.

Even if the massage therapist suspects that a client has a past history of sexual or physical abuse, not offering this as an interpretation or leading the client to this conclusion is very important. In the late 1980s and early 1990s, the psychotherapeutic community and society finally acknowledged sexual and physical abuse as serious and recurrent problems. Although this acknowledgment finally validated the experience of many victims of abuse, it also led to an imposition of that theory onto many individuals who had ambiguous symptoms. As much as the acknowledgment of abuse helped scores of people, misdiagnosis also harmed others. Following your client's process of discovery is the surest path. Your client, while on the table, may have only fragments of vague body sensations or may experience complete memories. If your client is really struggling, a referral to a specialist is in order.

Massage therapy can be an effective adjunct to working with sexual and physical abuse if done in collaboration with a mental health professional who has specialized training in working with this condition. *In the case of sexual or physical abuse, the body is the medium for the psychological wound.* Therefore, helping the client feel safe and cared for on the body level may be an essential component to healing. Two studies showed that receiving massage therapy resulted in lower anxiety and stress levels in subjects who had been sexually abused (Field et al., 1997; Mattsson et al.).

CHRONIC PAIN

Chronic pain is pain that continues a month or more beyond the usual recovery period for its cause or pain that goes on over months or years because of a chronic condition. Sometimes, no initial cause of the pain is identifiable. Pain may be continuous or may come and go. Many conditions are coupled with chronic pain (Box 10.9). Approximately 90 million people in the United States have a chronic pain condition (Koestler and Myers).

Box 10.9

CONDITIONS CAUSING OR ASSOCIATED WITH CHRONIC PAIN

Many conditions can cause or are associated with chronic pain.
Most Common Causes

▶ Chronic low back pain
▶ Chronic headaches
▶ Fibromyalgia
▶ Rheumatoid arthritis, osteoarthritis, and other disorders of the muscles and joints

Other Common Causes

▶ Chronic neck pain from whiplash injuries
▶ Cancer
▶ Heart disease
▶ Sickle cell disease
▶ Lupus
▶ Interstitial cystitis and other chronic pelvic area pain problems
▶ Pain associated with gastrointestinal disorders (such as irritable bowel syndrome and Crohn's disease)

Less Common Causes

▶ Diseases of the nervous system including diabetic neuropathy, postherpetic neuralgia, tic douloureux (trigeminal neuralgia), and reflex sympathetic dystrophy

Psychologically, chronic pain also can disrupt one's sense of control and self-esteem, and occupational and family roles. Coworkers, friends, and family members may not understand the pain problem and become frustrated and frustrating in attempts to be helpful. Family members also may try to pick up the roles that chronic pain sufferers can no longer fulfill, leading possibly to resentments and family conflicts. As a consequence, chronic pain sufferers may become increasingly isolated. Old ways of dealing with problems may no longer be effective in managing their pain. If unable to work, then they often become engaged in struggles with their employer or disability provider. For some, taking increasing numbers or doses of medications raises the risk of drug dependence.

Chronic pain also has its own set of internal physical and psychological dynamics. Stress reactions and pain cause the mind and body to become aroused and ready for action. Increased emotional and physical tension accompany this state and may become chronic, resulting in a downward spiral of further increased pain, reduction of function, and increased risk of depression, anxiety, and anger. Chronic pain sufferers may find it difficult to focus on things other than their pain and may lose access to the satisfying activities they previously enjoyed. Others may find it difficult to reduce their expectations and may overdo things, resulting in further injuries or a cycle of overwork and disability.

Through learning to reduce emotional and physical tension, manage stress, and interrupt the pain cycle, people with chronic pain can learn active and effective ways of coping with pain and related sources of distress. Understanding what causes fluctuation in pain intensity, having a more restorative sleep pattern, communicating more effectively, adjusting to their losses, limiting overexertion, and dealing with the limitations that pain has caused are also helpful. These methods may be helpful for achieving goals of increased self-control, reduced medication dependency, increased enjoyment of activities and relationships, and increased functional capacity and quality of life (Box 10.10).

Massage can be beneficial for chronic pain because of its ability to reduce tension and stress, positively affect the pain cycle, strengthen the immune system, and promote health. However, to convey these benefits successfully, the massage therapist must be able to manage the particular set of challenges presented by chronic pain. If, as a massage therapist, you feel "stuck" with someone who suffers chronic pain, referring such a client to a mental health professional who is experienced in working with chronic pain sufferers may be advisable.

Another challenge is that working with clients with chronic pain can cause countertransference. For example, a massage therapist may have the expectation that massage therapy should be able to reduce chronic pain; this may cause the massage therapist to become frustrated with the slowness or inability of the client to respond to treatment or to suffer a loss of confidence in one's work. If this is the case, then supervision is warranted.

Box 10.10

FACTORS AFFECTING PAIN

Factors that increase pain levels and factors that decrease pain levels.

Increase Pain Levels	Decrease Pain Levels
▶ Increased disease activity	▶ Positive internal dialogue
▶ Overdoing	▶ Monitored exercise
▶ Stress	▶ Relaxation
▶ Focusing on pain	▶ Medication (if appropriate)
▶ Fatigue	▶ Distraction (not focusing on pain)
▶ Improper body mechanics	▶ Conditioning
▶ Anxiety	▶ Strengthening
▶ Depression	▶ Ice
▶ Negative internal dialogue	▶ Heat (nonacute pain)

(Adapted from Koestler, Angela, and Myers, Ann. *Understanding Chronic Pain.* Jackson, MS: University Press of Mississippi, 2002.)

Box 10.11

CHRONIC ILLNESSES

Types of chronic illness include (mental health disorders not included):

Alzheimer's disease	Hypertension
Arthritis	Irritable bowel syndrome
Asthma	Kidney disease
Cancer	Lupus
Chronic fatigue syndrome	Lyme disease
Chronic pain syndromes	Lymphedema
Crohn's disease	Multiple sclerosis
Cystic fibrosis	Muscular dystrophy
Dental/oral health problems (various)	Osteoporosis
Diabetes	Parkinson's disease
Epilepsy	Scoliosis
Fibromyalgia	Skin disorders (various)
Heart disease	Stroke
Hepatitis	Thyroid disorders (various)
HIV/AIDS	Ulcerative colitis

CHRONIC ILLNESS

How people deal with *chronic illness* depends on several factors. The first factor is the degree of severity. Chronic illness can range from mild to severe. For instance, some people with lifelong asthma are only occasionally bothered by it, whereas for others asthma is life threatening. Therefore, the massage therapist should ascertain the severity of the chronic illness both in terms of the physical treatment and in the understanding of what effect that living with this illness might have on the client (Box 10.11).

A second factor is management of the illness and how well the client is able to participate in the management. Some chronic illnesses such as hypothyroidism are easily manageable for certain individuals. For example, the management may consist only of taking a pill on an empty stomach. As the management becomes more complex and difficult or the disease less stable, the client usually has increasing difficulty complying with what needs to be done. In particular, adjustments in lifestyle might feel too difficult. For example, some adult-onset diabetes can be managed with a change in diet. However, some people who are encountering this disease find that they feel "unable" to make healthy dietary changes.

Clients with chronic illnesses may feel acceptance of their condition, or they may feel unfairly singled out by fate and burdened. Management of complex illnesses may take a lot of time, which the person may resent. This management may also involve activities that may make the ill person feel "different" from others, such as eating or sleeping differently. This sense of "difference" may create shame and make management less attractive. The type of chronic illness can be a source of shame, particularly with such illnesses as AIDS and cancer, which sometimes leads the person to hide his or her condition from others. If the massage therapist harbors any judgment about the type of illness that the client has, the therapist must seek supervision to help both him- or herself and the client.

Working with a client who has a chronic illness and is resisting caring for him- or herself may bring up countertransference issues. The massage therapist may feel the need to be a cheerleader, the health police, or the good mother or father in order to get the client to take care of him- or herself. Another possibility is that the therapist may respond to the client's defenses with attitudes such as lack of empathy, contempt, or superiority. Avoiding enmeshment in the client's dynamics may become difficult with clients for whom a highly unstable chronic illness is combined with poor self-management. Therefore, in working with clients with chronic illness, the massage therapist needs to understand both what it takes for the client to manage the disease and also that the massage therapist is not responsible. If countertransference issues develop, then supervision is likely needed.

The client's prognosis is another important factor in how a person deals with chronic illness. Although most chronic illness is stable, some chronic illnesses such as cancer, heart disease, diabetes, and others have the potential of becoming disabling or life threatening. It may be important for the massage therapist to understand what degree of threat the client is living with, if any. The potential for mortal danger can cause a high degree of stress. Indeed, chronic illness can bring up a variety of fears for the client (Box 10.12).

The massage therapist might also work with the caregivers of clients with chronic illness. The well-being of caregivers can often be forgotten because the illness takes center stage. However, caregiving can be extremely stressful and draining, depending on the severity of the disease. Caregivers may need a lot of room to talk during a massage about what they are going through. The massage therapist needs to be prepared to hear without judgment the caregiver express negative feelings about the situation and the chronically ill client. It is normal for these negative feelings to occur and need to be expressed. The massage therapist does not need to do anything about these feelings, other than to allow their expression.

Box 10.12

THE EIGHT FEARS OF CHRONIC ILLNESS

As therapists, we need to understand the fears associated with chronic conditions and be able to honor the reality of the fears of the client. These could also be applied to chronic pain.

1. **Fear of loss of control**
2. **Fear of loss of self-image**
3. **Fear of dependency**
4. **Fear of stigma**
5. **Fear of abandonment**
6. **Fear of expressing anger**
7. **Fear of isolation**
8. **Fear of death**

(Adapted from comments by Ray Moriyasu.)

UNCONTROLLABLE ANGER OR RAGE

Uncontrollable anger or rage is a condition that differs from an emotional release of anger or rage during massage. When someone has an emotional release, it is inherently uncontrolled. However, this section is referring to a situation in which a person is unable to control strong emotions in most situations. A person prone to uncontrollable anger often has a hypersensitivity to feeling slighted, challenged, disrespected, or thwarted. The reaction to these feelings seems out of proportion; that is, such people use a nuclear weapon when a flyswatter would do. Anger and rage with this type of person escalate quickly and easily; that is, they go from "zero to 60 in three seconds." People in relationships with these persons may feel intimidated and scared. Because the reactions are unpredictable, they do not know what will set them off.

The reason that uncontrollable anger is being mentioned here is because of the following. If a massage therapist encounters this condition, understanding that the cause may not be due to unresolved emotional blocks or emotional release, but can be caused by biochemical imbalances or a sign of a physical illness such as a brain tumor, is important. Usually, someone with uncontrollable rage does not get very far before encountering some kind of intervention. However, a more likely time when a massage therapist might encounter this would be while the condition is developing. In this case, if it is possible, referring the person for a complete physical examination may be best.

Uncontrollable anger or rage can also be the result of a psychological condition, for example, bipolar disorder, psychosis, dissociative disorder, or Tourette's syndrome. Domestic violence and abuse are excellent examples of situations that may involve this problem. Although deep emotional releases of anger can be helpful, what is really necessary is psychological counseling and work to manage and channel anger into appropriate expression. Therefore, a referral would be in order.

MARITAL PROBLEMS

Marital problems are included here because they can come up in the course of a session. Marital problems—which could be expanded to include problems in any intimate relationship—may seem to be everyday problems that do not seem like psychological problems, so the therapist may not feel as concerned about being careful with marital problems as with another type of problem. Such a mistaken attitude can lead to errors; for example, giving advice for such problems is often tempting. Not only is this not appropriate, if the advice does not work it may create bad feelings and damage trust on the part of the client and interfere with the massage therapy. If you are working with a client with marital problems, remain aware that clients are particularly vulnerable when having such problems, which can lead to transference and countertransference issues. Respecting and being sensitive to their vulnerability help to avoid possible complications in the therapeutic relationship. Marital problems should be treated as any other psychological problem would be and should be referred to an appropriate professional if and when an appropriate opportunity to do so presents itself.

In summary, a cardinal rule in all cases is: *when in doubt, DON'T.* Regarding possible psychological disorders, this means that whenever you feel you are working outside the scope of your abilities, you should not proceed. Instead, consult a colleague, supervisor, or a professional in another field, or refer the client to a professional who is qualified to work with such a problem or situation. To be able to best heed this cardinal rule, a therapist must have a clear understanding of the focus or scope of his/her work, that is, what kind of clients and problems he or she works with in the practice and what kinds he or she does not. Also, have a clear sense of the range of your capabilities, that is, what you are trained to do. For more information about the conditions and disorders discussed, consult the Resources section on p. 250.

Having reviewed mental health conditions and disorders, in Chapter 11 we discuss to whom you should refer clients who have these conditions and disorders.

REFERENCES

American Academy of Pain Medicine, American Pain Society, and American Society of Addiction Medicine. (2001). *Definitions related to the use of opioids for the treatment of pain.* Consensus document.

American Psychiatric Association.(1994). *Diagnostic and statistical manual for mental disorders* (4th ed.) (DSM-IV). Washington, DC: American Psychiatric Press.

American Psychiatric Association Work Group on Eating Disorders. (2000). *Practice guideline for the treatment of patients with eating disorders* (revision). American Journal of Psychiatry, *157* (Suppl. 1), 1–39.

Becker, A.E., Grinspoon, S.K., Klibanski, A. & Herzog, D.B. (1999). Eating disorders. *New England Journal of Medicine, 340* (14),1092–1098.

Blehar, M.D. & Oren, DA. (1997). Gender differences in depression. *Medscape Women's Health, 2,* 3.

Davidson, J.R. (2000). Trauma: The impact of post-traumatic stress disorder. *Journal of Psychopharmacology, 14* (Suppl 1), S5–S12.

Feeny, N.C., Zoellner, L.A., Fitzgibbons, L.A., et al. (2000). Exploring the roles of emotional numbing, depression, and dissociation in PTSD. *Journal of Traumatic Stress, 13* (3), 489–498.

Field T., Seligman S., Scafidi F. & Schanberg, S. (1996). Alleviating posttraumatic stress in children following hurricane Andrew. *Journal of Applied Developmental Psychology, 17,* 37–50.

Field, T., Quintino, O., Hernandez-Reif, M. & Koslovsky, G. Adolescents with attention deficit hyperactivity disorder benefit from massage therapy. *Adolescence, 33,* 103–108.

Field, T., Schanberg, S., Kuhn, C., et al. (1998). Bulimic adolescents benefit from massage therapy. *Adolescence, 33,* 555–563.

Field, T., Hernandez-Reif, M., Hart, S., Quintino, O., et al. (1997). Effects of sexual abuse are lessened by massage therapy. *Journal of Bodywork and Movement Therapies, 1,* 65–69.

Field, T., Grizzle, N., Scafidi, F. & Schanberg, S. (1996). Massage and relaxation therapies' effects on depressed adolescent mothers. *Adolescence, 31,* 903–911.

Field, T., Morrow, C., Valdeon, C., et al. (1992). Massage reduces anxiety in child and adolescent psychiatric patients. *Journal of the American Academy of Child & Adolescent Psychiatry, 31,* 125–131.

Hart, S., Field, T., Hernandez-Reif, M., et al. (2001). Anorexia nervosa symptoms are reduced by massage therapy. *Eating Disorders, 9,* 217–228.

Hyman, S.E. (2001). A 28-year-old man addicted to cocaine. *Journal of the American Medical Association, 286,* 2586–2594.

Hyman, S.E. & Rudorfer, M.V. (2000). Depressive and bipolar mood disorders. In: Dale, D.C. & Federman, D.D. (Eds.) *Scientific American*(r); *Medicine.* Vol. 3. New York: Healtheon/WebMD Corp. Sect. 13.

Hyman, S.E. (1999). Introduction to the complex genetics of mental disorders. *Biological Psychiatry, 45* (5), 518–21.

Koestler, A. & Myers, A. (2002). *Understanding chronic pain.* Jackson, MS: University Press of Mississippi.

Kroenke, K., Spitzer, R.L. & deGruy, F.V. (1998). A symptom checklist to screen for somatoform disorders in primary care. *Psychosomatics, 39* (3), 263–272.

Mattsson, M., Wikman, M., Dahlgren L, et al. (1997). Body awareness therapy with sexually abused women. *Journal of Bodywork and Movement Therapies, 1,* 280–288.

McMillen, M. (2002). Paying attention to adult ADHD. *The Washington Post.* F1. July 30.

Merck Laboratories. (1999). *Merck Manual,* Seventeenth Edition. Rahway, NJ.

Nathan, P., Gorman, J. & Salkind, N. (1999). *Treating mental disorders.* New York: Oxford University Press.

National Council on Alcoholism and Drug Dependence.(1996). *Definition of alcoholism.*

National Institute on Alcohol Abuse and Alcoholism. (2002). *Alcohol alert no.56: Screening for alcohol problems-an update.* Rockville, MD: NIAAA.

National Institute of Mental Health. (2001). *Alcoholism: Getting the facts.* Publication No. 96-4153. Bethesda, MD: NIMH.

National Institute of Mental Health. (1996). *Attention deficit hyperactivity disorder.* Publication No. 96-3572. Bethesda, MD: NIMH.

National Institute of Mental Health (2001). *Bipolar disorder.* Publication No. 01-3679. Bethesda, MD: NIMH.

National Institute of Mental Health. (2000). *Depression.* Publication No. 00-3561. Bethesda, MD: NIMH.

National Institute of Mental Health. (2001). *Eating disorders.* Publication No. 01-4901. Bethesda, MD: NIMH.

National Institute of Mental Health. (2001). *Facts about anxiety disorders.* Publication No. OM-99 4152. Bethesda, MD: NIMH.

National Institute of Mental Health. (1999). *Obsessive-compulsive disorder.* Publication No. 99-3755. Bethesda, MD: NIMH.

National Institute of Mental Health. (2001). *Reliving trauma: Post-traumatic stress disorder.* Publication No. 01-4597. Bethesda, MD: NIMH.

National Institute of Mental Health. (1999). *Schizophrenia.* Publication No. 99-3517. Bethesda, MD: NIMH.

National Institute of Mental Health. (1995). *The physician's guide to helping patients with alcohol problems.* Publication No. 95-3769. Bethesda, MD: NIMH.

National Institute of Mental Health. (1995). *Understanding panic disorder.* Publication No. 95-3509. Bethesda, MD: NIMH.

Pursch, J. (1998). Is there a common basis for all addictions? *Psychiatric Times, 15,* 4.

Robins, L.N. & Regier, D.A. (Eds). (1990). *Psychiatric disorders in America: The epidemiologic catchment area study.* New York: The Free Press.

Saeed, S. & Bruce, T. (1998). Seasonal affective disorders. *American Family Physician.* 1340–1357.

Szamraj, L. (1999). Understanding the dynamics of addiction. *Positive Living,* May.

Widom, C.S. (1999). Posttraumatic stress disorder in abused and neglected children grown up. *American Journal of Psychiatry, 156* (8),1223–1229.

RESOURCES

General Anxiety, Phobias, Panic Disorder
The Anxiety Network
http://www.anxietynetwork.com/

The Panic Disorder Home Page
http://www.mentalhealth.com/dis/p20-an01.html

The Anxiety/Panic Resource
http://www.algy.com/anxiety

National Panic/Anxiety Disorder Association
1718 Burgundy Place, Suite B
Santa Rosa, CA 95403
707-527-5738

Anxiety Disorder Association of America
11900 Parklawn Drive, Suite 100
Rockville, MD 20852
301-231-9350

Obsessive-Compulsive Disorder
OCD Reading List
http://www.suncompsvc.com/ocd/reading.htm

The Obsessive Compulsive Disorder Forum
http://www.nibmusnet.com/wwwboard/ocdboard.html

Obsessive Compulsive Foundation
P.O. Box 70
Milford, CT 06460
203-878-5669

Post-Traumatic Stress Disorder
The National Center for Post-Traumatic Stress Disorder
http://www.dartmouth.edu/dms/ptsd/

David Baldwin's Trauma Information Pages
http://www.trama-pages.com/

National Center for Post-Traumatic Stress Disorder
Rural Route 3
White River Junction, VT 05009
802-296-5132

Attention-Deficit and Hyperactivity Disorder
The School of Education at Virginia
http://teis.virginia.edu/go/cise/ose/categories/add.html

National Attention Deficit Disorder Association
http://www.add.org

Substance Abuse
The National Clearing House for Alcohol and Drug Information
http://www.health.org/aboutn.htm

Online Intergroup of Alcoholics Anonymous
http://www.aa-intergroup.org/index.html

Center for Substance Abuse Prevention
5600 Fishers Lane
Rockville, MD 20857
301-443-0365

Eating Disorders

The Eating Disorders – Diagnosis and Treatment Web Site
http://home.planetinternet.be/~elombaer/ased/dia.htm#bulimia

American Anorexia/Bulimia Association
http://www.social.com/health/nhic/data/hr0100/hr0123.html

Cath's Links to Eating Disorders on the Internet
http://www.stud.unit.no/studorg/ikstrh/ed/

National Association of Anorexia Nervosa and Associated Disorders
P.O. Box 7
Highland Park, IL 60035
847-831-3438

Depression and Bipolar Disorder

Dr. Ivan's Page
http://www.psycom.net/depression.central.html

Mood Disorders
http://www.psych.helsinki.fi/~janne/mood/mood.html

Depression.com
http://depression.com

Depression and Bipolar Support Alliance
(formerly the National Depressive and Manic-Depressive Association)
730 North Franklin, Suite 501
Chicago, IL 60610
1-800-82-NDMDA

The National Foundation for Depressive Illness
P.O. Box 2257
New York, NY 10116
1-800-248-4344

Schizophrenia

The Schizophrenia Home Page
http://www.schizophrenia.com

National Alliance for Research on Schizophrenia and Depression
http://www.mhsource.com/advocacy/narsad/schiz.html

NARSAD Research
60 Cutter Mill Road, Suite 404
Great Neck, NY 11021
800-829-8289

Sexual Abuse

Sexual Offense Recovery Online
http://www.sexualoffenserecovery.com/

The Wounded Healer Journal
http://idealist.com/wounded_healer/index.shtml

Chronic Pain

Pain.com
http://www/pain.com

American Chronic Pain Association
P.O. Box 850
Rocklin, CA 95677
916-632-0922
http://www.theacpa.org

National Chronic Pain Outreach Association
7979 Old Georgetown Road
Bethesda, MD 20814
301-652-49480

Chronic Illness
Chronicillnet
www.chronicillnet.org/

HealingWell.com - Guide to Diseases, Disorders and Chronic Illness
www.healingwell.com/

Marital Problems
Marital Problems Website Review
www.abcparenting.com/index.cfm?cat=49

Working With Mental Health Professionals

Chapter 11

T

o be prepared to contact and work with mental health professionals, massage therapists need to thoroughly research the mental health practitioners and methods available in their area and find mental health practitioners who are compatible with both the massage therapist's and the client's philosophy and approach toward healing and therapy. Therefore, being aware of and going beyond one's prejudices and biases—positive or negative—regarding mental health methods is critical for massage therapists. Doing this includes being reasonably knowledgeable about psychology and the mental health field. Personal knowledge and anecdotal information are not enough to rely on. What is disastrous for some individuals is life saving for others, and vice versa.

The mental health field offers an array of methods to help people, depending on their situation. The massage therapy profession is in a very similar situation with its broad variety of methods; therefore, massage therapists should have a natural appreciation for the effort that goes into selecting the right therapist and method.

SITUATIONS THAT MAY REQUIRE REFERRAL

Three basic situations are likely to bring a massage therapist into contact with mental health professionals. One is a situation in which a massage therapist finds that problems presented by a client are beyond the massage therapist's scope of practice to work with or beyond the therapist's ability to handle, and a referral to a mental health professional is in order. For instance, the massage therapist may recognize signs of a mental health condition that should be treated by a mental health professional, or the massage therapist may be faced with a situation presented by a client that the therapist does not know how to handle; that is, the massage therapist feels "in over his or her head." This can happen either during the initial interview or during the course of therapy. Neither the massage therapist nor the client is at fault or has failed if and when this happens. It is simply the right thing to do, as portrayed in the case study.

Gwen and Peggy

Gwen had been working with Peggy as her client, who came for massage because friends of Peggy's suggested that massage would help her "feel better." Gwen had noticed that Peggy had often seemed anxious and distracted, but they had never discussed it. The massages seemed to help Peggy, and Peggy always said that she felt better afterward. About 3 months after beginning massage, Gwen moved the draping from Peggy's inner thigh to begin work on this area for the first time and noticed three long, thin parallel cuts there. Almost automatically, Gwen said, "Oh, did your cat scratch you?"

Peggy became visibly uncomfortable and said, "I don't have a cat."

Gwen said, "Oh, I saw the scratches on your thigh and thought you might have a feisty cat."

"No," said Peggy, "I can't remember how I got those."

Gwen thought about times when she herself had bumps or bruises that she could not remember either and went on with the massage. A couple months later, when working on the interior surface of Peggy's upper arm, Gwen noticed the same kind of scratches. "Here are those scratches again," remarked Gwen, "They are really quite uniform. How did you get them?"

Peggy turned her head toward the wall, saying, "I'd rather not talk about it."

Something about Peggy's tone alarmed Gwen. She said, "I really understand that you might not want to talk about it, but this seems pretty important because I'm getting the impression it wasn't an accident. Could that be true?" Peggy murmured something so quietly that Gwen could not understand what she was saying. "What did you say?" Gwen asked.

"I said, *I* put them there," Peggy said in much louder voice.

Internally, Gwen was shocked and taken aback, but was able to keep a warm, empathetic connection to Peggy. "Oh, you must have felt really bad to have done that to yourself," Gwen empathized.

"I felt bad, *and* I felt numb. I just felt I had to do it," explained Peggy.

Gwen responded, "It sounds to me as if things have gotten to that point inside of you, that you may need help in addition to massage therapy . . . such as help from someone who understands what you may be going through that would lead you to cut yourself. I have a really great network of psychotherapists and we can find someone who can help you and that you'll feel you can work with."

Peggy replied, "I feel bad that you know about this, but on the other hand I feel good that someone knows."

As massage therapists, we are not able to work with every situation with every client, no matter how healthy we are, how much work we have done on ourselves, how much knowledge we have absorbed, or how good we are at our work. From time to time, there are clients and situations to which we have strong personal reactions or are beyond our abilities. Being able to refer a client when the massage therapist realizes that something about the situation compromises his or her ability to do the best work is a mark of maturity.

Discomfort or uneasiness on the part of the massage therapist may be a signal that the therapist is "out of his or her depth." When this happens, it is time to talk to someone about this discomfort. It may mean that the therapist is underconfident about his or her abilities. In this case, a massage therapist may need to either look at his or her self-esteem as a therapist or get some support. On the other hand, such discomfort may be a signal that the massage therapist really does not know what to do and is dealing with something outside his or her capabilities. Knowing and accepting limits and dealing with the situation appropriately are essential.

An example of such a situation would be a client who begins to have indeterminate memories on the table that you as the massage therapist believe may be connected to past sexual abuse. In this case, without offering any diagnosis, you should suggest that the client visit a psychotherapist to explore where the memories are coming from. You may continue to work physically with the client, but a person qualified to work with such issues should work with and monitor the psychological aspects of the client's experience. When you are dealing with a mental health issue, it is not very much different from a situation in which you notice a mole or skin lesion on a client's back that could be cancerous and you need to refer the client to a dermatologist or another type of physician.

The second situation involving referral is when a mental health professional refers one of his or her clients to a massage therapist. Such a referral can happen in several forms. One is a very general recommendation from the mental health professional that the client go for massage therapy. In this case, the massage therapist should not expect to communicate with the mental health professional unless the client requests it or unless a specific situation arises that necessitates consulting with the mental health professional. If this happens, both the massage therapist and the mental health professional need written authorization to consult with each other (authorization to consult is discussed later in this chapter).

Another referral situation is general and includes a specific reason, such as that the client go for massage for stress reduction or to be more in touch with his or her body. In this case, because a specific reason for massage therapy was given, the massage therapist may have a stronger reason to consult with the mental health professional, such as to clarify what was meant. In this situation, you can bring this up with the client by saying, "Did you or your psychotherapist expect me to consult about the goals of our work together?" Putting it this way rather than saying something like, "I need to talk to your psychotherapist," gives the client more autonomy over both the massage therapy and psychotherapy processes and may feel less intrusive. The need for authorization is the same as explained in the preceding paragraph.

Another type of referral is specific in that the mental health professional suggests that the client make an appointment with a specific massage therapist for a specific reason. In this case, the massage therapist should inquire about consulting with the mental health professional. There is a greater likelihood that the referring mental health professional has something specific in mind and may contact the massage therapist, so the massage therapist needs to prepare for this possibility and obtain an authorization.

Finally, the most specific referral situation is one in which the mental health professional refers the client to a specific massage therapist with whom he or she collaborates and consults about what he or she would like the massage therapist to work on with the client. In this case, an authorization is definitely needed. The mental health professional may be interested in receiving progress reports from the massage therapist, so this is something that the massage therapist may want to ask about and be prepared to discuss.

A third situation that may bring a massage therapist into contact with a mental health professional is when the massage therapist sees a mental health professional for personal reasons, such as for psychotherapy. If the mental health professional also sees anyone who is a client of the massage therapist, then remembering that the mental health professional cannot share any information with the massage therapist concerning any of the massage therapist's clients is important. However, the massage therapist is free to tell the mental health professional any personal or professional information, and it will remain confidential, assuming that the mental health professional effectively holds the frame.

A potential condition presented by such a situation involves whether the massage therapist and the mental health professional should have any clients in common. We suggest that this be avoided, if possible. The nature of this type of dual relationship presents potential difficulties regarding the ability to consult about clients in common. For example, such a dual relationship situation may set up unconscious conflicts of interest that are difficult to avoid despite how well-intentioned both parties may be. It can also undermine the massage therapist's ability to be open and candid in his or her own therapy with the mental health professional. Ideally, a mental health professional would bring this up or not get into such a situation in the first place, but this is not always the reality. Although this kind of dual relationship happens in tight-knit communities, it should always be discussed, especially in terms of how it can best be handled.

PROFESSIONALS WITHIN THE MENTAL HEALTH FIELD

There are several types of mental health professionals, each of which has different areas of expertise and abilities. The following explanations are intended to help you to become familiar with them and to determine whom to contact or refer to.

Psychiatrists

Psychiatry is a branch of medicine specializing in the study, prevention, diagnosis, and treatment of mental disorders. A *psychiatrist* is a physician who has completed a residency in psychiatry. As a licensed physician, a psychiatrist can prescribe medication and hospitalize people. Some psychiatrists specialize in prescribing medication to treat mental disorders. Some do psychotherapy and prescribe medication. Yet others do only psychotherapy, and some further specialize in specific forms of psychotherapy, such as psychoanalysis. Psychiatrists often work with people who have severe mental illness, but may also see other people seeking mental health treatment. They may work in private practice, group practice, hospitals, long-term care facilities, and research centers.

In considering a psychiatrist, the following information is important:

1. Does the psychiatrist primarily prescribe medication, or does he or she provide psychotherapy as well? People seeing a psychiatrist for the first time often typically do not know what their needs are or appreciate the distinction.
2. What is the psychiatrist's philosophy of treatment? This includes attitudes toward medication, hospitalization, ECT (electroconvulsive shock treatment), addictions, alternative forms of treatment, and preferred methods of psychotherapy.
3. At what hospitals does the psychiatrist have privileges?
4. In the event that you are obtaining information for a specific client, what fee is charged, and are the services covered by the client's insurance?

Psychopharmacologists

Psychopharmacology is the study of the effects of drugs on behavior, combining methods of psychiatry and pharmacology. A *psychopharmacologist* is a psychiatrist who works with prescribing medications. A psychopharmacologist may see a patient for a long initial interview and, on prescribing medication, see the patient for short sessions of 15 to 30 minutes on a regular basis. Usually, what psychopharmacologist and patient do in the sessions is evaluate the medication(s), rather than provide psychotherapy. The psychopharmacologist may or may not refer a patient to a psychotherapist or counselor for therapy.

Psychologists

The basis of psychology is the scientific study of behavior and mental processes, such as feelings, motives, and thinking. The field of psychology is very broad, as exemplified by a list of chapter headings from a leading basic psychology textbook: Neuroscience, Genetics and Behavior, The Developing Child, Adolescence and Adulthood, Sensation, Perception, States of Consciousness, Learning, Memory, Thinking and Language, Intelligence, Motivation, Emotion, Personality, Psychological Disorders, Therapy, Stress and Health, and Social Psychology. *Psychologists* study the bases of behavior and mental processes. Under this broad general title, a variety of types are found, such as research psychologist, educational psychologist, organizational or industrial psychologist, and forensic psychologist.

Clinical Psychologists

The type of psychologist most likely to treat people with mental health problems is the *clinical psychologist.* Clinical psychology applies psychological principles to the assessment, diagnosis, treatment, and research of psychological distress, disability, dysfunctional behavior, and health risk behavior. Humanistic practitioners would include the enhancement of psychological and physical well-being and the realization of human potential in this description. Some areas of clinical psychology overlap with other fields, such as counseling psychology, as well as with some professional fields outside psychology, such as psychiatry, social work, and counseling. Clinical psychologists may specialize in research or clinical practice; some perform both.

A clinical psychologist generally has a Ph.D. in clinical psychology, however, other psychologists who work with people may have a Ph.D. or Ed.D. (doctor of education) in counseling psychology. Another more recently developed advanced degree is the Psy.D. (doctor of psychology). The difference between a Psy.D. and the other doctoral degrees is a candidate for a Psy.D. is not required to write a dissertation based on original research and is trained specifically to work clinically with people, rather than perform psychological research. In the United States, one of these degrees are usually required for licensure as a psychologist. However, not all states accept the Psy.D. degree for licensing.

According to the American Psychological Association, a generally accepted pattern is to refer to master's level positions as counselors, specialists, clinicians, and so forth (rather than as "psychologists," for which a Ph.D. is needed). At present, a psychologist may not prescribe medication, although psychologists are lobbying politically for this status. A psychologist may work in an individual or group practice or in hospitals, long-term treatment facilities, or schools.

Clinical Social Workers

There are many types of social workers. Clinical social work shares with all social work practice the goal of enhancement and maintenance of psychosocial functioning of individuals, families, and small groups. *Clinical social workers* apply social work theory and methods to the treatment and prevention of psychosocial dysfunction, disability, or impairment, including emotional and mental disorders. It is based on knowledge of one or more theories of human development within a psychosocial context.

Understanding the perspective of the situation in which a person is functioning is central to clinical social work practice. Clinical social work includes interventions directed toward interpersonal interactions, intrapsychic dynamics, and life support and management issues. Clinical social workers perform assessment; diagnosis; treatment, including psychotherapy and counseling; client-centered advocacy; consultation; and evaluation. In addition to having a Master of Social Work (M.S.W.) degree, a social worker who offers mental health treatment also has completed specified hours of supervision and internship to qualify for a Licensed Clinical Social Worker (L.C.S.W.) license. An L.C.S.W. may work in individual or group practice, hospitals, or long-term treatment facilities or may perform casework for an agency.

Counselors

Counseling is personal assistance provided by a professional for exploring attitudes, beliefs, feelings, values, interests, abilities, experiences, or goals in the context of addressing educational guidance, career development, life transitions, promoting mental and emotional wellness, personal growth, as well as personal problems and psychopathology. Considering the range of the description of counseling, there are several types of *counselors:* pastoral counselors, guidance counselors, career counselors, addiction counselors, marriage counselors, and mental health counselors.

According to the American Psychological Association, the objectives of counseling are to help individuals toward overcoming obstacles to their personal growth, wherever these may be encountered, and toward achieving optimum development of their personal resources. A counselor generally has earned a minimum of a master's degree in counseling or in a related relevant discipline. A gradual movement to license counselors is taking place, but this varies among states. The philosophical aspect regarding licensing of counselors is divided between those who believe unqualified practitioners may harm someone and those who believe a person should have the freedom to choose whomever they want to seek advice, guidance, and personal assistance. A counselor may be in individual or group practice or in schools or may work for an institution.

Psychotherapists

Definitions of psychotherapy are so varied and broad that going back to the origin of the term may be instructive. Psycho- comes from the Greek *psyche*, which means soul or mind, and from the Greek *therapeuo*, meaning to heal/to cure or to nurse/to care for. Therefore, in its original sense, psychotherapy means to heal or care for the mind or soul. In the most inclusive sense, psychotherapy involves the use of any technique or procedure that has a palliative or curative effect on any mental, emotional or behavioral disorder. In accordance with such a broad description, a vast variety of treatment approaches fall under the term psychotherapy. Many of these different schools of psychotherapy have developed with a focus of treatment on specific disorders (e.g., Interpersonal Therapy, and Cognitive Therapy, for depression), with a focus on specific problems (e.g., sexual dysfunction, addiction), or with a focus on specific theoretical approaches (e.g., psychoanalysis, Bioenergetics, Gestalt Therapy, Transactional Analysis). Psychotherapy, however, does not include drug therapy.

Given the nature of the term psychotherapy, *psychotherapist* is a more general title. Usually, a psychotherapist has a master's level degree or higher in psychology, social work, or counseling; or is a psychiatrist, clinical psychologist, marriage and family therapist, or psychiatric nurse specialist.

What is the difference between counseling and psychotherapy? This is a hotly debated question for which there is no consensus of opinion. The answer probably depends to some degree on whether one is looking at it from the point of view of who is the client, who is the practitioner, where one stands on issues (such as regulatory and legal, health care, or mental health), or one's job title and description. Most participants in the debate acknowledge that a fine line exists between counseling and psychotherapy, and a close look is required to distinguish whether there is a difference. Some believe the line is so fine that it either does not exist or is insignificant. However, most people on either side of the debate generally do agree that there are some aspects in which the two overlap and spill over into each other.

Counseling is defined as a "therapeutic experience for reasonably healthy persons, and psychotherapy as one for emotionally disturbed persons, or are referred for assistance with pathological problems. Thus, the primary difference is in the persons treated rather than the treatment process" (Ohlsen, p. 24). Consequently, the definition of counseling hinges on how the terms "healthy" and "emotionally disturbed" are defined. Another respectable definition of counseling is from the British Psychological Society's website: "[to] help people improve their sense of well being, alleviate their distress, resolve their crises and increase their ability to solve problems and make decisions for themselves." This suggests that someone who already has a sense of well-being can solve problems and make decisions, but who, in a time of crisis and distress may need a helping hand, will be helped by counseling. Both definitions say that counseling is for a person who is reasonably functional and healthy psychologically but who needs help solving or coping with nonpathological life problems. The level of adjustment or maladjustment of the client is the dividing issue.

These are orthodox definitions of counseling that are based on the "medical model" paradigm, which creates hierarchies of severity and complexity. Using the humanistic model, a reasonably healthy person is likely to benefit from the same type of in-depth work associated with psychotherapy that an emotionally disturbed person would. For example, if a person is grappling with a problem adjusting to a crisis in his or her life, it is useful to look at and work with the entire personality, rather than try to solve the only problem itself. Consequently, counseling and psychotherapy may involve performing the same work.

Perhaps a more practical distinction is that the growth model may be used in both psychotherapy and counseling, but certain conditions or situations are not amenable to an approach based on the growth model. These conditions may call for dealing with disturbances within the person in a manner for which a counselor is not trained, but a psychotherapist may be.

Marriage and Family Therapists

Marriage and family therapists (MFTs) broaden the traditional emphasis on the individual to attend to the nature and role of individuals in the primary relationship networks, such as marriage and family, in which the person is embedded. They treat a wide range of clinical problems including marital, individual, and child-parent problems. MFTs regularly practice short-term therapy, with 12 sessions as the average. About half of the treatment provided by MFTs is one on one; the other half is divided between marital/couple and family therapy or a combination of treatments.

MFTs have a master's or doctoral degree in marriage and family therapy and at least 2 years of clinical experience. MFTs are trained in psychotherapy and family systems; evaluate and treat mental and emotional disorders and other health and behavioral problems; and address a wide array of relationship issues within the context of marriage, couples, and family systems.

Body Psychotherapists

Given the subject of this book, a newer field called *body psychotherapy* merits inclusion. According to the United States Association for Body Psychotherapy, body psychotherapy is a distinct school of psychotherapy, with a connecting branch to the main body of psychotherapy and psychology.

Body psychotherapy involves a clearly different theory of mind-body functioning, which takes into account the complexity of the intersections and interactions between the body and the mind. The underlying assumption is that a functional unity exists between body and mind, but without establishing a hierarchical relationship between them. They are both functioning and interactive aspects of the whole person. Although other approaches in psychotherapy increasingly acknowledge and touch on this area, body psychotherapy considers this to be a fundamental principle.

Body psychotherapy also includes a developmental model; a theory of personality; hypotheses as to the origins of disturbances and alterations; and a rich variety of diagnostic and therapeutic techniques used within the framework of the therapeutic relationship. There are many different and sometimes quite separate approaches within body psychotherapy, as there are in the other main branches of psychotherapy. For example, some of these are Bioenergetics, Core Energetics, Orgonomy (Reichian), Organismic, Hakomi, Biosynthesis, Rubenfeld Synergy, and Radix (Box 5.2 in Chapter 5 gives explanations of several of these approaches). A wide variety of body-oriented techniques are used within body psychotherapy, generally involving touch, movement, and breathing. There is therefore a link with some massage therapies, bodywork, somatic educational methods, and some complementary alternative medical disciplines. However, although these therapies may also involve touch and movement, they are very distinct from body psychotherapy.

Directly or indirectly, *body psychotherapists* work with the person as an essential embodiment of mental, emotional, social, and spiritual life. In this sense, the practice of body psychotherapy is an integrative approach. Therapeutic goals include encouraging both internal self-regulative processes and the accurate perception of external reality. Through the work, the body psychotherapist makes it possible for alienated aspects of the person to become conscious, acknowledged, and integrated parts of the self. Body psychotherapists may have a doctoral or master's degree in one of the fields of mental health and have taken extensive training in one or more body psychotherapy approaches.

COLLABORATING WITH MENTAL HEALTH PROFESSIONALS

By collaboration between mental health professionals, we mean any consultation or discussion about a client that takes place between a massage therapist and a mental health professional, which may also involve agreeing on a treatment plan. Collaboration has several benefits. Most notably, the client benefits from the sharing of information and perceptions by both professionals. During consultation, new insights can be formed or gaps in information are filled in. Another benefit is that collaboration can keep both professionals from working at cross-purposes or duplicating efforts. The massage therapist can benefit from the perspective that the mental health professional offers, whereas the mental health professional can benefit from learning about the somatic perspective brought in by the massage therapist. This kind of collaboration, under the right circumstances, can lead to a relationship in which both parties become resources for each other about their respective fields.

Collaboration also has risks. The two most common risks, splitting and triangulation, arise out of the client's transference with either or both the massage therapist and the mental health professional. *Splitting* is an unconscious activity by the client that figuratively "splits" or divides the massage therapist and the mental health professional into two different roles that have polarized emotional significance. For example, the client may unconsciously split the two helping professionals into "good one" and "bad one" roles. The "good" and "bad" emotional attribution can take the form of one professional being more competent and one being less competent, one being more understanding and one being less understanding, one being more intelligent and one being less intelligent, one being more helpful and one being less helpful, and so on. The person playing the "good" role can at any given time be switched to the role of the "bad" one.

Splitting also occurs when the client unconsciously presents substantially different emotional and factual information to the massage therapist from what is presented to the mental health professional. For example, the client may provide contradictory information to each party or give important information to only one party. Another form of splitting can also occur when the client unconsciously presents him- or herself very differently to each party. For example, the client may appear to be very self-sufficient and independent with one party and needy and dependent with the other party.

Triangulation occurs when splitting becomes more active, thus creating three distinct roles in the triangle of the client and two helpers; this often results in the client attempting unconsciously to create conflict between the helping professionals. This usually results either in a "covering-up" or a "defusing" of the psychological issues at hand (Stierlin). A common origin of triangulation is the client's family situation in which the parents were pitted against each other and vied for the child's loyalty and love. This is a particularly thorny situation for children between the ages of 4 and 6 and for adolescents, when the child needs the love and attention of the parent of the opposite sex and may feel competitive with the parent of the same gender. In healthy families, children pass through this period with the support and love of both parents. In other words, the parents do not use the child's period of development as an arena for their own conflict. However, if the parents "triangulate" with the child, the child is prone to grow up believing unconsciously that one of the parties in a relationship must be rejected, demeaned, or sacrificed. As adults, they may seek out triangular situations and replay the situation of their childhood in their relationships. The following case study is an example of dealing with triangulation and splitting.

Fiona, Justine, and Angela

Fiona received a call from Justine, asking to make an appointment for massage. Justine said that her psychotherapist, Angela, felt it would be beneficial to have massage in conjunction with her psychotherapy. Fiona knew Angela because she had met Angela at a workshop, had spoken with her, and felt they shared similar values around psychotherapy and massage. When Justine came in, Fiona asked Justine if she could speak with Angela and had her sign an authorization. Fiona spoke briefly with Angela, who said that she had wanted Justine to come for massage therapy because she thought Justine was holding a lot of grief and that becoming more in touch with her body would help release it.

Fiona and Justine had several sessions that Justine clearly enjoyed. During the fourth session, a floodgate opened as Fiona worked with Justine's abdominal area. Justine cried for quite a while, and when the tears stopped she looked both relieved and radiant.

"I can't believe that happened! I can't believe that all *that* was in there!" said Justine, clearly feeling great relief and even greater energy. Fiona smiled and nodded. She, too, was happy with the session.

The next session Justine came in exclaiming, "You must be a magician. I've felt better all week. I've never felt this good when I left a session with Angela!"

Fiona felt flattered. Then a little light bulb went on in her head. She had taken a workshop on transference for massage therapists, so she suddenly realized that although she had done a good job, something else was happening with Justine to which she needed to pay careful attention. "Well, massage often helps

Fiona, Justine, and Angela

open something that the person has been working on for a long time. You and Angela may have been putting a lot of energy into exploring your feelings and the massage took it that extra mile. It would probably be good if you talked more about this with Angela."

"Okay," said Justine, "but I still think you're a magician."

By the time Justine came back, the euphoria of the initial emotional release had become more grounded. "Angela and I did talk, " said Justine. "We talked about how when I was a child, I always had to go to someone other than my mother to get comfort. I guess that kind of got mixed into this, but I'm really glad I know about it.

"Great!" said Fiona, "Let's see what we can work on today. What are you aware of in your body right now?"

Fiona recognized correctly that Justine was bidding to triangulate her relationship with Fiona and Angela. Fiona countered this by redirecting Justine's credit to Angela and by encouraging Justine to discuss her feelings with Angela, rather than only with Fiona. By suggesting that Justine "bring it back to therapy," Fiona also helped Justine keep from splitting her psychotherapy process.

When working with a client who is in psychotherapy or another form of mental health treatment, staying aware of the possibility of splitting and triangulation is important. This is particularly true when something as strongly charged as emotional release happens. For example, the client may have a strong emotional release during a massage concerning an issue he or she has been working on with the mental health professional for several years. If the client does not share what happened during the massage session with the mental health professional, then this has the effect of splitting the client's emotional process so that one piece is with the massage therapy and another piece is with the psychotherapy. Generally, good communication between the massage therapist and the mental health professional counteracts splitting and triangulation.

Effective Collaboration

Often when you are working with a client who is also working with a mental health professional, collaboration may not be needed. Relative to the psychotherapy or other mental health treatment, the massage work may be "invisible," meaning that little process material is generated by or during the massage, the massage therapist observes no troubling symptoms, and no transference difficulties develop. In other words, there is basically nothing that needs to be discussed.

If some potentially relevant psychological or medical material does comes up during massage therapy, encourage the client to bring this to the attention of his or her mental health professional or physician. Several different client responses are possible:

▶ If the client balks at the suggestion, then decide how important the material is. If it seems important, you should seek supervision as to how to proceed and what ethical or legal obligations exist.

▶ If the client pleads ignorance and wants you to communicate with the mental health professional, you must first get authorization in the form of a signed release, and then contact the mental health professional.

▶ If the client appears to have no insight or has an odd reaction to the suggestion, then you can offer to be a conduit of clinical information, which also requires getting a release.

▶ If the client is presenting worrisome symptoms of transference that is difficult to manage, or is provocative in a way that makes the massage work diffcult, you should consider either supervision or asking permission to call the mental health professional (a written release still is needed even if verbal permission is given) and consult. This assumes you can formulate the reason for talking to the mental health professional in an honest way that is not offensive to the client. While consulting with the mental health professional, you can pass the information on and maybe get some guidance for managing the situation. With such clients, making sure that proper procedure is followed is always a good idea.

If the mental health professional has made the referral and you are not absolutely clear as to the purpose of the referral, then you should consider requesting permission from the client to call and ask the mental health professional exactly that question. The mental health professional's agenda may not be the same as the client's, and it may be worth noting the difference for all three parties. You may want medical information if it is relevant to massage (e.g., musculoskeletal conditions, cardiovascular conditions), but this is a judgment call on your part.

If you have referred the client to the mental health professional, then you need to ask the client to sign a release so that you can at least leave a message for the mental health professional as to the reason for the referral, which may differ from the reason given by the client to the mental health professional. This may not be necessary if the client is ready, willing, and able to present him- or herself accurately.

You should *not* second-guess the psychotherapeutic or medical treatment. All concerns of this nature should be directed back to the mental health professional. Avoiding second-guessing with the client is doubly important to prevent splitting or undermining the therapy. For example, if the client is having some sort of disagreement with the psychotherapist, he or she may consciously or unconsciously be trying to generate opposing data with the massage therapist, allowing the client to avoid facing the conflict directly. For this reason, you should generally be very careful about discussing any of the client's therapists, even previous ones, because you may otherwise end up unwittingly colluding with the client's transference issues.

If you know the mental health professional personally, you should not discuss with the client the details of the mental health professional's life. If the client seems particularly curious, suggest that the client ask the mental health professional about whatever it is that he or she is curious. However, it is certainly okay to acknowledge that you and the mental health professional are friends, colleagues, or whatever else that applies. However, some mental health professionals prefer even that information to be kept private. If the mental health professional also is your client, then let the mental health professional decide whether to disclose this to the client.

The overall principle is to respect all three sets of boundaries—the client's, the mental health professional's, and your own—while at the same time facilitating the flow of important information to the proper person and place.

Obtaining Releases

Communication requires consent and authorization, preferably in the form of a written release. In all cases, permission must be granted by the client, and confidentiality must be preserved (where, when, and how you talk). The only exception to obtaining consent is when the client is clearly a danger to him- or herself or others and is not willing to take appropriate action, for example, if the client develops a visual impairment, but refuses not to drive. Seeking legal consultation for particularly tricky situations may even be advisable. Usually, a supervisory consultation with an experienced colleague is helpful. Concerning supervision, generally a release is not necessary for discussing your cases with your supervisor because your supervisor has the same confidentiality obligations with you as you do with your client. However, you may want to check this with your supervisor.

If the client refuses to sign a release, then you cannot proceed to discuss anything about your client with anyone else. In this instance, you may want to consider whether you think that obtaining this release is essential to your work with the client. If you do, then you would need to consider whether the absence of a release would prevent you from obtaining or providing critical information that could affect the outcome of the work.

Obtaining a release is quite straightforward. You need to develop a form that you are satisfied with, and then both you and your client need to complete the form and sign it. We have provided a sample release form that we find effective (Box 11.1). The completed and signed release should be kept on file. Before you can proceed, you should see a copy of the release granted to the other party, such as psychotherapist, psychiatrist, any other physician, or massage therapist. If you are dealing with a particularly difficult client, such as a client with trust issues, be particularly diligent in carrying out the formality of the release properly.

If the client is unfamiliar with the concept of a release, then you need to explain its purpose. First, inform the client why you feel you need to communicate with the other professional involved. At this point, the client may have questions concerning this necessity or what you might talk about. On another level, transference issues could be affected. For example, this could bring up feelings about being talked about "behind one's back," feeling special as the center of such attention, fear of being labeled or analyzed, feeling cared about, or feeling disempowered because the client is "left out" of the discussion. You do not have to do anything about the transference issues, but it may help to be aware of them. Second,

---

Box 11.1

SAMPLE AUTHORIZATION FOR RELEASE OF INFORMATION FORM

Authorization for Release of Information

I, _____, do hereby

authorize _____
to:

release written records to

_____

communicate verbally with

_____

This communication is:

☐ not limited
☐ limited to the following subjects:

_____

_____

☐ I wish the content of said communication to be communicated to me.

This authorization is valid between the dates of _____ and

_____

Signature of Client

_____(Date)_____

Signature of Therapist

_____(Date)_____

you may need to address privacy concerns, such as whether any of the information will go to an insurance company, an employer, or any other outside party.

NETWORKING WITH OTHER PROFESSIONALS

A massage therapist is likely to make a referral to a mental health professional in two situations in particular. One situation is when, during the initial interview, the massage therapist determines that the prospective client is seeking help for problems that are more appropriate for a mental health practitioner. The other is when, in the course of massage therapy, issues arise that require the attention of someone other than the massage therapist and who is qualified to work with such a problem. Either way, a massage therapist needs to be prepared to make a referral and needs to have a network or list of other professionals available to refer to.

Your network should include one or more of the following mental health professionals: physicians, psychiatrists, psychologists, clinical social workers, psychotherapists, or counselors who are compatible with massage therapy. Your network could also include specialists who work with specific conditions, such as addiction, marriage and family counseling, gender identity and sexual preferences, domestic violence, chronic illness and pain, death and dying, eating disorders, and sexual dysfunctions. You may also need other resources for your network, including Alcoholics Anonymous, Al-Anon, Narcotics Anonymous and other 12-step anonymous support groups, AIDS treatment and support centers, refuge houses for domestic violence, and hospices. You also need to know how to contact social service and human resource agencies in your area. In a sense, this would form an ideal referral network.

Building a network may seem like a formidable task, but it is usually done over time. Although you may not be able to make personal contact with everyone in your referral network, you can develop such a list by contacting the social service agencies in your area and asking how you might find these services. Social service agencies are listed in the phone book, usually in the government listings. Websites are another source. In addition, asking other massage therapists and professionals you respect about whom they have in their network might be useful. The most important thing is to anticipate whom you might need. You can do this by discussing with your colleagues, mentor, or supervisor the situations for which they have had to refer. After a few such discussions, note which situations have arisen and how frequently these seem to appear in a massage practice.

Contacting mental health professionals for the purpose of forming your network may seem daunting. A good way to start is with mental health professionals whom you have reason to believe are receptive to massage therapy and forms of somatic practice. Personal contact is usually the best way to find out whether your approaches and values are congruent. Phone calls, coffee dates, and attending lectures or presentations provide ways to make personal contact. We suggest that in the initial contact you simply explain why you are speaking with them; for example, you are forming a list of professionals that you can refer to if and when needed. In the course of the discussion, make it clear that you are not promoting your practice or seeking referrals in return as a *quid pro quo*. In our experience, most people are very responsive to such queries.

These suggestions would go far in forming a model network, so if you do not have every element of the suggested network in place, that is okay. You may rarely use the network, but when you do it will probably be very important for your client.

Another aspect of networking exists on the community level. The local community of massage therapists, bodyworkers, and somatic educators that you are part of may have a good relationship with the mental health community and be open to connecting. Alternatively, members of a massage therapy community may feel very suspicious of mental health and tend to reject such connections.

A possible reason for such uneasiness may be a perception that psychiatrists—and psychologists who function within a medical model—are likely to treat patients with pharmaceuticals. A continuing debate exists about whether some of these drugs suppress symptoms rather than get to the root cause of a problem or create a base of support for therapeutic work or cure the condition. On top of this, society in general, along with a substantial portion of the medical community, questions the scientific basis for many of the methods used in psychological and psychotherapeutic treatment. In addition, although being in some form of psychotherapy or counseling has become far more acceptable, cultural prejudices that consider being in psychotherapy as a form of weakness and self-indulgence persist.

In a community that is prejudiced in some way against mental health, practitioners have a tendency to avoid referrals or collaboration. Sometimes this can be to the detriment to the client, because referrals or collaboration do not happen when they should. Massage therapists also may develop a greater tendency to go outside their scope of practice rather than work with mental health professionals.

On the other hand, in a situation in which the massage community is well connected with the mental health community and psychological treatment methods are well accepted, a problem more likely may rest with a tendency to "psychologize" massage (to overuse psychological interpretation) and to refer clients excessively to psychotherapy, counseling, and growth workshops. A massage therapist may impose a psychological model on clients, rather than being aware of the true psychological needs emerging from clients.

Ideally, massage therapists have a balanced approach, understanding their scope of practice and making referrals when authentic psychological issues arise that are outside their scope of practice.

REFERENCES

American Association for Marriage and Family Therapy. Website: www.aamft.org.

American Counseling Association. Website: www.counseling.org.

American Psychiatric Association. Website: www.psych.org.

American Psychological Association. Website: www.apa.org

British Association for Counselling. Website: www.bac.co.uk

Canadian Psychological Association. Website: www.cpa.ca.

Kennedy, E. (1993). *On becoming a counselor: A basic guide on non professional counseling.* New York: Continuum.

National Association of Social Workers. Website: www.naswdc.org.

Ohlsen, M. (1970). *Group counseling.* New York: Holt, Rinehart, and Winston.

Stierlin, H., Wynne, L. & Simon, F. (1985). *Language of family therapy: A systemic vocabulary and source book.* Rochester, NY: Family Process Press.

United States Association for Body Psychotherapy. Website: www.usabp.org.